The Elemen 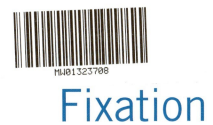 Fixation

The Elements of Fracture Fixation

Third Edition

Anand J. Thakur MS (Ortho), FCPS D Ortho
Consultant Orthopaedic Surgeon,
Hinduja Healthcare Surgical, Mumbai
Formerly, Consultant Orthopaedic Surgeon,
Cambridge Military Hospital, Aldershot, UK and RN Cooper
Municipal General Hospital, Juhu, Mumbai;
Professor of Orthopaedic Surgery, GS Medical College, Parel and
University of Bombay, Mumbai, India

Illustrations by the author

ELSEVIER

ELSEVIER

RELX India Private Limited (Formerly Reed Elsevier India Private Limited)
Registered Office: 818, 8th Floor, Indraprakash Building, 21, Barakhamba Road, New Delhi 110001
Corporate Office: 14th Floor, Building No. 10B, DLF Cyber City, Phase II, Gurgaon-122 002, Haryana, India

---

The Elements of Fracture Fixation, 3e, Anand J. Thakur

Copyright © 2015, by RELX India Private Limited (Formerly Reed Elsevier India Private Limited)
All rights reserved.

ISBN: 978-81-312-4236-0
e-Book ISBN: 978-81-312-4237-7

No part of this publication may be reproduced or transmitted in any form or by any means, electronic or mechanical, including photocopying, recording, or any information storage and retrieval system, without permission in writing from the publisher. Details on how to seek permission, further information about the Publisher's permissions policies and our arrangements with organizations such as the Copyright Clearance Center and the Copyright Licensing Agency, can be found at our website: www.elsevier.com/permissions.

This book and the individual contributions contained in it are protected under copyright by the Publisher (other than as may be noted herein).

Reprinted 2017

Notice

Knowledge and best practice in this field are constantly changing. As new research and experience broaden our understanding, changes in research methods, professional practices, or medical treatment may become necessary.

Practitioners and researchers must always rely on their own experience and knowledge in evaluating and using any information, methods, compounds, or experiments described herein. In using such information or methods they should be mindful of their own safety and the safety of others, including parties for whom they have a professional responsibility.

With respect to any drug or pharmaceutical products identified, readers are advised to check the most current information provided (i) on procedures featured or (ii) by the manufacturer of each product to be administered, to verify the recommended dose or formula, the method and duration of administration, and contraindications. It is the responsibility of practitioners, relying on their own experience and knowledge of their patients, to make diagnoses, to determine dosages and the best treatment for each individual patient, and to take all appropriate safety precautions.

To the fullest extent of the law, neither the Publisher nor the authors, contributors, or editors, assume any liability for any injury and/or damage to persons or property as a matter of product liability, negligence or otherwise, or from any use or operation of any methods, products, instructions, or ideas contained in the material herein.

Although all advertising material is expected to conform to ethical (medical) standards, inclusion in this publication does not constitute a guarantee or endorsement of the quality or value of such product or of the claims made of it by its manufacturer.

Please consult full prescribing information before issuing prescription for any product mentioned in this publication.

Content Strategist: Dr. Renu Rawat
Sr Project Manager—Education Solutions: Shabina Nasim
Content Development Specialist: Shravan Kumar
Project Manager: Athmanathan Nayagi
Cover Designer: Milind Majgaonkar

Laser typeset by GW India

Printed in India by Rajkamal Electric Press, Kundli, Haryana.

To my
Parents
Dr J G Thakur and Dr (Mrs) Vimal J. Thakur
Wife
Urmila
Sons
Nikhil & Kanishka

Foreword

I am pleased to welcome the reader to this third edition of Professor Anand Thakur's successful and well-regarded textbook, ***The Elements of Fracture Fixation***. This work provides an in-depth introduction to the amply stocked tool-box of today's fracture surgeon. It also provides helpful and current principles of when and how a particular device or technique might best be used. Unlike most medical texts, this is the work of a single author (doubling as illustrator!). It offers an accomplished senior surgeon's view of the technology now available for fracture fixation. The perspective and presentation of a single author provide clarity and directness, potentially missing when a team of editors assemble the work of multiple authors. However, single-author texts may not be as well suited for presentation of differing viewpoints and controversial issues. Professor Thakur skillfully navigates such treacherous waters, but occasionally the reader will wisely notice words of caution, like "The indications for these plates remain undefined", with regard to the Advantages of Locking Internal Fixator Plates (Chapter 4, p. 158). Such a statement exposes the state of our art – we still lack the strong evidence, necessary for confident and comprehensive recommendations. Nonetheless, most fracture surgeons recognize that we have ingenious new tools, which seem to provide solutions for real clinical problems. As a community, we share the responsibility of clarifying indications and techniques. The promise of new approaches, such as Glatt's "reverse dynamization" to stimulate bone growth in large bone defects (Chapter 8, p. 348) is supported by tantalizing laboratory evidence, but its safety and efficacy in humans remain to be established. While some might object to the topic's inclusion, I mention it as an example of the author's enthusiastic awareness of our advancing field, and an indication of cutting-edge coverage provided by this new edition. Similar timeliness is shown by sections on fracture healing, especially with regard to mechanical environment – the fourth side of Giannoudis and colleagues' "diamond concept." In addition to the section devoted specifically to fracture healing, you will find an excellent example, in the problem of asymmetric callus suppression in distal femur fractures treated with Locking Internal Fixator plates, and how this can be addressed with screw modifications that slightly reduce excessive stability of the fracture underlying the plate.

This book is both an introduction and a reference for advanced students and practitioners of fracture treatment. It succeeds in these regards. Although well-illustrated, clearly explained examples of clinical use are abundant, we must recognize that the book's topic is, indeed, ***The Elements of Fracture Fixation***. It does not attempt to provide a complete summary of fracture treatment. Do not expect to find discussions of diagnosis, classifications, indications, surgical exposure, peri-operative care, and rehabilitation. Reduction techniques might seem a bit outside the scope of the text. But they are nicely, extensively, and most appropriately presented in the timely new chapter (Number 10) on Minimally Invasive Osteosynthesis.

The author demonstrates over and again his understanding that fracture fixation involves construction of a composite of bone and fixation implants, in a way that preserves the healing potential of the bone tissue, while achieving optimal stability for fracture healing and rehabilitation. The fracture surgeon will find in this book elegantly illustrated and lucidly explained presentations of today's fracture fixation devices, often with consideration of how current implants have been devised to address shortcomings of their predecessors. I encourage the reader to browse these chapters, guided by the contents tables at their beginning. You will find much that is interesting, stimulating, and useful.

Peter G. Trafton MD
Emeritus Professor of Orthopaedic Surgery
Brown University
Providence, Rhode Island, USA
June 24, 2015

Preface to the Third Edition

"For your own satisfaction and for mine, please read this preface"
– **St Francis de Sales**
(1609, In Preface to *Introduction to the Devout Life*)

I am obliged to quote this because a reviewer of the second edition has taken exception to use of different fonts for emphasis*. Had the learned critic followed what St. Francis de Sales had urged four centuries ago, he would have appreciated the typographical finesse. I had in fact clearly mentioned the purpose of using distinctive fonts thus: "In situations where an average reader may be inclined to skip the paragraph, I have used a smaller type and refrained from omitting such esoteric material as 'principles of cutting instruments' or 'factors enhancing the efficiency of screw insertion', details which may be of interest to a reader with more scholastic leanings". This edition does away with use of two fonts. I am appreciative of the reviewer for another reason; he observed that without discussion of fracture biology the information on fixation was incomplete and the reader will be only partially informed about the bone healing, which is the motive for fracture fixation. I have become more aware of the importance of understanding the bone healing process since writing my third book 'Locking Plates—Concepts and Applications'. True, it is impossible to explain the reasons for change in bone plate's mechanics without highlighting the biological process of fracture repair and its sensitivity to mechanical environment surrounding the fracture.

In the new edition, I have added details of bone healing process to help the reader in understanding application of an individual process of fracture fixation, e.g., less number of screws in plating a comminuted fracture to generate relative stability and to encourage abundant callus formation. I have also added information on factors that impede or enhance bone healing process. Currently, a variety of new materials are being introduced in fracture healing; information on some of these has been included. Plate and screw designs and their uses have undergone a sea change; inevitably a large section of the book has been devoted to the new entities. Even though the evidence is lacking to recommend outright use of locking plate technology, its usage is exponentially increasing and the reader will benefit from the material included. In chapter 5, I have described the mechanical basis of positioning Poller screws, which will change the current arbitrary approach. The earlier edition had no information on usage of intramedullary devices for hip fracture fixation; this has been added. I have also drawn attention to hazards associated with use of a traction table. Chapter on wire, cable and pins is mostly unchanged and so is the chapter on external fixator; however, I have provided some biological perspective in the later, which will improve the understanding of certain configurations. The chapter on osteoporosis has been removed because most of its content has been assimilated in other sections. Two new chapters titled MIPO and Spinal Instrumentation have been added. While the chapter on MIPO should be useful for surgeons at all levels, the section on Spinal Instrumentation is aimed solely at the new entrant in orthopaedic speciality. There are two other visual changes. The publishers had received a feedback to

---

*Laurence M. Book Review: *The Elements of Fracture Fixation*, Second ed. A. J. Thakur Pp. 326. New-Delhi: Elsevier, 2007. ISBN: 978-81-318-0338-5 *J Bone Joint Surg [Br]* 2008;90-B:980.

include radiographic examples, and I have included several appropriate ones. My graphic skills have evolved and I have been able to add colour to simple line sketches. The book has proved useful for postgraduate students and newly qualified orthopaedic surgeons (had to be reprinted in 2011, 2012, 2013). With additional information and several new illustrations, it will be further useful for the student community and established members of the specialty.

I take this opportunity to thank my two friends, Vikas Agashe and Anil Karkhanis for marking out deficiencies in the second edition and making valuable suggestions for improvement. Similarly, I thank Ram Chaddha, Bhauk Garg, Swapnil Kenny, and Mandar Agashe for constructive recommendations and contributions towards building up the Third edition. My son Nikhil, now a spine surgeon in Andover, Mass, USA helped me to plan the new chapter on spinal instruments. In spite of indifferent health, Dr Rajeshwar Singh, Medical writer, Mumbai took keen interest and ensured that I was writing clearly and concisely. Kirit Kumar, my friend from medical college days and renowned urologist in Detroit, MI, USA used his 'Photoshopping' skills to bring out the best visuals from several archived radiographs and clinical pictures. My younger daughter-in-law Meghna, Assistant Professor of Medicine in University of California at San Francisco helped me in procuring references in quick time. My wife Urmila needs special thanks for allowing me to work at the computer during social hours and tolerating my indifference towards family matters as I strived to complete the writing in Elsevier imposed timelines. Renu Rawat, Shravan Kumar and Shabina Naseem of Elseiver have been very understanding and supportive during the revision phase.

Anand J. Thakur
Mumbai
thakurajt@gmail.com
14 June 2015

Acknowledgement

Several of my friends, acquaintances and fellow specialists have extended help in collating radiographs for this edition. I am listing their names in alphabetical order and specifying their contribution for copyright clarity.

Agashe VM—*Fig. 1.8, 4.68B, 4.71D, E; 5.17B*. Agashe MV—*Fig. 4.82B, 4.84A to C, 5.25H, 5.26C, D, E; 7.22, 9.22*. Ahire P—*Fig. 4.79A to C*. Ajgaonkar A—*Fig. 4.75D to G*. Aroojis A—*Fig. 5.27D*. Barhate S—*Fig. 6.20D*. Bemelman M—*Fig. 4.81B*. Bottlang M—*Fig. 4.56A,B*. Chaddha R—*Fig. 9.7B, 9.12A*. Chaudhary R—*Fig. 1.15A & B*. Dalvie S—*Fig. 9.3B, 9.9B*. Damle A—*Fig. 4.26F, 5.17D, 7.6D*. Gadegone WM—*Fig. 6.15B, C*. Ganesh Y—*Fig. 7.6B, 10.21*. Gupta RK—*Fig. 6.10F*. Hass N—*Fig. 4.56C*. Holz U—*Fig. 4.9C, 4.63A*. Jagiasi J—*Fig. 4.80D, E*. Jain M—*Fig. 10.16*. Jupiter JB—*Fig. 4.78E, F*. Kothadia P—*Fig. 10.4B, D*. Kulkarni GS—*Fig. 4.83C, D; 5.14B*. Kurupad S—*Fig. 6.9D*. Mehta R—*Fig. 2-6A, B; 5.25J, 5.26*. Modi S—*Fig. 6.9E*. Mohanty S—*Fig. 7.6A, 7.7D*. Mukhopadhyaya J—*Fig. 10.1*. Nadra A—*Fig. 6.9C*. Patankar H—*Fig. 7.7B, 7.22D, 7.27G to I; 7.28E to K*. Patwardhan S—*Fig. 5.27C*. Parihar M—*Fig. 8.1, 8.18A, D; 8.23A, 8.24G*. Pletka J—*Fig. 3.33A, 4.72C*. Puri A—*Fig. 1.15C*. Ruch D—*Fig. 4.77B to D*. Shivshankar B—*Fig. 1.17A to C; 5.9*. Tanna DD—*Fig. 1.17E, 4.9, 4.10D, 4.13D, 4.50B, 4.59C, D; 4.63B, C; 4.70F, 4.72E*. Tepic S—*Fig. 8.38*. Thakkar A—*Fig. 1.6B*. Thakur NA—*Fig. 9.1, 9.2, 9.6, 9.7, 9.8, 9.9, 9.10, 9.14, 9.15, 9.17*. Vasudevan PN—*Fig. 8.14C, 8.15, 8.28B*.

Preface to the First Edition

In fixation of fractures, the operating orthopaedic surgeon becomes a structural engineer as he creates a new structure from the wreckage of the old. Bone screws, bone plates, nails, wires and components of external fixation systems are the basic 'elements' which help an orthopaedic surgeon to reconstruct a fractured bone.

Surgery can be performed mechanically without any knowledge of anatomy and physiology, but this would be considered outrageous. Similarly, it would be reprehensible for an orthopaedic trainee not to know the biomechanical aspects of the tools of his trade. It is said that the true cause of internal fixation failure is not the failure of the device but in fact the failure of the surgeon to understand the principles of fixation and limitations of the implant. Information on these implants is scarce and scattered, often tucked away in a small section in the large books on fracture treatment and orthopaedic biomechanics. Some of it is available only in journals or in implant manufacturers' publications. New trainees in the specialty cannot get all of it in a concise form at the beginning of their careers when they need it most and have little time for large tomes.

This book describes the essential biomechanical and clinical aspects of each 'element' and informs on different effective methods of use, highlighting the advantages. Since a trainee is usually required to assist in fracture surgery, the book aims at giving practical information to help the trainee understand what is likely to be seen during one's initial days in the specialty: the design and uses of fracture fixation devices. The text is not intended to be a comprehensive review but basic reading to prepare for more exhaustive books and manuals on osteosynthesis.

The book has eight chapters. The first two deal with essential terminology and metals used in fracture fixation. The remaining six deal with the 'elements' in some detail. In situations where an average reader may be inclined to skip the paragraph, I have used a smaller type and refrained from omitting such esoteric material as 'principles of cutting instruments' or 'factors enhancing the efficiency of screw insertion', details which may be of interest to a reader with more scholastic leanings. The material included in the book is basic and I have kept referencing to a minimum. The formal inclusion of references in the text is made principally to meet copyright obligations. The literature from which I have drawn extensively is catalogued at the end as a bibliography.

All the illustrations, with three exceptions, have been redrawn with modifications to highlight the topic under discussion.

I take this opportunity to thank my orthopaedic surgeon friends, Mr Praful D. Sutaria, FRCS of Greenwich District Hospital, London and Dr Vikas M. Agashe, MS(Ortho) of Kurla, Mumbai (Bombay), for reading the various drafts of the manuscript and making valuable suggestions for improvement. The task of making sure I have said what I wanted to was facilitated by another friend. Mr Rajeshwar Singh of Kalina, Mumbai. I am obliged to him for proof reading and editing the manuscript in its formative stage. I wish to thank Mr Geoffrey Nuttall, formerly of Churchill Livingstone, for his keen personal interest and encouragement in the early stages of the project and his able successor, Mr Gavin Smith, for continued support and advice enabling me to complete the manuscript and illustrations in a short time. The traditional thanks to the artist and the secretary are missing because I have typed the manuscript and drawn all the illustrations on a PC.

Mumbai
January 1997

Anand J. Thakur
189 Swami Vivekanand Road, Irla
Vile Parle/West Mumbai (Bombay) 400056
India

Contents

Foreword vii
Preface to the Third Edition ix
Acknowledgements xi
Preface to the First Edition xiii

CHAPTER 1	Lexicon of Fracture Fixation 1
CHAPTER 2	Bone and Materials in Fracture Fixation 24
CHAPTER 3	Bone Screws 64
CHAPTER 4	Bone Plates 107
CHAPTER 5	Intramedullary Nailing 196
CHAPTER 6	Hip Fixation 239
CHAPTER 7	Wire, Cable and Pins 276
CHAPTER 8	External Fixators 313
CHAPTER 9	Spinal Instrumentation 360
CHAPTER 10	Minimal Invasive Osteosynthesis 377

Index 397

CHAPTER 1

LEXICON OF FRACTURE FIXATION

'As is our biomechanics, so is our orthopaedics'
— with apologies to **William Osler.**

Force
Types and Effects of Loading
   Bending
   Torsion
Loading Modes and Fracture Patterns
   Tension Load
   Compression Load
   Bending Load
   Bending and Axial Compression
   Torsion
   Torsion, Bending and Axial Compression
Useful Definitions
   Stress and Strain
   Moment, Moment of Inertia
   Polar and Area Moment of Inertia
   Stress Risers
   Stress Shielding

Column Loading and Tension Band Principle
Fracture Fixation Construct
Compression
Stiffness
Near and Far Cortex
Stable Fixation
Strength
Elasticity
Plasticity
Ductility
Toughness
Brittleness
Spiral
Helix
Working Length
Wolff's Law
von Mises Stress

To start a textbook on fracture fixation with definitions and concepts may seem uninviting but each specialty has its basics that must be mastered. In order to study and practice fracture fixation, understanding of basic terms such as force, tension, tension band, compression and working length is essential. Since the terminology of fracture fixation is heavily dependent on elementary mechanics, it is tantamount to learning a language foreign to medicine. To understand a few essential terms and concepts, one should start at the beginning of mechanics – the force.

FORCE

To change the state of motion of an object, an outside force is essential. A force is something that causes acceleration of a moving body or when it is blocked, which cause its deformation. Mechanical forces can be visualized easily as 'push or pull' applied to an object, or in the language of mechanics, to a 'body' or a 'particle'.

In mechanics, normal always means 'perpendicular to' (Fig. 1.1). A normal force represents a tension or compression applied perpendicular to a surface or a plane within an object. Shear indicates a force parallel to a surface or a plane within an object and tends to cause relative displacement of two parallel objects or of parallel planes within an object. Axial denotes 'along an axis'. An axial force applied to a body at a point on or along a central axis tends to cause its linear displacement.

A moment is the effect of force acting on a lever arm. It acts as a bending moment or as torque. Torque represents the turning, twisting or rotational effect of force.

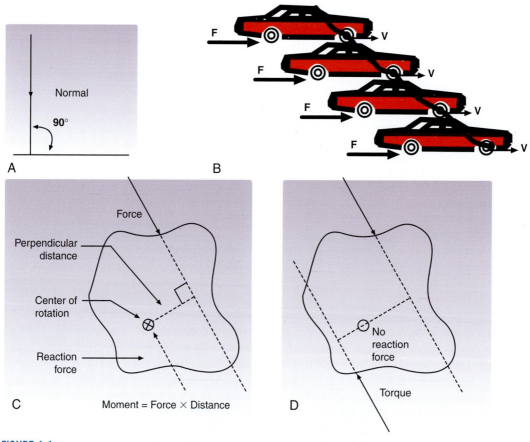

FIGURE 1.1

(**A**) A force acting perpendicular to any surface is referred to as normal. (**B**) A force causes acceleration. (**C**) The moment, or turning force, depends on the perpendicular distance of the line of action of the applied force from the centre of rotation (a fixed pivot point), as well as the magnitude of the force. There must be a reaction force at the centre of rotation to counteract the applied force. (**D**) If two equal and opposite forces act on the mass, a torque or couple is produced, with no net reaction force.[1]

Any force acting at a distance from an axis (about a point) produces a moment (Fig. 1.1B). A moment is an entity that is considered separately from a force; it represents the product of a force and the distance over which it acts (force × distance). Torque sometimes is used more specifically with reference to circular motion; e.g. the moment caused by a force applied tangentially to a wheel or a cylinder (Fig. 1.1C). In a clinical environment, a muscle applies both force and moment to a joint. The moment rotates the limb and force compresses the joint surfaces.

TYPES AND EFFECTS OF LOADING

A beam is a long piece of material with unaltered cross-section along its long axis. A piece of wood or a metal bar in a building are examples of a beam. Engineers refer to the application of a force to an object (e.g. a beam) as loading. There are five types of loading (Fig. 1.2). Axial load may be applied in tension (traction or pulling apart) or compression (pressing together). When the compression is applied in the center of a column it is called pure (centric) axial loading (see Fig. 1.16A and B). When an eccentric compressing load is applied, the deformation within the column is complex and bending is produced.

For clinicians, effects of bending are more important than effects of axial load. A bending load may act in a simple three-point, four-point or a cantilever mode. For clinicians, effects of bending are more important than effects of axial load. Torsion (twisting), direct shear and contact load are the remaining forms. When a long bone is loaded in torsion, overloading results in spiral fracture. A body under load

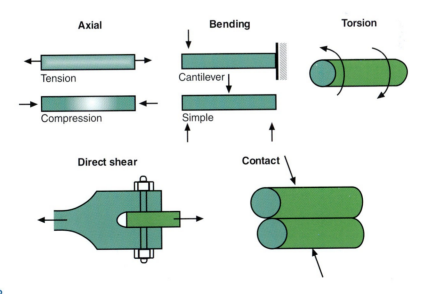

FIGURE 1.2

Five patterns of load, which are imposed upon surgical implants.[2]

reacts in two ways: it deforms (changes its shape) and it generates internal forces. Strain is a technical term used to express deformation. Force (load) that deforms an object is called surface force and may be either normal or shear. Normal force (one applied perpendicular to a body) causes either compression or tension, whereas shear force tends to cause sliding between parallel planes of an object (Fig. 1.3A). Accordingly, there are three corresponding types of strain.

Compressive strain is represented by the decrease in the length of a straight edge or a line drawn on a body. Tensile strain is represented by the increase in length of a straight edge or line drawn on a body. Shear strain is represented by a change in the angular relationship of the two lines drawn on the surface (Fig. 1.3B).

Reactionary force develops within the loaded material to maintain equilibrium by limiting deformation. The internal force resisting deformation is called stress. Like strain there are three basic types of stresses: compressive, tensile and shear (Fig. 1.3C).

As a person stands, the tibia does not collapse, but every particle within it deforms to a minute extent and strain develops. As the bone deforms, there are forces of molecular cohesion holding it together and resisting the applied load. This force that resists deformation is known as stress, as

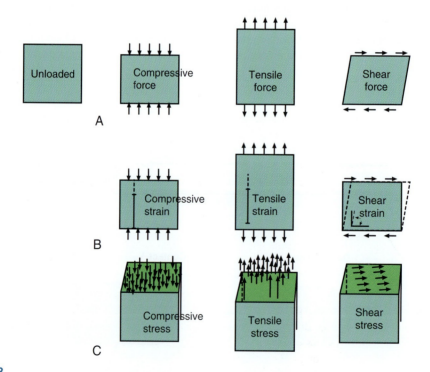

FIGURE 1.3

Three fundamental force components acting on a body. **(A)** Application of force to a body[1]; **(B)** deformation (strain) of the body in response to the applied force; **(C)** body's reactionary force – stress.[3]

mentioned above. If the load is too great and exceeds these intermolecular forces, this equilibrium is destroyed and the bone breaks.

Mechanical Properties of Beams

A beam, a shaft, a column, is a structure designed to support load (Fig. 1.4A–C). Implant/bone structures may act as complex beams, columns or shafts depending upon the loads applied to them. Axial compression, tension, bending and torsion overloads can cause a fracture. The last two, being the most common causative loads, are discussed in some detail.

Bending

Bending is the effect of a force applied perpendicularly to the axis of a beam. It may be applied to a beam by three methods: in three-point bending, in four-point bending and in cantilever form to a beam embedded within a wall (Fig. 1.4D–F). In many situations, long bones may be considered as beams, and their mechanical characteristics become highly relevant to fracture mechanics. As a beam bends under a load, one surface becomes convex, the other concave (Fig. 1.4G). Tensile strain develops at the convex surface, which tends to get longer, and planes of tensile stress develop perpendicular (i.e. normal) to the surface. Compressive strain and stress also develop in a similar fashion at the concave surface. These stresses are maximal at each surface and diminish towards the centre, where there is a transition from one to the other on a 'neutral plane', upon which the stresses are zero. The stress at the surface is often referred to as the maximal or extreme (outer) 'fibre' stress, as on an imaginary fibre of material at the surface. If the cross-section is symmetrical, the neutral plane will be central, and the tensile or compressive stresses will also be symmetrical. The strains along a beam axis follow linear bending theory; that is in three point bending a load is applied somewhere along the beam, while in four-point loading it is applied at two places. A bumper fracture of the tibia results from a three- or four-point bending. Four-point bending is clinically important because between the two internal points of load, the bending moment is constant. This property is significant for the assessment of bone healing, callus stiffness or the quality of osteogenesis; four-point bending test does not depend upon the exact position of the fracture or the callus. In clinics, four-point bending is similar to manipulation of a fracture (Fig. 1.4H).

A fracture of the distal third of the tibia may occur consequent to a blow to its upper end while the foot is firmly on the ground, as in standing; this is an example of a fracture in cantilever loading.

Torsion

Torsion results from torque (twisting force) applied to a cylinder; it depicts twisting of the structure about its long axis so that parallel lines drawn on the surface become helical (Fig. 1.5). In a bone, which is cylindrical in shape, torsion induces shear and tensile forces (Fig. 1.5A–C). The shear forces are in two planes, one transverse and one longitudinal through the bone axis, with maximal shear stress at the bone surface. The tensile stresses exist on a 45° plane to the axis of the bone. The bone tends to be weaker in shear than in tension and a spiral fracture starts with a shear failure parallel to the neutral axis and near the bone surface where the shear stress is highest; it then propagates along the 45° tension plane (Fig. 1.5D).

CHAPTER 1 LEXICON OF FRACTURE FIXATION

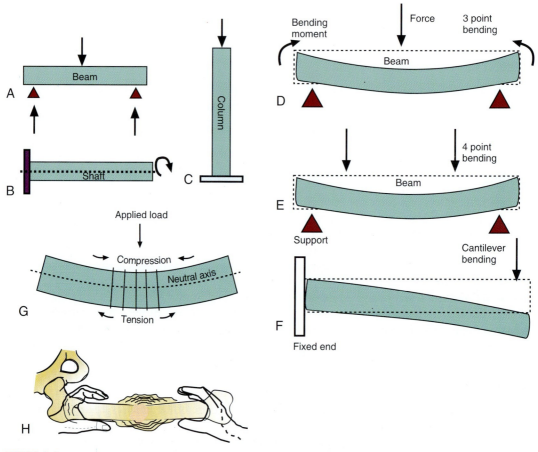

FIGURE 1.4

Three types of load bearing structures. **(A)** A beam sustains load between two supports; **(B)** a shaft resists torsion; **(C)** a column supports compressive loads. A beam can be loaded in **(D)** three point, **(E)** four point or **(F)** cantilever bending mode. A cantilever has a support only at one end and may be loaded at any point along its length. **(G)** Linear bending theory states that a plane perpendicular to the beam axis remains a plane perpendicular to this axis after bending. A bending moment is the load that deforms a beam into a curved shape. When a three point bending load is applied to a beam, the top (concave) surface shortens, resulting in compressive stress, while the bottom (convex) surface lengthens, resulting in tensile stress. At some point within the beam there is a transition between compressive and tensile stresses. This is termed the neutral axis.[1] **(H)** A clinician manipulating a fracture is four-point bending. This test to assess bone healing, callus stiffness or the quality of osteogenesis does not depend on the exact position of the fracture or the callus.[4]

LOADING MODES AND FRACTURE PATTERNS

Each load type creates a predictable and characteristic fracture pattern and these can be correlated in retrospect.

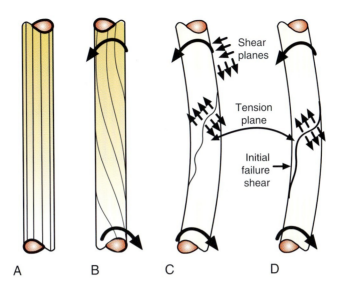

FIGURE 1.5

(**A and B**) Under torsion the parallel lines on a cylinder appear twisted. (**C**) Shear forces are indicated by the upper set of arrows and the tensile forces by the set in the centre. (**D**) At the beginning, the fracture line is parallel to the bone surface and then veers along a 45° plane.[3]

Tension Load

A fracture due to tension load is the simplest to explain in mechanical terms. Bone is placed under pure tension primarily by muscle action.

A tension fracture extends transversely, perpendicular to the load and bone axis, and involves cortico-cancellous bone (Fig. 1.6A). The fracture line disrupts the trabeculae in the cancellous bone; in the cortical bone, on the other hand, separation at cement lines and pulling out of osteons is seen. Tension fractures are avulsion of muscle origins or insertions, or occur in sesamoid bones, including the patella.

Compression Load

In a long bone, an axially applied compression load usually drives the diaphyseal bone, with its thick rigid cortex, into the thin metaphyseal bone like a battering ram. A diaphyseal impaction fracture results; this is the most frequent fracture pattern eventuating from axial loading of the long bones (Fig. 1.6B). Examples of this fracture pattern are supracondylar femoral fractures, tibial 'plafond' and comminuted tibial plateau fractures.

Bending Load

A bending load applied to a long bone induces two types of forces: the cortex on the concavity of the bone is subjected to compression forces, and the cortex on the convexity to tension forces (Fig. 1.7).

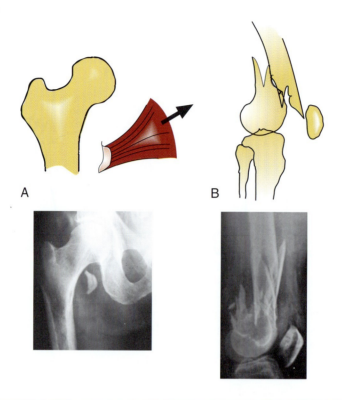

FIGURE 1.6
(**A**) Pure tension fracture. (**B**) Compression fractures are common in knee area.

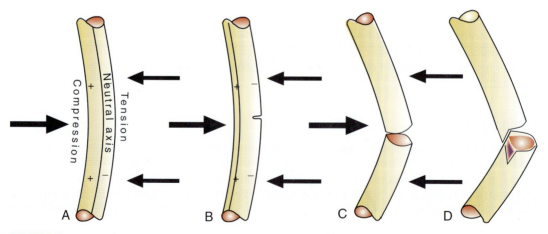

FIGURE 1.7
(**A**) Bending loads subject a long bone to tensile and compressive forces. (**B**) The neutral axis shifts towards to the concavity as the crack extends. (**C**) A typical transverse fracture or (**D**) its variation results.[3]

Cortical bone is weaker in tension than in compression, hence it generally fails in tension before it fails in compression. The crack begins on the tensile convex side of the cortex, and when the outer layer of the bone fails, the layer immediately under it is subjected to maximal stress and also fails. As successive layers fail, the crack propagates at right angles to the long axis of the cylindrical bone and produces a transverse fracture line (Fig. 1.7C). At some point, it may occasionally veer away from the transverse line on an oblique course (Fig. 1.7D). This is due to a progressive shift in the point of maximal compression as the crack propagates, as well as to factors related to energy dissipation. As the crack extends across the bone, the neutral axis shifts towards the concavity.

Bending and Axial Compression

A combination of bending and axial compression forces causes oblique transverse and butterfly fractures (Fig. 1.8). Pure axial loading produces a uniform compression force throughout the bone, whereas bending produces compression force on one side and tension force on the other. When axial and bending loads are combined, the net result is to add to the compressive force on the concavity and subtract from the tension force on the convexity. This fracture pattern is partially oblique (representing failure in compression) and partially transverse (tension failure). The butterfly fracture is a sequel to the oblique transverse pattern. As the fragments continue to angulate due to the bending load, the fragment containing the oblique segment (beak) impacts against the other fragment. Consequently the beak is sheared off, producing the classic butterfly fracture.

Torsion

High shear and tensile stresses develop in response to torsional loading and cause a spiral fracture. The bone tends to be weaker in shear and a spiral fracture initiates with shear failure parallel to the neutral axis and near the bone surface, where shear stress is highest; it then propagates along the 45° tension plane (see Fig. 1.5D).

Torsion, Bending and Axial Compression

A combination of torsion, compression and bending loads results in an oblique fracture, compression and torsion being the dominant components. The summation of these three forces is equivalent to a bending load about an oblique axis. The oblique fracture represents a higher energy injury than does the simple spiral fracture, and hence more soft tissue injury; consequently delays in healing may be anticipated. Different fracture patterns resulting from diverse loading modes, and their combinations are illustrated in Fig. 1.9.

USEFUL DEFINITIONS

"The more precisely we speak, the more effectively we are able to communicate our meaning to others. ... individual words have definitions to facilitate effective communication".

– **EC Halperin** (*Int J Radiation Oncol Biol Phys* 1987;13:143.)

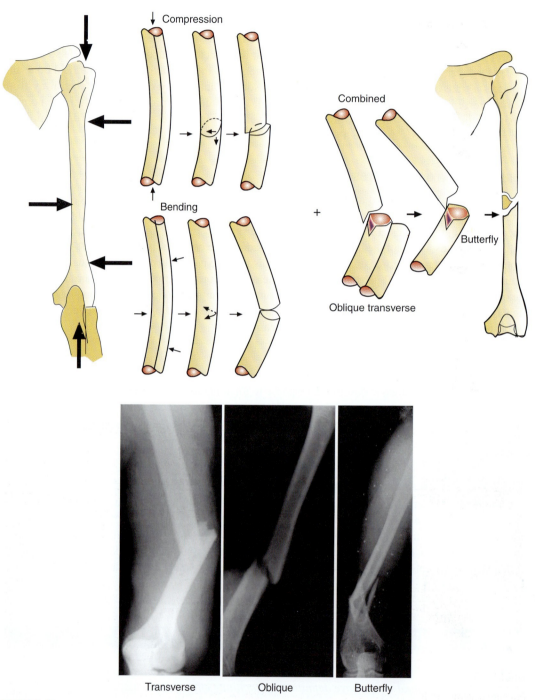

FIGURE 1.8
A combination of axial compression and bending loads produces an oblique fracture and a butterfly fragment.[5]

USEFUL DEFINITIONS

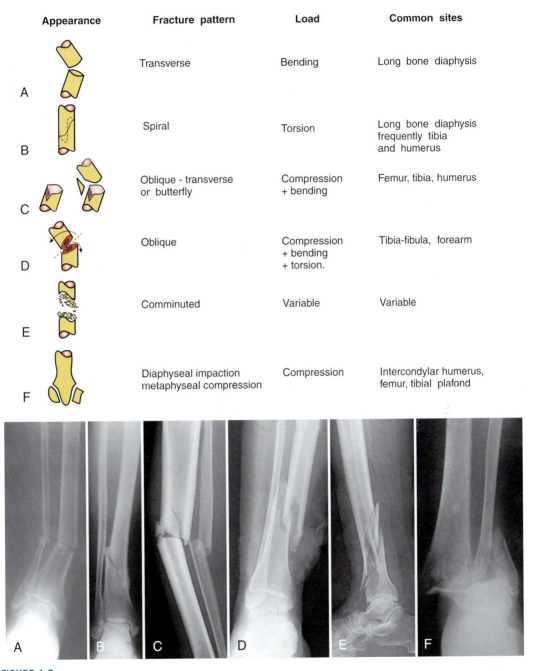

FIGURE 1.9
Fracture patterns resulting from different types of load.[5] Alphabetical labelling of sketches match clinical examples.

Stress and Strain

Stress and strain are values derived from application of force to a material and its resultant deformation. Its main utility is to compare results of experiments carried out under different settings.

Stress is the force applied to a cross-section of a material, divided by the area of that cross-section. Strain is the change in length of an object divided by its original length.

Elastic modulus (Young) is the ratio of stress to strain, and derived from an experimental plot (Fig. 1.10). Relative values of materials used in fracture fixation and orthopaedics are shown in Fig. 1.11.

Moment

It is a measure of the ability of a force to generate rotational motion. The axis the object rotates about is called the instantaneous axis of rotation (IAR).

Moment arm is the shortest distance between the IAR and the point of load application.

The magnitude of the moment generated by a force is the magnitude of the force times its moment arm. The SI unit for the moment is the Newton-meter (N·m)

Moment of Inertia (or Mass Moment of Inertia)

It is the inertia of a rotating body with respect to its rotation.

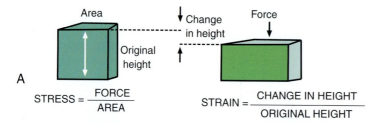

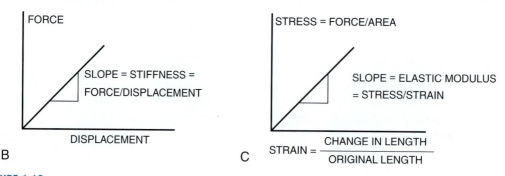

FIGURE 1.10

(A) Stress is calculated by applied force divided by area of the cross-section. **(B)** Value of strain is arrived by dividing change in height by original height. **(C)** Likewise the stress-strain graph can be drawn; load-deflection values and the slope of this line is the elastic modulus.

USEFUL DEFINITIONS   13

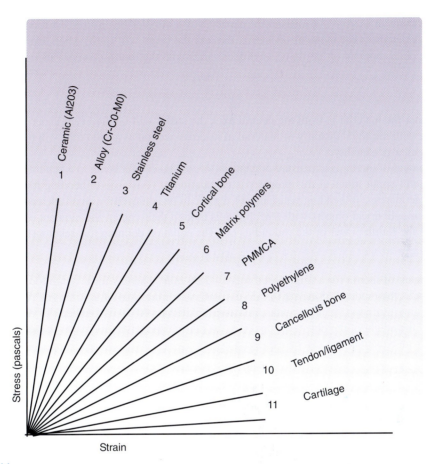

FIGURE 1.11
Relative values of Young's modulus of elasticity.[6] 1. Ceramic (Al₂O₃); 2. Co-Cr-Mo alloy; 3. Stainless steel; 4. Titanium; 5. Cortical bone; 6. Matrix polymers; 7. PMMA; 8. Polyethylene; 9. Cancellous bone; 10. Tendon/ligament; 11. Cartilage.

Polar and Area Moment of Inertia

The polar and area moment of inertia are related to the cross-sectional properties of a section and are fundamental geometric property of a structure (section is the cross-section of a piece; the property being described is for the section; when length is involved, it is the property of a member; several members acting together constitute a structure); the property measures the distribution of the material of a beam around its cross-section.[7] It describes the spatial distribution of material within a structure with respect to a particular axis of rotation or bending. The equation is expressed as:

$$I = \sum m_1 r_1^2$$

– the sum of each elemental mass (m_1) that is located at a distance (r_1) from the neutral or selected axis. Moment of inertia is a structural property only and is not related to the material used.

Polar moment of inertia is a measure of capacity of a circular beam to resist torsion or twisting force. The larger the polar moment of inertia, the less the beam will twist, when exposed to a given torque. The polar moment of inertia of a cylinder varies with the fourth power of its radius.

$$J_0 = \frac{\pi}{2} r^4$$

The further the material is from the neutral axis, the stiffer will be the beam under a given load; a hollow tube with the equal quantity of material in its cross-section as a solid tube will be stiffer; a long bone has similar personality.

Area moment of inertia is a measure of capacity of resistance of a beam to a bending force. One of the most useful applications of this property is calculation of resistance to bending for various structures. A large increase in bending resistance of a rod can be achieved by small increases in the rod's diameter. For cylindrical objects with a neutral axis though their center, the moment of inertia is proportional to the fourth power of the rod radius (r). The equation defining this relationship is:

$$I = (\Pi / 4) \times r^4$$

The moment of inertia for a 4-mm solid rod is 12.56 mm^4 whereas for a 7-mm rod it is 118 mm^4. In other words, the moment of inertia for a 7-mm rod is 10 times that of a 4-mm rod (Fig. 1.12).

The bending stiffness for rectangular objects is related to the height cubed. To a lesser degree, increases in the height of the object (or thickness) result in exponential increases in the bending resistance. Using an equation, this can be expressed as:

$$I = b \times h^3 / 12$$

The base (b) refers to the length of the plate, whereas the height (h) refers to the thickness.

In general, the further the mass is located away from the central axis, the higher the polar and area moment of inertia, i.e. a cylinder with a larger radius has a higher resistance to twisting and bending forces than one with a smaller radius. This helps to explain why tibial fractures are more frequent in the mid-lower segment than the upper third. The tibia, like most other long bones, resembles a cylinder. The mid-lower segment of the tibia has a smaller radius than the upper segment. The mid-lower tibial segment offers lesser resistance to torsional and bending forces than the upper third of the tibia. Under a specified load the mid-lower segment will deform more than the upper segment of the tibia and fail (Fig. 1.13).

The cortical index of a diaphyseal bone is defined as the cortical thickness divided by the bone diameter; there is a significant correlation between the cortical index and bone density.[8] The index is a coefficient ranging between 0 and 1 and demonstrates the importance of the medullary cavity: 0 for an empty tube and 1 for a solid bar. For diaphyseal bone, it varies between 0.35 and 0.6. With regard to the polar moment of inertia of a solid bar, the reduction is less than 5% for a thick tube ('normal' bone), and nearly 20% for a thin tube (very porotic bone): the outer part of cross-section plays a role in stiffness.

Dia. (mm)	Type	I (mm)	Stiffness = ∞|∞R^4
4	Solid	12.56	
5	Solid	30.65	
6	Solid	63.5	
7	Solid	118.0	

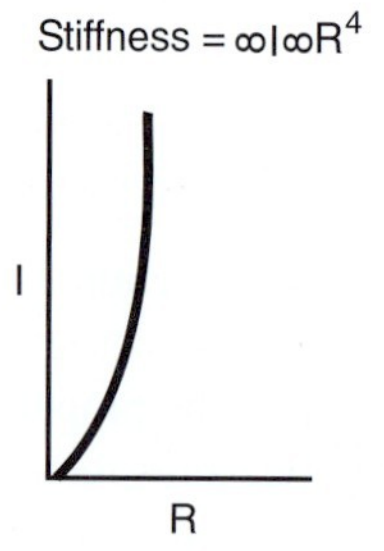

FIGURE 1.12

Small increase in radius manifests large increase in the stiffness of a rod and construct as the moment of inertia for a cylindrical rod is proportional to the fourth power of the radius

Stress Risers

A point at which the stress is appreciably higher than elsewhere due to the geometry of the stressed object is called a stress riser. The stresses, which result from loading, can be compared to the flow of water in a river. In the quiet part of a river, the flow is uniform, but around a large rock it is disturbed due to an increase in velocity and a rise in pressure in order to overcome the obstruction. Similarly the parallel stress lines in a structure are concentrated in the area of stress risers (Fig. 1.14A).

In a structure, a change in shape induces a variation in stress distribution. Stresses concentrate around discontinuities such as holes, sharp angles, notches, grooves, threads and any other sudden transitions in a structure. These discontinuities are also known as stress risers (Fig. 1.14B).

A cylinder with a slot on one side (open section) is weaker than one without it in resisting torsional loads. In an intact cylinder, all of the developed stresses resist the applied load: in an open section, only a fraction does so. If the stresses are represented as arrows resisting the applied load, the open section reverses their direction on the inner wall (Fig. 1.14C). The induced weakness is independent of the width of the slot. Bone and metal are similarly affected.

All stress risers greatly weaken a structure; stress risers (stress concentrators) produce increased local stresses, which may be several times higher than those in the bulk of the material and may lead to local failure. A drill hole in an intact tibia acts as a stress riser (Fig. 1.14D).

The presence of a screw does not diminish the weakening effect. Removal of a cortical bone graft creates a stress riser as well as an open section. The open section effect is more weakening than the stress concentration; moreover, open section greatly reduces bone's resistance to torsion (polar moment). Any reduction in stress concentration gained by rounding the corners of a square cut-out is overshadowed by the open section effect. A fracture may initiate at a screw hole in a bone or at a window created by removal of a cortical graft. Other clinical examples of stress-riser-induced break are a pathological fracture through a tumour, a re-fracture near an area of callus, and fracture at the end of a rigid bone plate (Fig. 1.15).

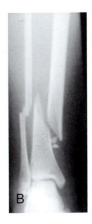

FIGURE 1.13

(**A**) Upper end of the tibia has a larger cross-section and higher polar moment of inertia than the mid-lower segment; as a result mid-lower segment is more prone to fracture than the upper end as it offers a lesser degree of resistance to torsional and bending forces. (**B**) Spiral fracture of lower end of the tibia in a 27-year-old woman.

Stress Shielding

Bone reacts to reduction in functional load by becoming less dense or weak.

Column Loading and Tension Band Principle

A column, when loaded along its central axis, displays a stress pattern, compression, which is evenly distributed over its horizontal cross-section (Fig. 1.16A and B). When the load is applied off-centre, the stress pattern changes. In addition to the direct compression, there are elements of compression and

16 CHAPTER 1 LEXICON OF FRACTURE FIXATION

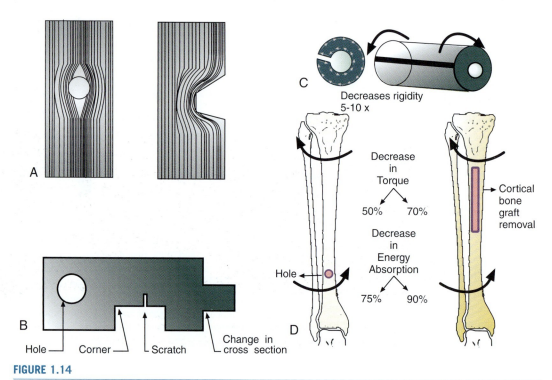

FIGURE 1.14

(**A**) Stress is concentrated at the equator of the hole and at the bottom of the notch. A sharp notch would concentrate the stress further.[9] (**B**) Stress concentrators may result from corners, holes, scratches or, changes in cross-section, or may be due to gouging between moving components.[1] (**C**).Open section reverses the direction of the stresses on the inner wall. (**D**) The tibia is considerably weakened by the presence of a drill hole or an open section but to different degrees.[3]

tension due to bending. This eccentric column loading is common in the skeleton. The more eccentric the loading, the more important the bending component, and the higher the stresses. The tibia and femur act as columns supporting the body weight and as beams resisting bending moments. If the foot twists then these bones act as shafts resisting torsion. The femoral stress distribution is illustrated in Fig. 1.16C.

The tensile forces produced by eccentric loading can be converted to compressive forces and used to some advantage in fracture fixation by application of a tension band. The tension band principle is explained in Fig. 1.16D to G.

Cables, metal wires, non-absorbable sutures and bone plates are used as 'bands' and function according to the tension band principle. A plate is able to resist very large amounts of tensile force. All of these implants are frequently utilized in fracture fixation.

Fracture Fixation Construct

A nail-bone or plate-bone construct is an arrangement or configuration of fixation implants applied to a fractured bone.

USEFUL DEFINITIONS 17

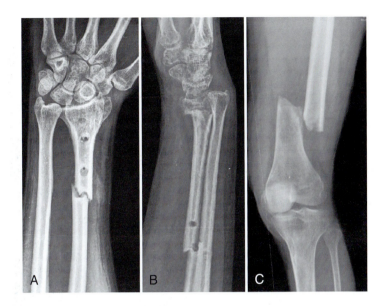

FIGURE 1.15

Radiographs showing instances of stress risers. (**A**) After removal of plate the distal most screw hole. (**B**) After removal of Schanz pin. (**C**) Tumor in the diaphyseal zone acts as a stress riser.

Compression

This is an act of pressing together that results in deformation, a shortening like that in a spring and an improvement in, or creation of, stability. In fracture fixation, compression is mainly used to provide stability to the bone-implant construct. Accurate reduction and application of a plate under compression improves the load sharing capacity of the construct. An implant may not break when bone shares a part of the load. Such a situation protects the implant and creates favourable mechanical conditions for bone healing. Compression also helps in the application of the tension band principle to restore dynamic loading of the bone fragments.

Stiffness

Stiffness is the resistance of a structure to deformation; in other words it is a term used to describe the force needed to achieve a certain deformation of a structure. There are many variables in application of load and points of application to a structure; the term 'stiffness' of a structure always requires an exact description of the load configuration, exact localization and the kind of deformation being measured. In absence of these details the calculated values from different experiments cannot be compared. The higher the stiffness of an implant the smaller the deformation; the smaller the displacement of the fracture fragments, the smaller the strain on the repairing tissue. A reduction in strain, but not its complete absence, promotes healing.

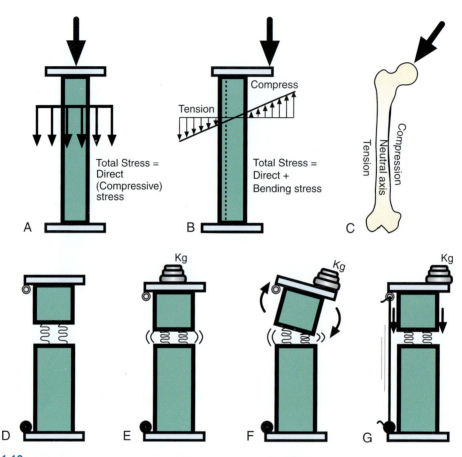

FIGURE 1.16

(**A**) Uniaxial column loading showing even distribution of compressive stress. (**B**) Eccentric loading of the same column generates additional bending stress.[3] (**C**) Stress pattern in a weight bearing bone like the femur.[5] (**D**) The tension band principle. An interrupted I-beam connected by two springs. (**E**) The I-beam is loaded with a weight (kg) placed over the central axis of the beam; there is uniform compression of both springs at the interruption. (**F**) When the I-beam is loaded eccentrically by placement of the weight at a distance from the central axis of the beam, the spring on the same side compresses, whereas the spring on the opposite side is placed in tension and stretches. (**G**) If a tension band is applied prior to the eccentric loading, it resists the tension that would otherwise stretch the opposite spring and thus causes uniform compression of both springs.[10]

Near and Far Cortex

The cortex nearest the plate and the one farthest away from it are named accordingly.

Stable Fixation

A stable fixation is characterized by lack of motion at the fracture site (i.e. a little or no displacement between the fragments of a fracture). It is also described as a fixation that keeps the fragments of a fracture motionless even during joint movement. Clinical examples of devices offering increasing levels of stable fixation is shown in Fig. 1.17. While unstable fixation produces pain with any attempt to move the limb, stable fixation allows early painless mobilization.

The term absolute stability describes an exceptional condition; it defines complete absence of relative displacement between compressed fracture surface. The definition of absolute stability applies only to a given time and a given site; some areas may displace in relation to each other, other areas of a fracture may not, and different areas may exhibit different displacement at different times. Within the same fracture surface, areas of absolute and relative stability may be present simultaneously. Practically the only method of achieving absolute stability consists in the application of interfragmental compression. The compression stabilizes by preloading and by producing friction.

Rigidity

Rigidity when used in context of fracture fixation describes an implant or of a bone-implant construct's physical property of resisting deformation under load.

Strength[11]

The ability of a material to resist an applied force without rupture.

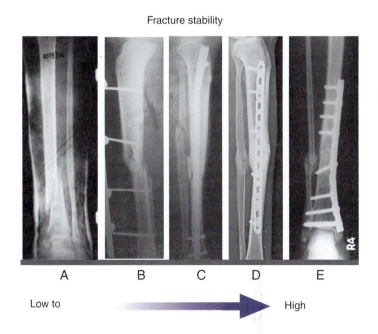

FIGURE 1.17

The term stability in fracture fixation is used to describe motion (or lack of it) between fracture fragments. **(A)** A plaster cast offers minimum stability. **(B)** External fixator and **(C)** intramedullary nail impart increasingly higher levels of stability, while **(D)** a plate fixation confers relative stability **(E)** only an interfragmental screw through the plate bestows absolute stability.

Elasticity

It is the ability of a material to recover its original shape after deformation. The physical reasons for elastic behavior differs from material to material; in metals the atomic lattice changes size and shape when forces are applied and returns to original state when forces are withdrawn; in rubbers the elasticity results by the stretching of polymer chains when the forces are active.

Plasticity

The ability of a material to be formed to a new shape without fracture and retain that shape after load removal.

Ductility

The ability of solid material is to be deformed under tensile stress and be stretched into a wire without fracture; it also bestows capacity to be shaped, e.g. construction of bone plates.

Toughness

The ability of a material to withstand suddenly applied forces without fracture.

Brittleness

The opposite of toughness; usually there is no evidence of plasticity prior to fracture.

Spiral

A curve on a plane that winds around a fixed point while moving even farther and farther from that point. (Fig. 1.18A).

Helix

A three-dimensional curve generated by a point that while turning around a straight line (axis) moves at a constant or continuously varying in one direction parallel to the axial line (Fig. 1.18B).

Working Length

The distance between the two points of fixation (one on either side of the fracture) along an implant, usually an intramedullary nail and the bone. It is not the overall length of an intramedullary nail or a bone plate that counts, but rather the length of the implant between the proximal and distal points of firm fixation to the bone on either side of a fracture; this is referred to as the working length of the implant.

The quantum of motion at the fracture site is directly proportional to the working length of the construct: the shorter the working length, the lesser the motion at the fracture site. The working length of construct is variable; it changes with the type of loading and differs in bending and torsion. The working

USEFUL DEFINITIONS

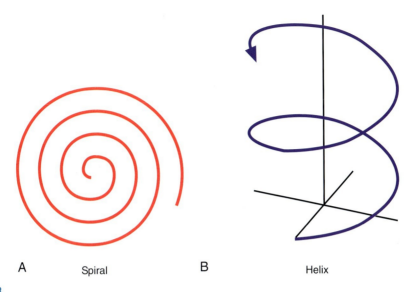

FIGURE 1.18

(A) A spiral is a curve in a one plane. (B) A helix is a curve with three-dimensions.

length in bending is determined by points of bone-plate fixation on either side of the fracture and changes with the direction of the bending force (Fig. 1.19A and B). The rigidity of a construct in bending is inversely proportional to the square of the working length.

For an intramedullary nail, working length in bending is smaller for a simple transverse fracture than for a comminuted fracture (Fig. 1.20A); in torsional loading, its working length is determined by the points at which interlocking is present between the bone and the nail (Fig. 1.20B). The torsional rigidity is inversely proportional to the working length. In an original Küntscher nail, there is no resistance to torsion and the concept is not applicable.

Wolff's Law

'The shape of the bone being given, the amount and the structure of bone adapts itself to the (dynamic) physiological loads applied to it'.[13]

Bones develop the structure best suited to resisting the forces acting on them. Any changes in either the form or function of a bone are followed by specific changes in its internal architecture and secondary

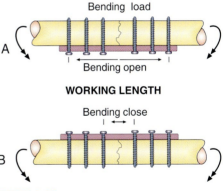

FIGURE 1.19

(A) The working length of a plate is greater in bending open than in bending close situation. The plated bone is particularly weak under loads that tend to bend open the fracture. The outer screws bear highest stresses as the direction of the load is towards the plate. (B) When a plate is applied as a tension band in the bending close construct, the working length of the plate in bending is minimal, since it is in contact with bone on either side of the fracture.

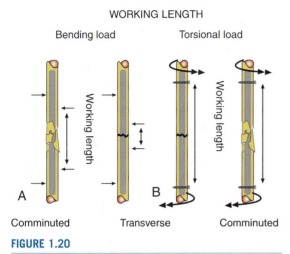

FIGURE 1.20

(A) In intramedullary nailing of a transverse fracture, the working length for bending load is smaller than in fixation of a comminuted fracture. (B) The torsional working length of an interlocked nail varies with the distance between the proximal and distal locking points.[12]

alterations in its external shapes-changes usually involving responses to alterations in weight-bearing stresses (form follows function). This applies only to long-lasting unloading.[14]

von Mises Stress[15]

This refers to a theory called the 'von Mises–Hencky criterion for ductile failure'. It is a formula for calculating whether the stress combination at a given point will cause failure. At given point in an elastic body, three calculable principal stresses are known to exist and act in x, y and z axes. von Mises discovered that the combined effect of these often-undersized stresses could cause failure of the material. The combination of three stresses is often referred to as 'equivalent stresses'; the term von Mises stress is short name for equivalent stress. It is a number that is used as an index. When 'von Mises stress exceeds failure stress (yield stress) of a material, the material exists in a failure condition. The formula below is used to calculate von Mises stress:

$$(S_1 - S_2)^2 + (S_2 - S_3)^2 + (S_3 - S_1)^2 = 2S_e^2$$

Where S_1, S_2 and S_3 are the principal stresses and S_e is the equivalent stress, or 'von Mises Stress'.

REFERENCES

1. Tencer AF, Johnson KD. Biomechanics in orthopaedic trauma: bone fracture and fixation. London: Martin Dunitz; 1994.
2. Mears DC. Materials and orthopaedic surgery. Baltimore: Williams & Wilkins; 1979.
3. Cochran GVB. A primer of orthopaedic biomechanics. New York: Churchill Livingstone; 1982.
4. Cordey J. Introduction: basic concepts and definitions in mechanics. Injury 2000;31:S-B 6–7.
5. Gozna ER, Harrington IJ, Evans DC. Biomechanics of musculoskeletal injury. Baltimore: Williams & Wilkins; 1982.
6. Karadsheh M. Bone material properties: material properties, Available at: http://www.orthobullets.com/basic-science/9062/material-properties; 2014 [accessed 14.08.22, 9.08 am].
7. Maher TR, Valdevit A, Caruiso S. Spinal biomechanics. In: Bono CM, Garfin SR, editors. Spine. Philadelphia: Lippincott Williams & Wilkins; 2004.
8. Virtama P, Telkkae A. Cortical thickness as an estimate of mineral content of human humerus and femur. Br J Radiol 1962;35:632–3.
9. Radin EL, Rose RM, Blaha JD, Litsky AS. Practical biomechanics for the orthopaedic surgeon. 2nd ed. New York: Churchill Livingstone; 1992.

10. Browner BD, Mast J, Mendes M. Principles of internal fixation. In: Browner B, editor. Biomechanics of fractures in skeletal trauma-fracture, dislocation and ligamentous injury. Philadelphia: WB Saunders; 1992. p. 243–68.
11. Green M, Nokes LDM, editors. Engineering theory in orthopaedics: an introduction. Chichester: Ellis Horwood; 1988. p. 14.
12. Hipp JA, Cheal EJ, Hayes WC. Biomechanics of fractures. In: Browner B, editor. Biomechanics of fractures in skeletal trauma - fracture, dislocation and ligamentous injury. Philadelphia: WB Saunders; 1992. p. 95–125.
13. Cordey J. Introduction: basic concepts and definitions in mechanics. Injury 2000;31:S–B2.
14. Wagner M, Frigg R. Internal fixators. Davos Platz, Switzerland: AO Publishing; 2006. p. 5.
15. Kazimi SMA. Solid mechanics. New Delhi, India: Tata McGraw-Hill; 1982. ISBN 0-07-451715-5.

CHAPTER 2

BONE AND MATERIALS IN FRACTURE FIXATION

Immobilization does not favour the formation of callus, movement does.
– **Just Lucas-Championnière, 1910.**

Bone as Material
   Biomechanical Properties of Bone
   Tensile Strength and Elasticity
Four Steps of Fracture Healing
Healing of a Treated Fracture
   Perren Hypothesis
   Healing Process
      Callus Formation and Internal Fixation
      Osteonal and Non Osteonal Healing
   Diamond Concept
Conventional Plate and Bone Vascularity
Adverse Clinical Conditions Delaying Bone Healing
   Chronic Inflammation
   Diabetes
   Hypovitaminosis
   Ageing
      Muscular Mass
      Diet, Alcohol and Smoking
   Polytrauma
   NSAIDs
Enhancement of Bone Healing
   Parathyroid Hormone Therapy
Orthobiologics and Tissue Engineering
   Natural Bone-Based Bone Graft Substitute
      Autogenous Bone Grafts
      Bone Marrow
         Reamer–Irrigator–Aspirator
      Allogenic Bone Grafts
      Demineralized Bone Matrix
   Growth Factor-Based Bone Graft Substitutes
      BMPs and Other Growth Factors
      Platelet-Rich Plasma (PRP) or Autologous Platelet Concentrate
   Cell-Based Bone Graft Substitutes
      Stem Cells
      Collagen
      Gene Therapy
   Ceramic-Based Bone Graft Substitutes
      Calcium Hydroxyapatite and Tricalcium Phosphate (TCP)
      β-TCP
      Bioactive Glass Ceramices (Bioglass)
   Polymer-Based Bone Graft Substitutes
   Coral-Based Bone Graft Substitutes
      Coralline Hydroxyapatite
Other Modalities to Enhance Bone Healing
   Electromagnetic Stimulation
   Shock Wave Therapy
   Ultrasound
Materials in Fracture Fixation
   Metals in Orthopaedic Use
      Stainless Steel
      Cobalt–Chromium Alloys
      Titanium Alloys
      Comparison of Stainless Steel and Titanium for Fracture Fixation
   Shape Memory Alloy
      Nickel–Titanium Alloy
Polymers
   Bioresorbable Polymers
      Mechanical Properties
      Fracture Fixation
   PEEK

Functionally Graded Material
   Clinical Relevance
      Metal Failure
      Metal Removal
      Mixing of Implants
Standards Organizations
Metal Working Methods and Their Effects on Implants
   Forging
   Casting
   Rolling and Drawing
   Milling
   Cold Working
   Annealing
   Case Hardening
   Machining
   Broaching
   Surface Treatment
      Polishing and Passivation
      Nitriding
   Fabrication of Implants
Corrosion
   Galvanic Corrosion
   Crevice Corrosion
   Pitting Corrosion
   Fretting Corrosion
   Stress Corrosion
   Intergranular Corrosion
   Ion Release

BONE AS MATERIAL

Biomechanical Properties of Bone

Bone is categorized as long bone and flat bone. On macroscopic level, cortical and cancellous types exist, which are described as lamellar and woven bone at microscopic level. Cortical bone exists in 80% of the skeleton. It is made of Haversian systems, which have osteons and Haversian canals; canals contain arterioles, venules, capillaries and nerves. The region between osteons is filled with interstitial lamellae. Cortical bone has slow turnover rate and high Young's modulus. Cancellous bone is organized as a loose network of bony struts measuring approximately 200 μm. It is porous and contains bone marrow. Newly formed bone is known as 'woven' bone and has random arrangement of the tissues. It contains more osteocytes per unit of volume and higher turnover rate compared to lamellar bone. It is also more flexible and weaker than lamellar bone. When it is organized and oriented along the lines of stress, remodelled woven bone is known as lamellar bone. It is stronger and stiffer than the woven bone.

Bone is a composite of type I collagen, ground substance (organic matrix) and calcium and phosphate (inorganic mineral salts). The organic components make the bone hard and rigid whereas the inorganic components give bone its tensile strength and elasticity. Bone is viscoelastic i.e. when loaded at higher rates it is stiffer, stronger and stores more energy. Gross appearance of bone is cortical (compact) and cancellous (porous); both have similar constitution but varying degree of porosity and density. The apparent density of bone is calculated as the mass of bone tissue divided by the volume of the specimen; apparent density of cortical bone is 1.8 g/cm^3 while range of apparent density of cancellous bone is from 0.1 g/cm^3 to 1.0 g/cm^3. After the fifth decade progressive net loss of bone mass occurs, but in women it proceeds at a faster rate. This loss leads to diminished bone strength, a reduced modulus of elasticity and increased possibility of fractures. Nature's compensatory mechanism initiates remodelling of bone. Bone is absorbed from endosteal location and deposited in subperiosteal zone. This activity leads to an increase in bone diameter and subsequent higher moment of inertia. Thus, thinning of bone is compensated by increased diameter; the transition is smaller in women and predisposes them to an increased rate of fracture.

Tensile Strength and Elasticity

Bone is formed in two ways. Endochondral bone formation occurs in non-rigid fracture healing (secondary bone healing), longitudinal physeal growth and embryonic long bone formation. Chondrocytes produce cartilage, which is absorbed by osteoclasts. Osteoblasts lay down bone on cartilaginous framework; bone replaces cartilage; cartilage is not converted to bone. Chondrocytes play a significant role in endochondral bone formation throughout the formation of the cartilage intermediate. Intramembranous bone formation is the second method of bone formation, generally known as primary bone healing, contact healing and Haversian remodelling. Fetal bone formation (embryonic flat bones like skull, maxilla, mandible, pelvis, clavicle and subperiosteal surface of long bone) also takes place by intramembranous bone formation. The process is also associated with distraction osteogenesis and fracture healing with rigid fixation, and is a part of healing process in intramedullary nailing. Intramembranous bone formation commences with aggregation of undifferentiated mesenchymal cells that later differentiate into osteoblasts; simultaneously organic matrix is deposited.

FOUR STEPS OF FRACTURE HEALING

The entire process of diaphyseal fracture healing may be divided into four stages: inflammation, soft callus, hard callus and remodelling. Inflammation starts immediately after the fracture occurs and lasts for 7–10 days. Initial haematoma is gradually replaced by granulation tissue. Osteoclasts remove necrotic tissue from the bone ends. Soft callus is formed in 2–3 weeks after the fracture. Fragments are in a sticky state and there is sufficient stability to prevent shortening, but not angulation. Progenitor cells from the periosteum and endosteum mature to form osteoblasts. Bone growth takes place away from fracture gap and forms a cuff of woven bone at both subperiosteal and endosteal locations. Blood vessels grow into the callus. Mesenchymal cells in the fracture gap proliferate and differentiate into fibroblasts or chondrocytes producing characteristic extracellular matrix. Hard callus develops when the fracture ends are held together by soft callus. The process continues for 3–4 months. Ossification process commences at the periosteum as cartilage is converted into rigid calcified tissue by endochondral ossification. Thus, bony callus growth begins in the peripheral areas and slowly progress towards the gap. Osseous bridge is formed away from the cortex, either externally or in the medullary canal. Finally, through endochondral ossification, the soft tissue in the gap is converted. The fourth stage of remodelling commences after hard callus is well established. The osteoclasts ream out a tunnel in the dead cortical bone down that a blood vessel follows, bringing in the osteoblasts that lay down the lamellar bone. If the fractured bone ends are closely opposed then the osteoblasts penetrate directly into the opposite fragment to re-establish the cortical continuity. In cancellous bone the cells are close to blood vessels and the process of bone replacement takes on the surface of the trabeculae, a phenomenon referred to as 'creeping substitution'.[1]

The cancellous bone heals more quickly and reliably than cortical bone in healing process.

HEALING OF A TREATED FRACTURE[1]

A bone fractures when mechanically overloaded; the injury causes soft tissue damage and haematoma, and bone ends lose their blood supply. The avascular broken ends of the bone and injured soft tissue play an important part in stimulating bone healing in an effort to regain original bone integrity. The fracture healing is an extraordinary repair process in the body, as it does not leave a scar like other tissues and leads to an authentic reconstruction of damaged bone to its initial structure.

In the late 1950s, it was observed that the osteotomies fixed with rigid compression plating united directly by osteonal or Haversian remodelling in contact areas (contact healing). Subsequently, fracture healing has been recognized in two patterns: primary bone healing – healing with minimal callus formation (synonyms: direct healing, contact healing); secondary bone healing – healing with abundant callus formation (synonyms: secondary fracture healing, spontaneous fracture healing, non-contact fracture healing). The term 'primary bone union' is a radiographic definition, where the lack of external callus formation and the gradual disappearance of the narrow fracture line served as the main criteria and this terminology is clinically established. Accordingly, secondary bone union refers to a healing mechanism of substantial external callus formation seen on radiographs.

Perren Hypothesis

Fracture healing process is dependent on maintenance of the fracture haematoma, the perfusion of the surrounding soft tissues and bone, as well as the stability between the bone fragments. A fracture heals only if it is stable. The level of stability of fixation decides the extent of movement occurring at the fracture site – more the stability, lesser the movement. Perren's 'interfragmentary strain' hypothesis states that the local mechanical environment affects the tissue response.[2] The interfragmentary strain is defined as the ratio of the relative displacement of fracture ends versus the initial fracture gap width (Fig. 2.1). Interfragmentary strain governs the type of tissue that forms between the fracture fragments. According to the hypothesis, a balance between the local interfragmentary strain and the mechanical characteristics of the callus tissue is the determining factor in the course of both primary and secondary fracture healing. The interfragmentary strain is inversely proportional to the fracture gap size. In the presence of a small gap, moderate interfragmentary motion can increase the strain to the extent that the progress of tissue differentiation is not possible. To circumvent this situation, small sections of bone near the fracture gap may undergo resorption, thus making the fracture gap larger and reducing the overall strain.

As mentioned above, all healing tissues need stable conditions to grow. Treatment devices provide stability of varying degrees and fracture gap strain changes accordingly (Fig. 2.2). Primary (direct) bone healing occurs only if the movement at the fracture site is bare minimum, i.e. the strain level is kept to less than 2%, a state of absolute stability. When the tissue elongation is between 2% and 10%, a state of relative stability exists and secondary (indirect) bone healing occurs. If the stability is poor and strain level (movement at fracture site) is more than 10%, bone tissue does not grow. In contrast, granulation tissue tolerates greater level of elongation and grows in the face of 100% strain levels. Fibrous tissue, tendon and bone have decreasing tolerance for elongation; bone tissue has the least tolerance for elongation.

In any form of fracture fixation, bone fragments under load experience a certain amount of relative motion that, by yet unknown mechanisms, determines the morphologic features of fracture repair. Depending on the prevalent mechanical environment, bone will heal in one of the two

$$\text{Interfragmentary strain} = \frac{\text{Change in the fracture gap width}}{\text{Original fracture gap width}}$$

FIGURE 2.1

Interfragmentary strain is the ratio of change in the width of the fracture gap divided by the original width of the fracture gap.

CHAPTER 2 BONE AND MATERIALS IN FRACTURE FIXATION

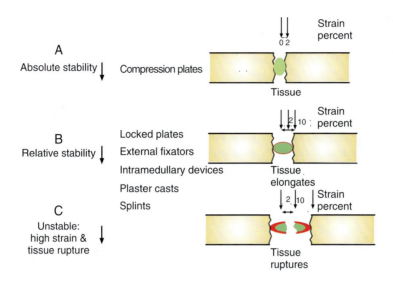

FIGURE 2.2

(A) Absolute stability creates a lower strain environment encouraging primary bone healing. (B) Relative stability creates an environment conducive to secondary bone healing. (C) High strain condition creates a situation where the gap elongation exceeds tissue compliance, which can lead to its rupture and cessation of fracture healing.

ways: indirect (secondary) or direct (primary). Indirect fracture healing results from conditions of relative stability. Indirect bone healing is the natural method of bone healing and requires granulation tissue and callus precursors. As callus forms and matures, the callus mass stiffens and fracture stability improves. The callus increases the diameter of the fracture site and the bone and this change improves the mechanical leverage. Callus formation paves way for effective bone healing and can be facilitated by splinting.

Healing Process
Callus Formation and Internal Fixation
Callus forms at three locations: 'gap' callus between the bone ends, 'medullary' (endosteal) callus along the medullary cavity and the 'periosteal' callus under periosteum (Fig. 2.3). Callus provides initial stability so that osteogenesis can commence. When an implant for fracture fixation provides absolute stability, there is no stimulation for the callus process, and healing by primary intention results. In indirect fracture healing, gap callus generated between well-reduced fracture ends is the weakest. Medullary callus provides some resistance to bending moments. The periosteal callus is most effective in providing resistance to bending and torsional forces, and resisting force is proportional to the fourth power of the radius of the cross-section of bone through the callus mass. Use of intramedullary nail minimizes medullary callus but periosteal callus is produced in abundance (Fig. 2.4). In plate fixation, there is plenty of medullary callus as well as periosteal callus on the opposite (compression) side of the plate. When a non-contact plate is used, callus appears even beneath the plate. Table 2.1 highlights different aspects of formation of callus, its behaviour and visibility on radiographs.

Osteonal and Non Osteonal Healing

Direct bone healing is a biological process of osteonal bone healing and can be achieved under conditions of absolute stability that is created only by surgical fixation (Fig. 2.5). It is a contact healing between two avascular bone surfaces and callus formation is lacking. In the initial days after surgery there is minimal activity near the bone ends. The haematoma is resorbed or transformed into repair tissue. Later the Haversian system internally remodels the bone. Haversian remodelling has two main functions: (a) the revascularization of necrotic fracture ends and (b) reconstitution of the intercortical union. There are three requirements for the Haversian remodelling across the fracture site: (a) exact reduction (axial alignment), (b) stable fixation and (c) sufficient blood supply. Subsequently, cutting cones reach the fracture site and cross it wherever there is bone contact, or the gap is minute, producing a multiple microbridging effect through newly formed osteons that cross the gap. Callus is not seen. Fracture gap does not widen. The ability to remodel is time limiting and is induced by biochemical signals.

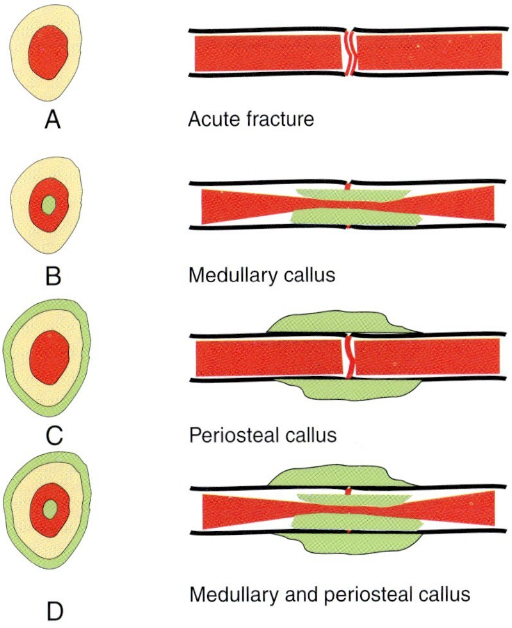

Simultaneously, gaps between imperfectly fitting fragment surfaces begin to fill; granulation tissue develops in small gaps, which then matures into lamellar and cortical bone and gap healing results (Fig. 2.5D). Bone resorption at fracture site also reduces strain if local motion does not tend to increase. In clinical set up, fracture gap strain is reduced by fracture comminution and imperfect reduction.

Each step in the healing cascade decreases the motion at the fracture gap, and therefore the gap strain, ultimately creating environment conducive to bone formation. Fig. 2.6 illustrates callus formation with different types of fixation.

To summarize, absolute stability leads to direct or primary bone healing; flexible fixation leads to indirect or secondary bone healing; variation in the fracture gap due to level of stability decides the progress of fracture healing; biologic fixation techniques are aimed at relative stability and secondary bone healing; bridging fixation obtained through casts, splint, external fixators, intramedullary nails and locked plate construct decrease gap strain by decreasing motion while tolerating increased gap length.

FIGURE 2.3
Callus formation at different sites. (**A**) Acute fracture. (**B**) Medullary callus. (**C**) Periosteal callus. (**D**) Medullary and periosteal callus. Callus that forms away from the cortex increases the bone diameter; thickened bone offers higher resistance to destabilizing forces.

Diamond Concept

Fracture healing is a complex physiological process and requires the spatial and timely coordinated action of several different cell types, proteins and the expression of hundreds of genes working towards restoring its structural integrity without scar formation. In this cascade of events, a vibrant cell population is most

CHAPTER 2 BONE AND MATERIALS IN FRACTURE FIXATION

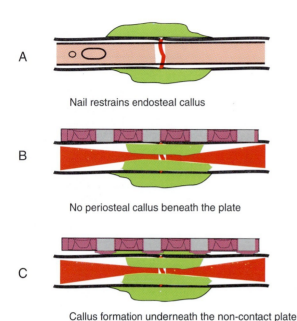

FIGURE 2.4

Callus formation with implants. **(A)** Nail inhibits endosteal callus but periosteal callus forms in abundance. **(B)** Conventional plate restrains periosteal callus formation but callus forms at the far cortex and at endosteal locations. **(C)** Callus forms underneath a non-contact plate.[3]

essential first element. Multipotent mesenchymal stem cells (MSCs) are enlisted at the fracture injury site or transferred to it with the blood circulation. The multipotent MSCs are transformed to osteoblasts.

The second constituent of the process is the fracture haematoma, which contributes signalling molecules (interleukins [IL-1, IL-6], tumour necrosis factor-α [TNF-α], fibroblast growth factor [FGF], insulin-like growth factor [IGF], platelet-derived growth factor [PDGF], vascular endothelial growth factor [VEGF] and the transforming growth factor-β [TGF-β] superfamily members). These factors are secreted by endothelial cells, platelets, macrophages, monocytes and also by the MSCs, the chondrocytes, the osteocytes and the osteoblasts themselves. These entities kick-start and sustain healing events.

The third factor in fracture healing, the extra-cellular matrix provides a natural scaffold for all the cellular events and interactions. Within the fracture haematoma, there forms a network of fibrin and reticulin fibrils; collagen fibrils are also present. Osteoclast in this environment removes necrotic bone at the fragment ends. The fracture haematoma is gradually replaced by granulation tissue and lays down the collagen fibres and the matrix that will later become mineralized to form the woven bone.

These three biological processes of fracture healing have been well recognized and studied. A less acknowledged fourth element, namely mechanical stability is a decisive factor for bone healing, and is indispensable for the formation of a callus that bridges the fracture site and progressively matures from woven to lamellar bone. Surgical treatments such as the application of systems of internal or external stabilization are designed to improve stability of fixation and there by enhance healing. These four vital elements of fracture healing are aptly called, 'the diamond concept'[6] (Fig. 2.7).

CONVENTIONAL PLATE AND BONE VASCULARITY

Although mechanical stability is essential, bone vitality is paramount in fracture healing because a dead bone cannot heal. In initial days of plate fixation, primary bone healing, also known as direct or osteonal healing was the golden aim and this was achieved only under an absolutely stable fixation. Wide exposure of the bone was necessary to gain access and to provide good visibility of the fracture zone to permit reduction and plate fixation. The bone fragments were extensively handled to accomplish perfect anatomical reduction and heavy implants were used. The screws had to be tightened to fix

Table 2.1 Different of Types and Locations of Callus in Fracture Healing[4]

Callus	Periosteal	Endosteal	Cortical (Gap Healing)	Cortical (No Fracture Gap)
Location	External surface of cortex and under periosteum	In the medullary cavity	In fracture gap <1 mm	Between two cortical surfaces under compression
Function	Stabilizes the fracture on emergent basis	Stabilizes the fracture with immature bone	Settles the fracture in initial phase 'gap healing'	Contact healing remodelling
Growth is stimulated	By fracture gap movements, elastic fixation	Appears after the peripheral callus grows Abundant in distraction osteogenesis (Ilizarov)	Rapid within 1 week of fracture	By absolute stability at fracture
Inhibited	Instability Soft tissue interposition	Mobility at fracture gap elastic fixation and instability	Instability	By mobility at fracture site
Duration	Limited time only in first 12 weeks	Slow to appear after peripheral callus grows Grows for unlimited period	In initial healing period	Slow process over several months
Visibility on radiographs	Seen in splinted fracture Casting Intramedullary nailing External fixation Plating	Difficult to see	In the small gaps between bone fragments	Not seen

and compress the plate onto the bone. Relative movement between fragments was eliminated by compression load and friction. Intramembranous bone formation, direct cortical remodelling and absence of external callus are characteristics of primary bone healing. In presence of absolute stability the blood vessels crossed the fracture line without disturbance and faster revascularization occurred. As there is no increase in bone diameter under direct osteonal healing, its load-bearing capacity does not increase and implant must be retained for longer time. Tightly fixed implants, as well as extensive bone and soft tissue handling, lead to a change in the bone which can be noted as porosis beneath the plate on early postoperative radiographs (Fig. 2.8).

This bone loss in the vicinity of a plate can be erroneously interpreted on the basis of Wolff's law as a reaction of living bone to mechanical unloading of the plated bone segment (stress protection); subsequent research has discovered its true avascular nature (Fig. 2.9). It was revealed that the compressive force under the plate prevents periosteal perfusion resulting in periosteum as well as bone necrosis deep to the plate and adjacent to the fracture site. Such episodes may occasionally lead to localized bone resorption at the screw threads and result in implant loosening.

It is also noted that the loss of vascularity is directly proportional to the contact area of the plate; the smaller the contact area of the plate, the lesser the vascular damage (Fig. 2.10). It is further postulated

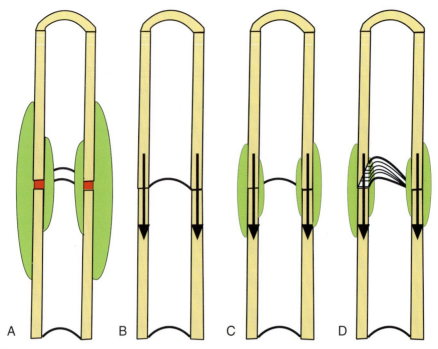

FIGURE 2.5

Schematic diagram illustrating non-osteonal and osteonal ways of fracture healing. **(A)** In non-osteonal fracture healing abundant periosteal plus small amount of endosteal callus formation is observed. No primary healing of the bone cortex is observed and remodeling processes are slow. The fracture union relies on maturation and remodeling of the periosteal osseous tissue with extensive remodeling processes of the fracture ends. The reasons for nonosteonal bone union are (1) axial malalignment (2) excessive fracture gap, or (3) unstable fixation in the presence of axial alignment. The critical gap size is not completely known but seems to be within the limit of I mm. Abundant callus is needed to reduce motion at the fracture site, which finally assists in remodeling and bone healing. Non-osteonal fracture healing is observed after cast immobilization where the fracture gap and the motion between the fragments are large. **(B)** Primary contact healing is characterized by direct cortical reconstruction but without substantial periosteal new bone formation. In a mechanically stable situation, as is the case in a rigid osteosynthesis, primary osteonal fracture healing takes place. Regenerating osteones migrate directly from one fragment through the fracture gap to the opposite fragment. No remodeling takes place and no callus is seen. Primary contact healing is possible only when the fragments are in direct contact. It takes place after rigid plate osteosynthesis with anatomical reduction and interfragmentary compression. **(C)** Secondary contact healing. Less rigid osteosynthesis results in micromotion at the fracture site. The fracture healing is initiated by periosteal and endosteal callus formation, followed by osteonal fracture healing. This is called secondary osteonal fracture healing. Remodeling processes are fast as long as the bone fragments are in direct contact or with only a small fracture gap. The bone-healing pattern is characterized by periosteal callus formation and direct cortical construction by secondary osteons. Secondary osteonal fracture healing is currently the preferred process. **(D)** Secondary gap healing. In spite of attaining a perfect reduction there are incongruencies with small gaps asymmetrically interspersed with contact areas or even within contact points that are located around the circumference of the bone cortex. Thus, contact healing does not imply that the entire cortex will undergo the contact healing mechanism. The growth of secondary osteons from one fracture fragment to another does not necessarily require intimate contact of fracture fragments. These gap regions are filled within weeks after fracture with no lag period, by direct lamellar or woven new bone formation (appositions bone formation). The boundary between the new bone and the original cortex is the weak link of the union process at this stage of healing. Secondary osteons use the gap tissue as a scaffolding to grow from one fragment to another. Although this step is crucial for the final union, the growth of secondary osteons results, paradoxically, in a transitory compulsory reduction of cortical bone density. The new bone in the gap also shows a similar porotic change as a part of the union process known as secondary gap healing.[5]

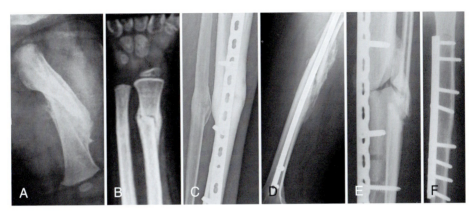

FIGURE 2.6
Periosteal callus is seen after treatment of fracture by (**A**) splinting, (**B**) cast fixation, (**C**) plating, (**D**) nailing. Gap healing (**E**) callus is seen bridging the gap between the butterfly fragment and shaft. In cortical or primary bone healing (**F**) no callus is seen due to osteonal (primary) fracture healing.

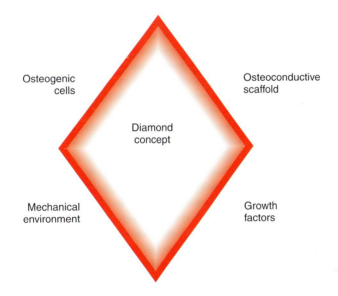

FIGURE 2.7
The four-sided model of bone fracture healing interactions. Bone producing cells under the influence of growth factors grow on a trellis that facilitates bone formation, provided these are placed in a mechanically stable environment.

that, by preserving the blood supply to bone, it would be possible to minimize or avoid delayed union, non-union and refracture after hardware removal as well as prevent development of infection into a sequestrum under the deep surface of the plate.

An undesirable consequence of the use of rigid compression plates is post-union osteopenia. This can translate into porotic transformation of the cortex beneath the plate with a net decrease of bone

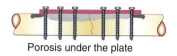

Porosis under the plate

FIGURE 2.8

Schematic representation of porosis beneath the plate seen on early postoperative radiographs due to reduced vascularity of the cortex.

mass and with impaired mechanical properties of the healed bone. It has been related to the occurrence of refractures after plate removal. Most investigators believe that the structural change is secondary to the overprotection of the underlying bone from normal stresses – stress protection. The prevalence of post-union osteopenia in plated human fractures is unknown and there is uncertainty about the mechanism causing post-union osteopenia. The bone density at the fracture site is marginally reduced but this bone loss is offset by an increase in the total area of the bone. There are three potential solutions to overcome these disadvantages: (a) continue to use rigid plates but modify the timing of plate removal, (b) the use of biologically degradable materials for internal fixation plates and (c) the use of a fracture fixation system of reduced rigidity.[7]

Once the true nature of these events was uncovered, the priorities have changed from mechanical stability to biology. It is known that external fixator causes least vascular damage in comparison to intramedullary nailing or conventional plate fixation. The fixator bridges the fracture gap and produces an environment of low stress of 2–10% that leads to more natural healing. The success of bridging fixation has spurred an interest in creation of an internal fixator. The Schuhli-Nut, Pc-Fix and Zespol plates are regarded as early attempts at creating an internal fixator. When the screws are firmly fixed to the plate, they function as threaded locked bolts and the plate–screw assembly could act as a fixed-angle implant.

Similar to the bars of an external fixator, plates are not applied directly to the bone, thereby providing elastic fixation, which facilitates more natural fracture union through secondary bone healing with callus formation. Free of the need to apply the plates directly to the bony surface, the locked plate can create a more biologic approach to the management of fractures. The new biological internal fixation or 'bio-buttress' fixation makes more sense from biological point of view.

The goal of a surgical treatment to fix bone fractures is to allow for full restoration of the function and pain-free mobility in shortest possible time. In extra-articular fractures, good clinical outcome can also be obtained with splints, such as nails, external fixators or bridging plates. When a splint sustains physiological load, it bends elastically, i.e. the original shape of the fracture fixation is restored when

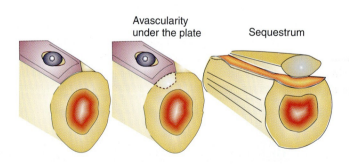

FIGURE 2.9

Observed patterns of bone loss beneath a plate did not correspond to the stress patterns of the corresponding bone segment.

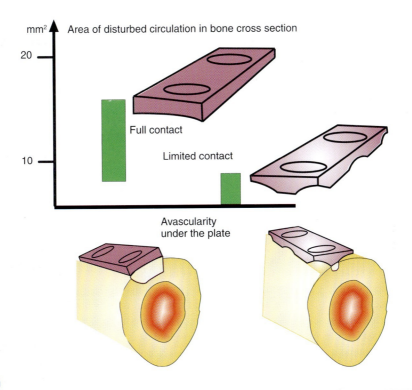

FIGURE 2.10

Loss of vascularity is proportional to the contact area of the plate. Smaller the contact area of the plate, the lesser the vascular damage.

the load subsides. This physical property allows for some inter-fragmentary bone movement that induces callus formation. An extreme overload results in irreversible, plastic deformation of the implant and leads to misalignment. New methods of internal fixation by compression plates have been developed to reduce the extent of trauma to the soft tissues. The steps like indirect fracture reduction while avoiding or minimizing its exposure, inserting the plate under the muscles and placing the screws through tiny incisions have helped to regain and maintain the bone length and alignment, and attain a relatively stable fixation. However, problems happen as conventional screws in plate holes lose hold on mobilization or in osteoporotic bones; malunion and fixation failure are encountered. Locking plate technology, a plate and screws system, where the screw can be locked in the plate have solved some of these issues.

ADVERSE CLINICAL CONDITIONS DELAYING BONE HEALING[8]

Fracture healing is not only a local phenomenon but several extrinsic factors influence the outcome. It is often difficult to isolate the role of a particular systemic factor in clinical situations. For example, impaired fracture healing in the elderly may be related to age, osteoporosis, drugs, malnutrition and/or anaemia. Other conditions like chronic inflammation, diabetes, hypovitaminosis, aging and polytrauma also delay fracture healing. This is a brief review of some of the ways by which these conditions negatively influence bone repair:

1. chronic inflammation,
2. diabetes,
3. hypovitaminosis,
4. aging,
5. polytrauma.

Chronic Inflammation

Prolonged inflammation subsequent to lingering inflammatory diseases, polytrauma or infection retards bone repair process. Lipopolysaccharide (LPS) endotoxins that may leak from injured gut are known to cause bone resorption. LPS prompt pro-inflammatory activity of macrophages which in turn stimulate hypertrophic and immature callus formation (Table 2.2).

The endotoxins possibly cause increased influx of neutrophils in fracture haematoma; the inflow dilutes local concentrations of growth and associated factors and retards bone repair process. Another theory proposes that the presence of excessive inflammatory mediators shorten the lives of chondrocytes and osteoblasts while prolonging the lives of osteoclasts. Contrary to this negative effect of inflammatory environment, 'inflammatory cytokine IL-12' could be used to immunomodulate the environment and aid bone formation.

Table 2.2 Algorithm Showing How Chronic Inflammation Delays Fracture Healing[8]

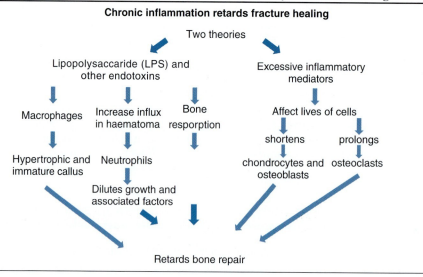

Diabetes

Bone union is delayed in diabetics mainly due vascular and neuropathy problems. Reduced formation of collagen in bone callus and marked reduction of cells involved at the repair process.

Activated platelets within a fracture haematoma release growth factors like PDGF, TGF-β, and VEGF to initiation of bone repair. In diabetics decreased localization of PDGF and decreased PDGF messenger RNA (mRNA) in the early fracture callus is believed to play a role in delayed bone repair. Correction of depleted levels may help in enhancing the bone healing speed.

Hypovitaminosis

Low vitamin D levels (25 (OH) vitamin D, 32 ng/mL) delay bone repair because its metabolites are critical for fracture healing; low values of the vitamin have been associated with secondary hypoparathyroidism. Besides, persons with <20 ng/mL vitamin D levels have a 1.77 times increased risk of fracture compared with individuals with normal vitamin D levels. Frequent causes of low values are decreased exposure to sunlight, inadequate vitamin D intake, malabsorption of vitamin D in the gut (Paan Masala, bariatric surgery) and antiepileptic medications.

Low vitamin C levels delay collagen synthesis, an important process in bone repair and ultimate bone strength. Individuals who daily consume 250–400 mg of vitamin C have lower incidence of fracture compared with those who did not regularly take vitamin C supplements.

Ageing

Women over 55 years of age are prone to delayed fracture union due to paucity of oestrogen. Clinical experience shows that bone heals slower in older patients compared with younger patients. This is explained at cellular level (Table 2.3). MSCs residing in bone marrow are the progenitors for osteoblasts and other cell types. The number of MSCs with osteogenic potential decreases with age. There is consequential decrease in the number of osteoblasts, reduction in bone formation and subsequent

Table 2.3 Table Showing Causes of Poor Quality of Bone Healing in the Elderly[8]

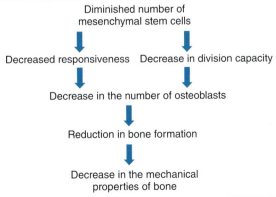

decrease in the mechanical properties of bone in elderly. It stands to reason that diminished number of MSCs and cells with osteogenic potential negatively influence bone repair in older patients. It is further specified that MSCs have a decreased responsiveness to signalling molecules and decrease in division capacity; in general, with aging there is decreased blood vessel formation, lower osteoinductive activity, and a decrease in the local and systemic levels of signalling molecules. Osteoporotic bone lacks the capacity to regenerate and regain valid biomechanical characteristics.

Muscular Mass[9]
Muscular atrophy negatively influences bone healing. Good muscle tone facilitates swift functional recovery leading to better biomechanical stability of the fracture.

Diet, Alcohol and Smoking
Diet poor in protein, calcium, phosphorus and vitamin D does not cause a significant delay in fracture union. Mostly it affects the mechanical strength of the bony callus itself, and thus requires a longer period of protection, until mineralization is completed.

Alcohol abuse delays fracture healing by inhibiting new bone formation. Smoking increases the risk of delayed fracture union and of pseudo-arthrosis. Nicotine is a vasoconstrictor and reduces tissue perfusion leading to hypoxia and ischemia. It also prevents cellular proliferation during the fracture healing and inhibits activity of osteoblasts.

Polytrauma
Multiple injuries to body's soft tissues, solid organs, appendicular and axial skeleton in polytrauma incite a substantial inflammatory response; this enhanced response particularly due to the increase in circulating inflammatory mediators, bone repair and generalized healing is delayed. Mediators like TNF-α, leukotrienes, VEGF, TGF-β and PDGF have a direct effect on fracture healing after trauma. Lack of TNF-α retards fracture healing as it has a regulatory role in endochondral cartilage absorption. Leukotrienes increase chondrocyte proliferation and promote early bone formation. Diminished levels of VEGF in clinical sepsis, adult respiratory distress syndrome and multiple organ failure retard bone formation. TGF-β, and PDGF are released from platelets and initiate fracture healing.

NSAIDs
NSAIDs (nonsteroidal anti-inflammatory drugs) delay fracture union when used in immediate postoperative period; the reduced osteoblastic activity and synthesis of prostaglandins lead to delay in formation of bone callus.

ENHANCEMENT OF BONE HEALING

Bone healing significantly depends on mechanical stability. Fracture repair can be improved by biophysical stimulations like shockwave, electromagnetic fields, ultrasound or biological substances like bone grafts, hormones or growth factors. In vitro several growth factors have been identified and have been shown to stimulate bone growth in various animal models.

Parathyroid Hormone Therapy[10]

Intermittent recombinant parathyroid hormone (PTH 1-34) treatment enhances and accelerates the skeletal repair process by its effect on MSCs, angiogenesis, chondrogenesis, bone formation and resorption. Furthermore, it also augments bone repair in animal models of aging, inflammatory arthritis and glucocorticoid-induced bone loss. Based on the preclinical success, it has been used in 'off-label' clinical situations. The therapy has improved healing in the patients who suffered from delayed or non-unions. There is anecdotal level IV (case series) evidence to support the premise that teriparatide therapy facilitated bony union in tibia and humerus shaft fractures in high energy trauma as well as in odontoid fractures in over 80-year-olds with osteoporosis, vitamin D deficiency and diabetes.

ORTHOBIOLOGICS AND TISSUE ENGINEERING

'Practically all classical operations of surgery have now been explored, and unless some revolutionary discovery is made which will put the control of osteogenesis in the surgeon's power, no great advance is likely to come from modification of their detail.'

– Sir John Charnley, circa 1950

Orthobiologics is an ill-defined term that may be described as the clinical application of biologically derived materials engineered to promote the repair or regeneration of musculoskeletal tissue. Current research seeks to identify the molecular and cellular constituents of osseous healing and to acquire the ability to manipulate their numerous interactions to gain direct control over the pathways of bone formation.[11]

Tissue engineering (TE) is an interdisciplinary field to restore, maintain or improve tissue function.[12] It applies the principles of engineering and the life sciences with an aim to create biological substitutes to repair or replace failing organs or tissues due to trauma or ageing. One of the more promising approaches in TE is to grow cells on biodegradable scaffolds that act as temporary supports for the cells to attach, proliferate and differentiate; after which the scaffold will degrade, leaving behind a healthy regenerated tissue.

Bone regeneration is an intricate, well-organized physiological process of bone formation seen during normal fracture healing and is seen as an ongoing process through out life in continuous bone remodelling. The process needs to be accelerated in situations like fracture healing, filling of large bone gap, atrophic non-unions due to trauma or ablative tumour surgery and infection; it is also needed in managing osteoporosis. Autologous bone graft is the 'gold standard' to augment the impaired or 'insufficient' bone-regeneration process; however, it is associated with morbidity and the stocks are limited. Other strategies like free fibula vascularised graft, allograft implantation and use of growth factors, osteoconductive scaffolds, osteoprogenitor cells and distraction osteogenesis exist and newer ones are being discovered. A short résumé of the available and future methods is presented.

Bone graft substitutes:

- Natural bone-based
- Growth factor-based
- Cell-based
- Ceramic-based
- Polymer-based

Natural Bone-Based Bone Graft Substitute

1. Autogenous bone grafts
2. Bone marrow
   Reamer–irrigator–aspirator (RIA)
3. Allogeneic bone grafts
4. Demineralised bone matrix (DBM)

Autogenous Bone Grafts

Autogenous bone grafts are being used since early 1930s and have been a standard treatment. All other substitutes are compared to autogenous bone graft for usefulness.

Bone Marrow

Use of bone marrow aspirate from the iliac crest has been used to stimulate bone formation by the transplantation of osteoprogenitors and MSCs with success. Collection and injection is a minimally invasive percutaneous procedure. Bone marrow injection is used as stand alone procedure or it is used as graft extender in combination with other procedures. Adding bone marrow to autograft increases osteogenic potential. It also has osteoinductive potential. Centrifuged at 400 times of the gravity for 10 minutes separates cells from plasma and reduces the volume for injection; on an average one in every 100,000 nucleated marrow cell is a stem cell. Injection of bone marrow is used to stimulate bone formation in skeletal defects and non-unions; it works in simple non-unions. It augments bone regeneration but does not reduce the healing time. There is no agreement on the quantity of marrow required to achieve the desired effect.

Reamer–Irrigator–Aspirator

The irrigation–suction technique with sequential reaming was introduced in 1986 by Stürmer and Tammen.[13] Reamer–irrigator–aspirator is a surgical instrument that works on minimally invasive principles and provides large amount of osteogenic material with minimal surgical insult. It consists of a disposable reamer head, a reusable drive shaft, a seal and tube.[14] After assembly, this device forms a reaming system that provides concomitant irrigation and suction of intramedullary contents. The mechanism, compared to conventional reamers, has less rise in intramedullary temperature and pressures and a lesser magnitude of adverse effect on immune system. The reaming particles, which are collected using a mesh screen or trap, centrifuged and reused as an ideal autograft in numerous applications in the field of trauma and orthopaedic surgery. These reaming by-products provide osteoinductive stimulus. Bone marrow provides haematopoietic and bone marrow stem cells. Haematopoietic stem cells form all types of blood cells; bone marrow stem cells have osteogenic properties and can generate bone, cartilage and fibrous tissue.

Allogenic Bone Grafts

Allogenic bone grafts are obtained from living donors or human cadavers. Allografts have mainly osteoconductive properties, reduced osteoinductive (bone morphogenetic proteins [BMPs]) properties, but no osteogenicity, since they are devitalized via irradiation or freeze drying processing and have no viable cells. Disease transmission and high cost of harvesting, processing and conservation of allografts are associated issues.

Demineralized Bone Matrix[15]

Acid extraction of bone removes the mineral content, leaving behind growth factors, non-collagenous proteins and collagen. The method used to process the cortical bone determines the biological activity of the final product. Demineralized bone matrix (DBM) is osteoconductive and also has osteoinductive potential because it contains osteoinductive and growth factors in the extracellular matrix that are freed to the host; it is devoid of antigenicity. DBM cannot provide structural support, but quickly revascularizes and is a suitable vehicle for autologous bone marrow aspirate. DBM is available as gel, putty, paste, flexible sheet, pulverized granules, crushed chips or a fine powder, and cortical chips within the matrix. It may be used to expand autologous cancellous bone grafts, with autologous bone marrow or with synthetic bone graft substitutes like calcium sulphate. DBM may transmit diseases and must be used only in stable fixations. It is used in repair of large bone defects and complex fractures.

Growth Factor-Based Bone Graft Substitutes

BMPs and Other Growth Factors

Several BMPs have been identified since their discovery by Urist in 1965. BMPs are potent osteoinductive factors. They induce the mitogenesis of MSCs and other osteoprogenitors, and their differentiation towards osteoblasts. With the use of recombinant DNA technology, BMP-2 and BMP-7 have been licensed for clinical use since 2001. Delivery of BMP at the target area is problematic because large dose is required in humans and it is quickly neutralized in body. Two systems have been used. In protein-based therapy a type-1 collagen carrier incorporates the desired characteristics; gene therapy is the second delivery strategy. Research is ongoing to develop injectable formulations for minimally invasive application, and/or novel carrier collagen that serves to retain the concentration and releases them consistently over time.

Clinical application of BMP-7 for recalcitrant non-union and off-label use of BMP-2 in bone grafting composites have demonstrated good performance and effect.[17] BMP-7 is used in fracture non-unions, augmentation of periprosthetic fracture treatment and osteotomies, enhancement of fracture healing, distraction osteogenesis, free fibular graft and arthrodesis of joints. With an overall success rate of 82%, no local or systemic adverse effects are reported.

In general BMPs are used for acute fracture treatment, defect healing, delayed and non-unions. In acute fracture care, it is uncertain whether the growth factor should be applied at the first surgery or later; the upper limit of size of defect is unknown. Their osteoinductive potential is beneficial for atrophic non-unions resulting from biological problems, but it might also be useful for the treatment of hypertrophic non-unions. However, the correct time and method of application is undecided. These growth factors are especially effective in metaphyseal and diaphyseal problems. In non-union of a bone, the mechanical stability is achieved and then the growth hormone is applied. Associated local and vascular problems of atrophic non-unions are resolved before application of the substance.

Other growth factors are also present and help in the processes required in bone regeneration like cell proliferation, chemotaxis and angiogenesis. Fibroblast growth factor (b-FGF) is produced locally in bone during the initial phase of fracture healing, has a powerful mitogenic factor and stimulates the differentiation of chondrocytes. VEGF improved healing in large bone defects. IGF-1 and TGF-β mostly modulate the synthesis of the cartilage matrix. PDGF has a stimulatory effect on fracture healing.

Platelet-Rich Plasma (PRP) or Autologous Platelet Concentrate

An increasingly popular therapy is the application of platelet-rich plasma (PRP) to enhance bone regeneration and soft-tissue healing. PRP is a quantity of plasma fraction of autologous blood with platelet concentrations above baseline, which is rich in many of the growth factors described earlier. These growth factors and cytokines are useful in many musculoskeletal conditions. Their degranulation and the release of growth factors namely, PDGF and TGF-β, to the fracture-healing site are well-known initial steps during the bone repair cascade. The effects of PRP on bone healing have been controversial in the literature, with ill-defined indications and no reliable evidence about the timing of therapy, the volume and frequency of treatment and the optimum vehicle for distribution of the PRP formulation that will allow for sustained growth factor and cytokine release.

Cell-Based Bone Graft Substitutes

Stem Cells

Stem cell is an 'immature' or undifferentiated cell which is capable of producing any identical twin cell. The main sources of stem cells include somatic (adult) and embryonic stem cells. Somatic stem cells include haematopoietic stem cells, bone marrow stromal MSCs, neural stem cells, dermal stem cells and several others. MSCs have a unique auto-renewing potential.

The MSCs derived from the bone marrow yield two types, the haematopoietic stem cells that give rise to the entire blood cell lineage and the MSCs from which various connective tissues are derived, such as bone and adipose tissues.

Cell harvesting, in vitro expansion and subsequent implantation of articular cartilage is being done successfully. However, the procedure adds substantial cost and risk of contamination, which may reduce the proliferative capacity of the cell. The process is time consuming and requires two-stage surgery. MSCs have also been identified and currently being used for the repair and regeneration of bone, cartilage, muscle, tendon and ligament. The role of MSCs in fracture repair is still in its infancy, largely due to a lack of studies into the biology of MSCs in vivo in the fracture environment. Recently in vivo phenotype of bone-marrow MSCs has been identified and these are fairly abundant in vivo in normal and pathological bone. This information opens up fresh approaches for the management of fracture non-union based on the biology of these key MSC reparative cells and would improve outcomes. Fig. 2.11 graphically shows relationship of factors involved in bone regeneration.

Collagen

Collagen is an osteoconductive material, but does not offer any structural support; its use in cell-based bone graft substitutes is as a carrier for growth and differentiation factors, especially BMPs. Extracellular bone matrix has abundant collagen that contributes to mineral deposition, vascular ingrowth and growth factor binding. Collagen can be used in combination with other osteoconductive carriers like hydroxy-apatite or tricalcium phosphate (TCP). Collagen is used only as a delivery system but not as a grafting material itself. It significantly enhances graft incorporation and can be also used as an autograft extender. There is no evidence that calcium–collagen graft materials can effectively substitute for autologous bone graft to stimulate healing of non-unions. This material with autologous bone marrow can be used as an alternative to autologous bone graft for acute long-bone fractures with significant comminution or cortical bone loss to require bone grafting when internal or external fixation is undertaken. It is not recommended

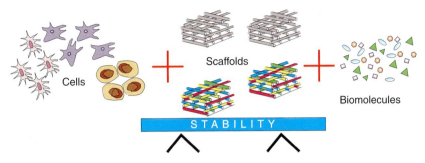

FIGURE 2.11

Graphic representation of elements of bone regeneration. Cells related to bone production multiply on a suitable scaffold under influence of growth factors in a mechanically stable environment. Absence of any one or more factors disturbs the equilibrium.

for the treatment of non-union (except as bone graft expander) or to fill metaphyseal bone defects resulting from intra-articular fractures, as it does not offer structural support.

Gene Therapy

Another upcoming method of growth-factor delivery is gene therapy, which transfers genetic material into the bone cells (targeted cell) to promote prolonged formation of specific protein (BMPs) from the cells themselves. Gene can be introduced directly into the non-union site or specific cells can be harvested from the patient, expanded genetically, manipulated in tissue culture, and then re-implanted. The direct method is easier than the indirect one. However, the indirect method is safer as the manipulations are under controlled conditions. Bone regeneration by gene therapy is successful in animals but biosafety, efficacy and cost are still a concern in humans.

Ceramic-Based Bone Graft Substitutes

1. Calcium hydroxyapatite (HA)
2. Tricalcium phosphate (TCP)
3. Bioactive glass
4. Calcium Sulphate
5. Injectable ceramic "cements"

Ceramics are synthetic scaffolds made from calcium phosphate (CP) and induce a biologic response similar to that of bone. The inorganic basic bone substance contributes to approximately two-thirds of the dry substances of osseous tissues. Its composition is, CP (85–90%), calcium carbonate (8–10%), magnesium phosphate (1.5%) and calcium fluoride (0.5%). In bone, minerals exist as apatite crystals. Hardness and resistance of bone are set by the connections between calcium hydroxyapatite (HA) and collagen fibres. These connections build hexagonal crystals, on the principle of space grids and exist both within and outside the collagen fibrils.

Calcium Hydroxyapatite and Tricalcium Phosphate (TCP)

HA is a highly crystalline hydroxylated CP salt with a high degree of hardness, which comprises the main component of inorganic substance in bones. HA is produced by osteoblasts from phosphate and calcium ions. HA are built into human bones; 70% of the bone volume is mineral in nature. HA ceramics and natural HA have great chemical similarity. Synthetic HA is a biocompatible form of CP. Its osteoconductive and biocompatibility is attributed to its chemical similarity to the mineralized phase of bone. HA is an excellent carrier for osteoinductive growth factors and osteogenic cells, making this material also useful as a graft extender. HA is a brittle material and undergoes slow resorption; and thus implants of this material can become a focus of mechanical stress. It is often modified and combined with other materials (HA/TCP alone or combined with autogenous bone) for improved outcome and faster resorption.

TCP ceramic is similar to amorphous bone precursors; its surface layer ceramic enhances bonding with the adjacent bone of the host. This stimulates osteoclastic resorption and osteoblastic new bone formation within the resorbed implant. When close to normal bone, osteoid is created straight onto the surfaces of the ceramic in absence of when soft tissue coverage is absent. Subsequently, the osteoid mineralizes and the new bone is formed which goes through remodelling process. TCP-ceramic and HA are greatly biocompatible but are different in their biological response at the host site HA/TCP (60/40) provide a scaffold which has a close interface with adjacent bone and has an application in the treatment of load-bearing segmental bone defects. Porous TCP is removed from the implant site as bone grows into the scaffold; the surface layers of TCP enhance bonding with adjacent host bone. This stimulates osteoclastic resorption and osteoblastic new bone formation within the resorbed implant. TCP show better degradation characteristics during bone regeneration when compared to HA; HA is more permanent. HA has been established as an excellent carrier of osteoinductive growth factors and osteogenic cell populations, which adds to their utility as bioactive delivery vehicles.

α-TCP and the corresponding beta-TCP (β-TCP) differ from each other in biological properties. Pure-phase α-TCP is made of porous granules that can replace bone and is absorbed in 24 months. Primarily α-TCP is soluble in body fluids but some α-TCP is converted to HA which can be seen at surgical site on radiographs for several years.

β-TCP

Ultraporous β-TCP is available in injectable formulation. It is an abundantly porous substance. The pores are interconnected and vary in size from 1 to 1000 µm. It was created to imitate the trabecular structure of cancellous bone. Its porosity facilitates activities of bone regenerating entities like bone-forming cells, nutrients and growth factors and supports their phagocytic action, resorption and infiltration. β-TCP (>99%) has good biological compatibility and bone conductivity; after implantation the material is quickly covered by blood vessels and is embedded in tissue. β-TCP is bone-conductive, microporous and has a homogeneous ceramic sintered structure. It is totally absorbed in a few months as new bone is formed at the surgical site.

This process of growth ends with the total metabolism of the implant material and the nearly total restoration of the compromised bone region. Seldom, due to rapid breakdown it may lead to inflammatory reactions and volume loss.

The porosity of ceramics plays a crucial role in bone integration. Ceramics with $CaO:P_2O_5$ ratios ranging from 2:1 to 4:1 have the best biocompatibility, while the optimal ratio is 3:1. This represents TCP-ceramics. The ideal pore size for a bioceramic material should be similar to that of spongious bone. Microporosity (pores <10 μm) allows body fluid circulation, while macroporosity (pores >50 μm) provides scaffold (pore size, 100–200 μm and porosity, 60–65%) for bone-cell colonization. A ceramic with higher porosity and lower density construct provides greater surface area for vascularisation, and bony ingrowth. Ceramic materials have also been used to coat and enhance osteointegration of implants.

Bioactive Glass Ceramices (Bioglass)

Bioactive glasses are hard, non-porous materials consisting of, calcium, phosphorus and silicon dioxide. By varying the proportions of sodium oxide, calcium oxide and silicon dioxide, a form ranging from soluble to non-resorbable can be produced. Bioglasses possess both osteointegrative and osteoconductive properties. Bioglasses possess an interconnective pore system and bioactivity of its surface enables the growth of osseous tissue. A mechanically strong bond between bioactive glass and bone forms eventually through HA crystals similar to that of bone. Bioglass is brittle and prone to fracture with cyclic loading. Incorporation of stainless steel fibres into bioglass increased its bending strength.

Calcium Sulphate

Calcium sulphate is osteoconductive bone-void filler. It is completely resorbed and substituted steadily as new bone remodels and restores the structural properties. It is biocompatible, bioactive and resorbable after 12 weeks. Indications for calcium sulphate graft material are: filling of a bone cysts, benign bone lesions and cavitary or segmental bone defect; as a grafts expander in spinal fusion, and for filling of bone graft harvesting sites. It loses its strength upon degradation and is unsuitable for load-bearing applications.

Calcium sulphate has been combined with various heat-stable antibiotics to create a resorbable delivery system for bone and soft-tissue infections.

Polymer-Based Bone Graft Substitutes

Polymers differ from those of the other bone graft substitutes and have been discussed in detail (see page 51). Scaffolds for bone regeneration are made from polymers. Polymers are combined with CP to improve mechanical strength and organic integration; mixing bestows radio-opacity on the scaffold. Polymers are useful for drug delivery systems as well.

Coral-Based Bone Graft Substitutes

Coralline Hydroxyapatite

Coralline hydroxyapatite is based on natural material derived from sea coral. Sea coral species produce a porous structure made of CP (coralline). This is processed to produce crystalline hydroxyapatite with pore diameters between 200 and 500 μm and in a pattern very similar to that of human trabecular bone. This is suitable as osteoconductive substitute for bone grafting. It is brittle with low tensile strength but has high strength against compressive forces. As filler, it has shown results as good as the autogenous bone graft and has been used in treatment of tibial plateau fractures. It is also been used as a carrier for BMP and other growth factors.

OTHER MODALITIES TO ENHANCE BONE HEALING

Electromagnetic Stimulation

Bone tissue has electrical potential, known as bioelectrical potential (BE). In the growth or healing area the BE is electronegative. BE returns to neutral or electropositive as healing progresses. In areas of tension, BE is electropositive and in compression it is electronegative.

Electromagnetic stimulation of bone to promote healing may be carried in one of the following ways:

- Direct current delivered through implanted electrodes (DCES – direct current electric stimulation)
- Alternating current delivered through an external coil used intermittently for promoting bone healing (PEMF – pulsed electromagnetic field)
- Current delivered between two plates that form a magnetic field used continuously for promoting bone healing (CCS – capacitively coupled electrical stimulation)

It is unclear as yet how electromagnetic stimulation acts; it is likely that each type listed here acts differently.

Shock Wave Therapy

Shock wave therapy is used in hypertrophic non-unions. The waves create microfractures in the hypertrophic tissue, leads to neovascularization and osteoinduction; reported results are contentious.

Ultrasound

Low intensity ultrasound also may further bone healing.

MATERIALS IN FRACTURE FIXATION

A variety of metals has been used in the past for fracture fixation; Lane (circa 1905) used bone plates made from vanadium steel. The 18-8 type of stainless steel was invented in 1926. 'Vitallium' was introduced for dental use in 1929. Titanium was first used in bone surgery in the 1950s. The implants for fracture fixation are commonly made of stainless steel and titanium alloys; alloys are materials composed of two or more elements, one of which is a metal. Alloys of the same metal containing different quantities and types of elements will have different physical, mechanical and chemical properties.

Composition of an alloy is regulated by specifications set down by standards institutions. Various metal working methods are employed in implant manufacture and these affect the mechanical properties of the implant. The biocompatibility of a metal is directly related to its corrosion resistance.

The actual mechanical properties of the metal are a function partly of its composition and partly of its grain structure[18] (Fig. 2.12). In general, a metal with finer grain is both stronger and more ductile – useful attributes in fracture implants, which are frequently shaped in the operating room. Grain structure is affected by the method of fabrication of the metal into its finished shape.

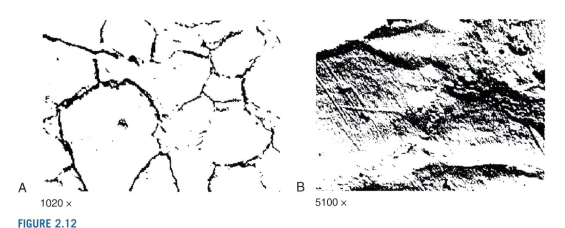

FIGURE 2.12

Microscopic views of the surface of a metallic implant show the interlocking metallic grains. The example shows carbide precipitations within the grain boundaries of the surface of a fixation plate. (**A**) × 1020. (**B**) × 5100.

The terms 'alpha' and 'beta' form of a metal are commonly used to describe different phases of the alloy having different properties. Some properties of metal deserve special mention. Ductility is the ability of a material to absorb relatively large amounts of plastic deformation before failing. It is an important property for implants such as wires or plates that have to be contoured during the operative procedure. The ductility of metals provides a safety factor and an opportunity to detect overloaded implants by radiographs. But ductility must be combined with adequate stiffness and a high enough yield point so that the material can meet routine loading demands. A high yield point of a metal used in fracture fixation means that a relatively high stress is required to cause permanent deformation. Beyond this point, however, these metals are ductile, i.e. they can bend to a reasonable extent without breaking.

Metals in Orthopaedic Use

An ideal implant material should be inert, non-toxic to the body, and absolutely corrosion-proof. It should be inexpensive, easily worked and mouldable in a variety of shapes without expensive manufacturing techniques. It should have great strength and high resistance to fatigue. Such a material is not available at present.

Stainless Steel

There are at least 50 alloys and grades of alloys identified as commercial stainless steel. Only a few are useful as implant biomaterial in fracture surgery.

Stainless steel designated as ASTM F-55, -56 (grades 316 and 316L) are used extensively for fracture fixation implants. Type 316L stainless steel is an iron-based alloy. Its composition is shown in Fig. 2.13. Alloying with chromium generates a protective, self-regenerating chromium oxide layer which provides a major protection against corrosion.

The addition of molybdenum decreases the rate of slow, passive dissolution of the chromium oxide layer by up to 1000 times. Molybdenum further protects against pitting corrosion. Nickel imparts

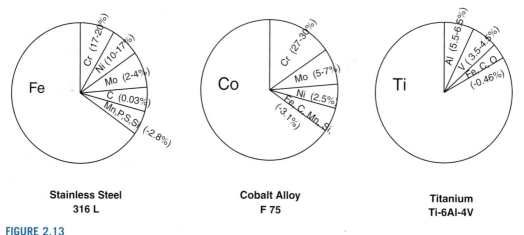

FIGURE 2.13

Composition of common orthopaedic alloys (pie cuts not to scale).[19]

further corrosion resistance and facilitates the production process, while limited quantities of manganese and silicon are added to control some manufacturing problems.

The carbon component increases the strength, but its presence in the alloy is undesirable. Under certain conditions created as a result of improper heat treatment, the carbon segregates from the major elements of the alloy, taking with it a substantial amount of chromium in the form of chromium carbide precipitates. Carbides form at grain boundaries, where corrosion selectively occurs. Furthermore, the carbides degrade the mechanical properties of the material. Mixing of small quantities of titanium or niobium reduces the formation of intergranular carbides by competing for carbon.

Type 316L stainless steel has a very low permissible level of carbon to minimize this problem. To increase the resistance to fatigue failure, 316L stainless steel is available in a special grade with smaller and more widely spaced inclusions. This grade, designated as AISI 316LVM and specified by ASTM F-138, is produced by a special method called 'vacuum-melting', which results in a cleaner metal. The strength of 316L can be greatly altered by the method of manufacture, and it can be made extremely ductile (up to 55% strain to failure). The alloy designated F-745 is a high strength casting material, while 22-13-5 has much greater yield strength than 316L for the same treatment method.

Though it is a strong, stiff and biocompatible material, 316L stainless steel has a slow but finite corrosion rate. Concerns about the long-term effects of nickel ions, however, prevail. Stainless steel is best suited for short-term implantation in the body as in fracture fixation. Stainless steel is frequently used because the base materials are cheap, the alloy can be formed using common techniques, and its mechanical properties can be controlled over a wide range for strength and ductility. The elastic modulus of stainless steel is approximately 12 times higher than the elastic modulus of cortical bone.

Composition of alloy F-90	
Cobalt	55–65%
Chromium	19–21%
Tungsten	14–16%
Nickel	9–11%
Carbon	0.05–0.15%

Cobalt–Chromium Alloys

The cobalt–chromium–tungsten–nickel alloy (ASTM F-90) employed for the manufacture of fracture fixation implants is very different from the F-75 alloy used for a femoral prosthesis. The alloy can be hot forged or cold drawn. It is quite ductile and strong. It is available in a wide range of yield strength, ultimate tensile strength and strain to failure. Its yield strength can be controlled by processing. In clinical practice, it is used to make wire and internal fixation devices including plates, intramedullary rods and screws.

Titanium Alloys

Titanium is the ninth most common element in the earth's crust, where it forms oxidic minerals (rutile, ilmenite). The pure element is very reactive; it is the only element that burns in nitrogen. However, the metal rapidly becomes coated with an oxide layer, making it physiologically inert and resistant to most chemicals. Titanium is used for making orthopaedic implants in two forms: commercially pure and a variety of alloys.

Titanium–aluminium–vanadium alloy (ASTM F-136) is commonly referred to as Ti6Al4V. This alloy is widely used to manufacture implants. Impurities such as oxygen, hydrogen and nitrogen tend to make it brittle, which explains why only minimal amounts are acceptable in titanium alloys used in surgical implants. ASTM F-136 limits the oxygen concentration to an especially low level of 0.13%, known as the ELI (extra low interstitial) grade. Limiting the level of dissolved oxygen improves the mechanical properties of the material, particularly increasing its fatigue life. Aluminium stabilizes the alpha form of the material while vanadium stabilizes the beta form. Combination of both components forms a two phase alloy with good strength properties and one that can be heat treated. Ti6Al4V ELI is frequently used for making orthopaedic implants.

Commercially pure titanium is not a single chemical element, but is alloyed by a level of oxygen dissolved into the metal. It also has traces of iron, nitrogen, carbon and hydrogen. The presence of all these trace elements influences the mechanical properties of the titanium. International standard ISO 5832/2 defines the level of permissible impurities.

Titanium has an elastic modulus approximately half that of the stainless steel and cobalt–chromium alloys. The lower stiffness of bone plate made of titanium reduces the severity of stress shielding and cortical osteoporosis. Another advantage of lower stiffness is that a titanium plate is less prone to fatigue failure than a stainless steel plate. The elastic properties of titanium require that contouring be achieved by slight over bending: it is important, however, that no metal should be bent or twisted repeatedly at the same location. The modulus of elasticity of titanium is still roughly 6 times that of cortical bone. The ductility of titanium alloy is considerably lower than that of most stainless steels. Due to this difference a surgeon requires some adaptation of his feel when determining the optimal amount of torque to be applied to the screws. The feel should be acquired before starting to use these screws in clinical practice.

The corrosion resistance of pure titanium is outstanding because a very dense and stable layer of titanium oxide (TiO_2) is formed. This protective oxide layer may be destroyed mechanically during implantation by instruments such as bending pliers. The passive layer is restored spontaneously, rapidly and effectively (re-passivation). In the presence of unstable fixation, the titanium components of an internal fixation system are subjected to fretting conditions and produce metal debris. Such debris causes grey or black colouration of the surrounding tissues. This discolouration, which is not a result of corrosion, is harmless. Special surface treatment of the implant reduces such discolouration.

Comparison of Stainless Steel and Titanium for Fracture Fixation

Both materials have relative benefits and deficiencies. Stainless steel can be produced with a higher elastic modulus and ductility than titanium alloys, but with similar endurance limits (mean stress at which fatigue failure does not occur). The machinability and relative cost of the base metals mean that stainless steel implants are potentially cheaper. The more significant advantage of titanium alloy is its corrosion resistance and the lack of potentially toxic ions such as chromium and nickel which are found in stainless steels. Another advantage is that it does not cause allergic reactions in individuals sensitive to nickel and chromium. These properties make it possible to leave the titanium implants in situ wherever there is no mechanical hindrance to soft tissues. The mechanical properties of titanium are closer to bone than those of steel. The high cost of titanium implants is compensated for by the fact that a second operation is often unnecessary and prolonged absence from work is avoided.

Shape Memory Alloy

Nickel–Titanium Alloy

Nickel–titanium alloy, or Nitinol, a shape memory alloy (SMA) was discovered in 1965. Nitinol is an acronym for Nickel Titanium Naval Ordnance Laboratory, where the alloy's remarkable properties were discovered. The alloy contains nearly equal numbers of nickel and titanium atoms, leading to its common compositional representation as NiTi. The relative amounts of Ni and Ti can be varied by a few percent in order to control the temperature of the phase change responsible for its 'smart' behaviour. A more accurate representation of its composition is Ni_xTi_{1-x} where x represents the percentage of Ni in the alloy. Since the discovery of Ni–Ti, at least 15 different alloy types have been discovered that exhibit shape changes and unusual elastic properties consequent to deformation.

SMA can be 'trained' to take on a predetermined shape in response to a stimulus such as a change in temperature. Implant made from SMA has the ability to return to its original shape after the environment temperature rises to a certain level (e.g. 37°C). Its shape can be changed easily at low temperature (e.g. 0–5°C). SMA can be bent, compressed or deformed in many other ways, but can then be made to recover its original shape by heating.

The material has been used in many orthopaedic areas (Fig. 2.14). Compressive staples for osteotomy fixation, scaphoid and tarsal bone fractures[20] bone plates for mandible fractures, and intramedullary nails with retractable fins are commercially available. In spinal surgery NiTi rods are used in corrective scoliosis surgery; intervertebral disc replacement is

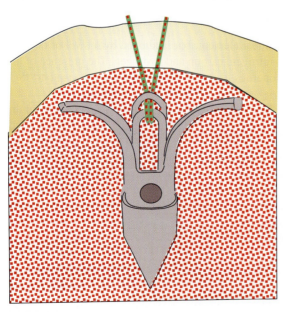

FIGURE 2.14

Suture anchor made from SMA (shape memory alloy). The anchor is stored in refrigerator and is introduced with folded fins which fan out as the implant acquires the original shape when it achieves body temperature.

another use of NiTi. Porous NiTi, characterized by low density, high surface area, high permeability, high strength relatively low stiffness, high toughness and by a shape-recovery behaviour, is beneficial for osteointegration processes of joint prosthesis. It has been verified that porous NiTi gives a higher stimulus for bone tissue growth and a bone deposit velocity two orders higher than traditional materials like titanium, stainless steel and chromium–cobalt.[21] The metal is also useful in physiotherapy of partially atrophied muscles; wired glove fingers can be flexed or extended with change in temperature.

POLYMERS

Polymers are large molecules made from amalgamation of monomers, smaller molecules. The chemical structure, molecular weight of the monomers and the way monomers are attached to each other (physical structure) dictate polymer's properties. Besides these factors, orientation of atoms (isomerism) and the packing of polymeric chains in orderly atomic arrays (crystallinity) are other dominating factors.

Bioresorbable Polymers

Biodegradable, bioresorbable, bioabsorbable and bioerodable are confusing terms; however, their clear definitions are on hand:

Biodegradables are solid polymeric materials and devices which break down due to macromolecular degradation with dispersion in vivo but no proof for the elimination from the body (this definition excludes environmental, fungi or bacterial degradation). Biodegradable polymeric systems or devices can be attacked by biological elements so that the integrity of the system, and in some cases but not necessarily, of the macromolecules themselves, is affected and gives fragments or other degradation by-products. Such fragments can move away from their site of action but not necessarily from the body.

Bioresorbables are solid polymeric materials and devices which show bulk degradation and further resorb in vivo; i.e. polymers which are eliminated through natural pathways either because of simple filtration of degradation by-products or after their metabolization. Bioresorption is thus a concept which reflects total elimination of the initial foreign material and of bulk degradation by-products (low molecular weight compounds) with no residual side effects. The use of the word 'bioresorbable' assumes that elimination is shown conclusively.

Bioerodibles are solid polymeric materials or devices, which show surface degradation and further, resorb in vivo. Bioerosion is thus a concept, too, which reflects total elimination of the initial foreign material and of surface degradation by-products (low molecular weight compounds) with no residual side effects.

Bioabsorbables are solid polymeric materials or devices, which can dissolve in body fluids without any polymer chain cleavage or molecular mass decrease. For example, it is the case of slow dissolution of water-soluble implants in body fluids. A bioabsorbable polymer can be bioresorbable if the dispersed macromolecules are excreted.

Improvements in polymer science have led to more frequent use of bioabsorbable implants in orthopaedic surgical procedures for fracture fixation of as well as for soft-tissue reattachment (Table 2.4). The chief advantage of these implants is that initially there is adequate stability for healing and then it is gradually resorbed after biologic healing is achieved. These implants limit stress shielding of bone and as they degrade, gradually transfer load to the healing tissue, eliminate the need for hardware removal, and offer radiolucency that facilitates postoperative evaluation by radiography and other imaging modalities.

Table 2.4 Table Listing Various Bioresorbable Polymers, Indications for Their Clinical Use, Names of the Available Commercial Products and Time These Take to Dissolve in the Tissue[23]

Polymers	Degeneration time in months	Applications	Commercial product	
Poly (lactide)	6 to 12	Orthopaedic surgery Oral and Maxillofacial surgery	Fixsob® Neifix® Arthrex: Linvatec: Zimmer:	(screws, nails, pins) (screws, nails, pins) Bio-Tendesis® interference screw. Bio-corkscrew® suture anchor SmartScrew® SmartNail® SmartTack® SmartPin BioScrew® Bio-statak® (suture anchor) bone cement plug, prosthetic stent
Poly (glycolide)	> 24	Orthopaedic surgery General surgery	Bioscience: Dexon® Bondek® Valtrac™	Biofix® screws sutures, mesh suture anastomosis ring, prosthetic stent
Polycaprolactone	> 24	Drug delivery Sutures	Ethicon:	Capronor Monocryl sutures
Poly (D,L-lactide-co-glycolide) Poly (D,L-lactide-co-glycolide 85/15 Poly (D,L-lactide-co-glycolide) 82/18 Poly (L-lactide-co-glycolide) 1090	5 to 6	Sutures Drug delivery Maxillofacial surgery General surgery Orthopaedic surgery	Polysorb™ Makar: Biomet: Sulzer:	 Biologically Quiet™ Interference Screw, suture Lactosorb®, plates, screw, Staple 85/15 mesh, pins, anchor surgicalclip, VicrylMesh Vicrylsuture, Phusisline® interference Screw Sysorb Screw (50/50) ResorPin® 70/30
Poly (L-lactide-co-D,L-lactide) 98/2 Poly (L-lactide-co-D,L-lactide) 50/50 Poly (L-lactide-co-D,L-lactide) 70/30 Poly (D-lactide-co-D,L-lactide-coL-lactide)	12 to 16			Geistlich biomaterials Macrosorb System (Screw, plates, mesh, nail, pins 70/30) Polypin® Zimmer : Leadfix BD Biosciences-No clinical approval BD™ 3D OPLA® (Open-cell Polylactic acid) scaffold
Polydioxanone	>24	Orthopaedic surgery General surgery		Ethipin Orthosorb™, Suture mesh foils Bone cement plug
Poly (D-L-lactide-co-caprolactone) 65/35	24	Nerve regeneration		Neurolac® Polyganics B.V., Groningen, The Netherlands
Polycaprolactone-based polyurethane				Tissue reinforcement Torn tendon replacement patch Interpositional space in osteoarthritis Artelon® sportmesh™ Arteleon® CMC spacer Arthro
Lactide co caprolactone		To prevent adhesion		Mesofol

Polylactic acid (PLA), polyglycolic acid (PGA) and polydioxanone (PDS) belong to a group of polymers known as alpha-polyesters or poly-(alpha-hydroxy) acids.[22] A mix of these polymers improves their biomechanical properties for a specific biomedical use. Change in manufacturing process like a change in temperatures and rates of cooling change the pattern of crystallinity, which in turn influences material's biomechanical strength and degradation character.

Polymers used in orthopaedics are viscoelastic in nature; therefore, their physical properties change with the rate of load application and are time dependent. In general, high- to average-molecular weight polymers are highly viscous and biodegrade gradually than those of lesser molecular weight and viscosity. The glass-transition temperature (Tg) is defined as the one below which a polymer is firm and tough and above which it is yielding and rubbery. Tg changes with polymer's composition, molecular weight and the portion of amorphous polymer. Polymers in biomedical use have a Tg above body temperature, which enables them to withstand higher loads.

PLA, PGA and PDS are frequently used bioabsorbables in orthopaedics. Lactic acid, which leads a significant role in energy production at cellular level, has a three-carbon molecule, which is hydrophobic and small in size.

Its two laevo and dextro forms, whose mechanical and degradation properties differ markedly, are PLLA (Poly-L-lactid) that is highly crystalline and PDLLA (Poly-D-lactid) being more amorphous. Polyglycolic acid is popularly used in orthopaedic implants as its self-reinforced form is unyielding than all other polymers. It is hydrophilic and stronger than most polymers in use. It degenerates faster and cause more synovitic reactions than PLA.

Monomer para-dioxanone is polymerized to produce PDS, which is a colourless crystalline polymer. Violet dye is added to get its characteristic colour. Polymer granules are melt-extruded through violet dye to produce PDS sutures. These sutures are inherently stiff, easily go through suture passers and are extensively used in arthroscopic repairs.

Polycaprolactone (PCL) was one of the earliest polymers synthesized in early 1930s.[23] It was being used in 1970s and 1980s for drug delivery devices. It did attract attention during then but was soon overwhelmed by popularity of more rapidly resorbable polymers such as polylactides and polyglycolides. PCL is of greater interest in the TE field as it has superior rheological and viscoelastic properties over many other polymers; these properties make it easy to manufacture and manipulate PCL into a large range of scaffolds. It is economical to manufacture PCL and many regulatory bodies have approved its clinical use. The material can last in the tissues for 2–4 years, but this time may be shortened by blending it with lactones or glycoide/lactides. It is biocompatible and has not shown any immunogenic, carcinogenic or thrombogenic response. PCL is useful in many drug delivery systems as micro and nanospheres, as suture material, wound dressings, fixation devices; in tissue, bone, cartilage engineering, nerve regeneration, artificial blood vessels and contraceptive devices.

Bioabsorbable implants degrade in an anticipatable format. The speed of breakdown depends on polymer's starting molecular weight, its crystallinity, the composition, porosity of the implant, its loading conditions and local vascularity. The breakdown starts with loss of molecular weight leading to reduction of strength and lastly decrease in the quantity of the matter. Initially chemical breakdown occurs which is followed by biological activity and subsequent disappearance of the implant. The material loses strength much before its complete absorption.

Water molecules enter the implanted material and initiate degradation by hydrolysis, causing sharp division of the monomeric molecular bonds. This splits the larger polymer chains into smaller ones and decreases their molecular weight. Mechanical strength of this material depends on its molecular weight. Reduction in molecular weight weakens the implant. An implant's porosity regulates the speed of autocatalysis; low porosity blocks the clearance of degradation products inside the material leading to increased acidity and brisk scission of the molecules. As the implant loses its coherence and disintegrates, it is removed by biological processes.

The rapid degradation of these implants causes marked foreign-body reactions, synovitis and even activation of the complement cascade. PGA degrades rapidly and most symptomatic foreign-body reactions are associated with it but reactions to PLLA have also been described. The most common soft-tissue complications related to use of these materials are sterile sinus tract formation, hypertrophic fibrous encapsulation and osteolysis. These inflammatory responses occur in fewer than 10% of patients, but may be severe enough to require surgery for resolution of the reaction. The rates of degradation of these materials are optimized for biologic fixation by changing the polymer ratios of PGA and PLLA.

Mechanical Properties

Bioabsorbable orthopaedic implants are initially exposed to high loads that slowly diminish as healing progresses. These implants are more viscoelastic than stainless steel implants and show superior properties of creep and stress relaxation. Property of stress relaxation is responsible for loss of 20% of its compressive force after 20 minutes of insertion of an interfragmentary screws made of bioabsorbable polymer. There is evidence that degradation rates are more rapid with in vivo testing secondary to enzymatic contributions. Areas of high tissue metabolism and blood flow facilitate material degradation. Furthermore, implants under load tend to degrade faster, possibly secondary to microfracture.

Mechanical strength of bioabsorbable implants can be improved by reinforcing techniques. Screws made from this material have been used in fracture fixation. The original strength of self-reinforced PGA is higher than that of stainless steel but is quickly lost as the material breaks down.

In animal studies, the PDS suture retained 74% of its non-implanted strength at 2 weeks, but by 6 and 8 weeks that value had dropped to 41% and 14%, respectively. Similarly, PGA materials weaken by 6–8 weeks. The mechanical qualities decay at different pace; bending strength is lost first and is followed by shear strength at slower rate. Such materials are suited for fracture fixation in areas where high shear loads exists, e.g. fractures in periarticular cancellous bone. In degradation of self-reinforced materials, reinforcing elements lose strength slowly as compared to matrix material.

Fracture Fixation

Although bioabsorbable fracture fixation devices appear to have obvious advantages over metal implants, these materials have not gained popularity due to apprehension about the commencing fixation strength. Fixation materials must have the strength to stabilize the bone fragments while healing process is completed. Manufacturing process is important; self-reinforced materials are more useful in fracture fixation as they are stronger than melt-molded polymers. Compared with metallic fixation, absorbable fixation has shown a lower incidence of infection.

It is an attractive proposal to use bioabsorbable implants for paediatric patients because implant removal is unnecessary. In experimental studies, the presence of an absorbable implant and an empty drill hole across a growth plate has similar effect on activities of a growth plate. Bioabsorbable implants have shown acceptable results, except for supracondylar humerus fractures where the displacement forces encountered overwhelm the mechanical properties of the absorbable pins, resulting in displacement. Reported complications with the use of these materials include sterile sinus tract formation, osteolysis, synovitis and hypertrophic fibrous encapsulation. Complications associated with the use of these materials have diminished with the development of newer, self-reinforced polymers.

The application of bioabsorbable implants in musculoskeletal procedures is gaining acceptance. Plates and screws for fixation of fractures of lower end of radius, fractures of small bones of hand, ankle fractures and pins for children's fractures are now available. Bioabsorbable intramedullary inserts improve hold of a screw in porotic bone. While most commonly utilized in the field of sports medicine for soft-tissue fixation, these implants may have additional applications in other aspects of orthopaedics like a protective perforated membrane for bone grafts in a gap non-union or as carriers for osteogenic substance to enhance bone healing without interference with imaging.

PEEK

PEEK (polyether ether ketone) is a colourless, linear aromatic organic polymer that belongs to the family of polyaryletherketone (PAEK).[24] Its properties (like toughness, superior strength, biocompatibility, ideal imaging properties, optimal modulus, excellent chemical resistance and ability to be sterilized repeatedly without degradation of its mechanical properties) make it one of the most adaptable biomaterials for long-term implants. While metals/ceramics are preferred for hard tissue applications, polymers are suitable for soft tissue applications. The modulus of implantable-grade PEEK can be adapted in contrast to metals and ceramics and therefore prevent the stress shielding effect. With the fibre reinforced PEEK; it is possible to enhance its mechanical strength and physical performance. It has been used in the finger joints, bone screws and pins.

Porous and bioactive PEEK scaffolds have been designed and manufactured to enhance osteointegration and permanent fixation in load-bearing interbody spinal fusion cages.[25] Radiolucent PEEK enables postoperative radiographic assessment of fusion and enhanced load transfer to tissue in the cage, both of which are inhibited by metals. PEEK scaffolds with 75–90% porosity, pore size ranging 200–500 μm and reinforced with 0–40% whisker-shaped hydroxyapatite crystals show promise as suitable material for interbody spinal fusion. However, the centre cavity of the cage needs to be filled with osteoinductive agents like autograft, BMP or DBM. PEEK rods are used in posterior spinal stabilization.

FUNCTIONALLY GRADED MATERIAL[26]

Functional gradation is one characteristic feature of the living tissue. Human tissues exhibit gradients across a spatial volume, in which each identifiable layer has specific functions to perform so that the whole tissue/organ can behave normally. Such a gradient is termed a functional gradient. Functionally graded materials (FGMs) are advanced biomimetic materials that have different properties as the dimension varies resembling human bone. For example, femur has porous cancellous metaphysis resembling a sponge while the diaphysis has compact bone that has less porosity. The properties of FGM are different than the individual material that forms it. This concept utilized more often in joint replacement is also useful in preparing scaffold for bone growth in problematic fracture healing. Functionally graded HAP–collagen I scaffolds are a suitable material for in vitro growth of bone. Appropriate pore size, porosity or material gradient create an optimized mechanical behaviour, as well as the intended improvement of the cell ingrowth.

Clinical Relevance

Metal Failure

Brittle, plastic and fatigue failures are the types of mechanical failure observed in clinical practice. A screw head made of material with poor ductility may demonstrate brittle failure when overloaded in torsion. In plastic deformation, the implant bends permanently because of loading beyond the yield strength of the material, causing loss of surgical alignment.

Inserting a metallic implant into a situation where the load is greater than the endurance limit triggers a competition between the completion of the implant's designated functional task and its fatigue failure. All metallic materials are subject to fatigue fracture under cyclic loading, a process that is hastened by body fluids. Such a repetitive loading may be experienced by implants used to fix a weight-bearing bone in the lower extremity. Fatigue fracture of an implant originates in the small flaws within the material. Cracks may begin at defects in the structure of the material (grain boundaries, voids, inclusions) or at mechanical defects on the surface (scratches, notches, bends); these progress with cyclic loading and the implant may fracture unless removed or unloaded. Only rarely do major intrinsic material defects play a significant role in the fatigue failure of orthopaedic implants. With modern fabrication techniques and manufacturing practices, quality control is excellent. Extrinsic defects, such as scratches, bends and divots from surgical clamps, act as stress risers and can decrease the fatigue life of an implant.

The fracture fixation device such as a bone plate or intramedullary nail is designed to share the load with the fractured bone. The bone is expected to heal and to assume a larger share of the load with the passage of time. This unloads the fracture fixation device and prolongs its fatigue life. Failure does occur when the loads are excessive, such as when the fracture is comminuted and the bone is unable to partake in load bearing. Fatigue failure also occurs when the period of load bearing is longer than the device was designed to endure. Fatigue life therefore can be important in cases of delayed union or non-union. Most fracture stabilization devices are over designed to minimize the occurrence of fatigue failures.

Metal Removal

There are drawbacks and benefits to both retention and removal of implants. The most obvious drawback of removal is the high cost and risk of a second operative procedure. The procedure may be complex because bone remodelling around implants makes removal difficult. On the other hand, the long-term effects of retention of the implant are unclear at the time of writing.

Stainless steel has a slow but finite corrosion rate; the concerns about the long-term effects of nickel ions are also well founded. Stainless steel is best suited for short-term implantation in the body, as in fracture fixation, and implants made from this material should be removed. Titanium implants may be left in the body indefinitely.

A plate may be removed as soon as healing is complete. This applies particularly to patients with normal bones. In the lower limb a plate must be removed; isolated screws, however, may be left permanently. In the upper limb a plate may be left in place. From a mechanical viewpoint, it is not necessary to remove a nail in a weight-bearing limb and it may be left indefinitely in the body. Removal of any implant initiated by patient request should be delayed for at least 18 months. A bony union on radiological examination is a prerequisite for such a removal.

Mixing of Implants

It is not uncommon to 'mix and match' implants from different manufacturers in fracture fixation. This is an unsound practice for a variety of reasons.[27]

Though implant materials of similar specifications must be compatible, it is only to be expected that slight variation in the material exists. The mixing of implants made of materials from different producers can lead to a high risk of corrosion. The mechanical strength of an implant varies according to the material used and manufacturing process employed. During milling, drilling or turning of an implant, energy dissipation raises the temperature and may cause drastic changes in the structural and mechanical properties and alter corrosion resistance. The final surface quality can be diminished by an incomplete or inappropriate manufacturing procedure which may again strongly influence its corrosion resistance. As different manufacturers do have different working methods, the mechanical properties of the implants would be different even if they were made of metals of the same specification. A combination of implants and instrumentation of different designs can lead to jamming, broken drills and taps, gaps, loose fits and loosening. When implants from various sources are mixed, no manufacturer will take the responsibility for implant failure – the surgeon alone would be blamed. It is therefore good clinical practice to use instruments and implants from one manufacturer.

STANDARDS ORGANIZATIONS

Several national and international organizations develop standards for implantable materials. The initials of one of these organizations are often imprinted on a material, so it is worthwhile getting to know them. For example, standards ASTM F-55 and F-56 describe the composition of stainless steel suitable for fracture fixation implants. ISO 5832/2 details the level of permissible impurities in commercially pure titanium. The organizations set specifications of minimum compositional requirements of the material and the maximum allowable percentage impurities, desirable mechanical properties and manufacturing standards. Manufacturers may have their trade names for the standard, alloys but must conform to these standards.

METAL WORKING METHODS AND THEIR EFFECTS ON IMPLANTS

Forging

Forging is essentially the art of the blacksmith. The metal is heated and hammered or squeezed into shape. A die is sometimes used; this is a mould to guide the flow the metal. Drop forging, the most commonly used forging method, means that the piece is formed in a mould consisting of two or more parts in an eccentric press. Forging produces an orientation of the grain flow, making the metal stronger.

Casting

Casting consists of heating the metal to a molten state and pouring it into a mould. Few fracture fixation implants, if any, are currently fabricated in this manner.

ASTM: American Society for Testing and Materials Committee f-4, Surgical Implants.
AMSI: American National Standards Institute.
AISI: American Iron and Steel Institute.
BIS: Bureau of Indian Standards.
BSI: British Standards Institute.
DIN: Deutsche Industrie Norm.
ISO: International Organization for Standardization Committee TC-150, Surgical Implants.
CE: conformite européenne.

Rolling and Drawing

Rolling (between rollers) and drawing (through a hole in a hardened plate) are used to form bar and wire.

The material is plastically deformed in the process and the grains become elongated in the direction of deformation.

Milling

Milling is a basic machining process in which material is removed by feeding the workpiece or the work (the core material from which a part of specified geometry and surface finish is to be fabricated) into a rotating cutter or by having the rotating cutter advance into a stationary workpiece. The cutter generally consists of multiple cutting teeth and material can thereby be removed at high rates. Milling provides good surface finish characteristics.

Cold Working

Cold working is a finishing process employed after the metal has been shaped by hot forging and is similar to it but the work is performed below the recrystallization temperature. The advantages of cold working are a smoother surface finish, higher tensile strength, uniform grain structure and superior dimension control. Cold working requires more energy compared to hot forging to deform the metal below its recrystallization temperature.

After forming, metal parts undergo heat treatment to alter their structure and properties. In particular, annealing and case hardening:

Annealing

Annealing is heating to about half the melting point, followed by controlled cooling. The process reverses the effects of work hardening and restores ductility and toughness to the metal. Annealing (heat treatment) of a forged piece reduces its internal stresses.

Case Hardening

Some products are also treated to cause the outside surface of the rod to be harder than the inner core. The advantage is that the harder outer surface will resist indentation while the core is able to absorb more energy.

Machining

Geometric features like holes and grooves require machining. This may work harden the surface of the material but its grain structure remains unchanged.

Broaching

Broaching is a machining process that is comparable to sawing except the cut is performed in a single pass of the broach. The geometry of the broach is the inverse geometry of the surface that is to be machined and consists of cutting teeth that run the full length of the tool. Generally broaches are used in the machining of non-circular holes, slots and other recesses of geometry that may be difficult to produce with other machining processes.

Surface Treatment

Polishing and Passivation

Implants are surface finished by grinding and polishing to a specified roughness. Polishing removes scratches, this could act as local stress risers. The implant is cleaned with a special cleaning agent.

The passivation process produces a protective oxide layer. It involves immersion of the device in a strong nitric acid solution for a specific time. The solution dissolves embedded iron particles left by the machining operations and generates a thin, transparent but dense oxide film on the surface of the alloy. This process is important in enhancing the corrosion resistance of the implant. Stainless steel forms a chromium oxide. Titanium and its alloys form a dioxide so that even the pure metal while active electrochemically, is quite inert in saline.

The passivation can be damaged by cold working, scratching and other mechanical trauma; care is therefore needed in handling implants. It may also be disturbed by metal fatigue induced in a saline environment. The protective layer is self-repairing to varying degrees in the presence of oxygen, a phenomenon called re-passivation. The cobalt–chromium alloys apparently do not form a distinct passivating layer in the same sense as do stainless steel and titanium; consequently their corrosion resistance, although not well understood, tends to be less susceptible to mechanical degradation.

Nitriding

Nitriding, or allowing the surface to react with ammonia or potassium cyanate, is used to harden the surface of titanium implants.

Fabrication of Implants

The manufacture of fracture fixation implants involves many of the metal-working methods described so far. A brief account of the fabrication process of some implants follows.

A bone screw is manufactured by very precise procedures from steel or titanium rod with a diameter of at least the width of a screw head. The cylinder or a blank if required, may be subjected to cannulation at this stage, which is added by gun drilling. Gun drilling is an exact procedure with minimum variation from the required dimensions. The special drill has a central channel for cooling fluid delivery and removal of metallic debris. The next step in screw production involves machining of the threads. The cutting flutes are first milled into the thread cylinder. The final bone thread can be machined by a number processes, e.g. turning, milling or grinding operations, or by using cutting dies. Grinding is among the most frequent techniques used for cutting threads in orthopaedic screws. To make the hexagonal socket, a hole is first drilled into the head and then to shape it, a hexagonal tool is pushed into the hole. Electro polishing and passivation are performed on the screw to clean the material after machining and increase the material's resistance to the corrosion.

A bone plate is produced from a bar that already has the profile of the plate. Specially shaped plates are cut out of titanium or steel sheets and holes are drilled or milled according to the design (round or self-compressing). The plate for a sliding hip screw is produced from a bar which is not uniform but has two distinct segments – one flattened and one quadratic. The quadratic section is bent to the desired angle (e.g. 135°, 140°, 145° and 150°). The barrel segment of the plate is turned on a lathe and the barrel hole is drilled and broached. The plate is than milled to obtain the correct profile. The plate's holes are milled and the product is finally finished. This is a labour-intensive job requiring advanced manual skills.

The Küntscher nail is produced by cold working. It is made from a flat sheet of stainless steel which is rolled into its final shape by cold working. The effect of cold working is twofold because of the two different diameters of arches present. The arch with the larger radius is less deformed, less cold worked and softer. The two tighter curved arches connecting the 'cloverleaf sections' are cold worked to a greater degree and are relatively harder.

An example of combined metal working techniques is the AO/ASIF nail (T Jeavons, 1995, personal communications). This is formed from a stainless steel which is welded into a tube and then annealed. The tube is then cold drawn and annealed several times to reduce the wall thickness and diameter of the tube. The cloverleaf profile is formed by rolling the tube. The longitudinal slot is then cut into the tube, and the drive is threaded. The locked Universal nail is made not from a sheet of stainless steel but from a stainless steel tube which is cold drawn and annealed several times to reduce the wall thickness and diameter. A longitudinal slot is then cut into the tube and, lastly, the threads are cut in the drive. A non-slotted nail is made from a solid bar of stainless steel. The central cannulation is produced by the gun drilling method.

The Ender nail is an example of a stainless steel rod that has been work hardened to high tensile strengths yet retains a reasonable amount of ductility for insertion into bone. Manufacturing consists of stretching the rod to shape while keeping the rod at a constant diameter. This type of cold working increases implant strength. Reduction in size requires many rolling and drawing operations; some of these are done while the material is hot to prevent overworking and cracking.

The Zickel nail is manufactured by a casting process and is made form cobalt–chromium alloy.

CORROSION

Corrosion is the gradual degradation of metals by electrochemical attack, and is therefore a concern when a metallic implant is placed in the electrolytic environment of the body. Metals used for orthopaedic implants depend on the existence of an inert protective layer to prevent corrosion. Initiation of corrosion depends on pH and oxygen tension at the implantation site. Generally, tissue conditions (pH 7.4) are such that the protective preformed oxide layer is stable but some tissue locations and occasional transient conditions, such as the acid pH shift associated with infection, may damage the oxide layer and produce corrosion. Corrosion weakens the implanted metal, changes the surface of the metal and releases metal ions into the body fluids.

Galvanic Corrosion

In general the components of a galvanic cell (two different electrically conducting solids, an electrically conductive path between them and an electrolyte solution containing free ions) are required to set up the corrosion process. Essentially, a battery is formed and any protective layer is destroyed. Even within a single metal a battery effect can be produced. Unintentional use of a stainless steel screw in a cobalt–chromium plate may be an obvious cause of corrosion. Galvanic corrosion may occur at the surface of an implant in which an impurity was accidentally included during manufacturing. At a more intrinsic level, separation of metal granules in different phases may start a corrosive process. At times, rubbing of implants and instruments (cold welding) may transfer metal, leading to corrosion. A significant amount of metal may be transferred from the screw driver to the screw head and from the drill bit to the plate. Use of an instrument set made from a material matching the composition of the implant eliminates this cause.

Crevice Corrosion

Metals and alloys that depend on an oxide film or passive layer for corrosion protection are particularly susceptible to crevice corrosion. In a narrow gap (crevice) between implants, e.g. screw head and plate, high concentrations of chloride or hydrogen ions destroy this film and local corrosion commences. Crevice corrosion can occur in a fatigue crack and in defects such as a scratch or macroscopic fissure, where oxygen tension becomes low, causing a reactive area. Lack of oxygen also inhibits repair of the passivation layer. Molybdenum tends to limit crevice corrosion.

Pitting Corrosion

This is a localized reaction similar to crevice corrosion. Starting as a defect in the passive surface layer, corrosion proceeds into the metal, setting up self-accelerating concentration gradients. Chromium, nickel and molybdenum are added to stainless steel to increase the resistance to pitting corrosion. Titanium and its alloys can quickly re-passivate to regain protection against pitting corrosion.

Fretting Corrosion

Fretting corrosion results from very small oscillating movements, vibrations or a slip between the components of a device, causing abrasive damage to the passivating layer and permitting initiation of the reaction. A multicomponent weight-bearing implant may be affected by fretting corrosion.

Stress Corrosion

High mechanical stresses may alter the activity of a metal and rupture a protective passive surface layer thereby increasing its susceptibility to corrosion. Stress corrosion involves both mechanical and chemical effects. A scratch or crack can act both as stress concentrator and as a small corrosion cell. If conditions are right, the material may re-passivate, forming a new protecting oxide. Cyclic loading and the presence of organic molecules, either singly or together may interfere with this process. Localized corrosion can enhance stress concentration and premature failure.

Intergranular Corrosion

If impurities aggregate between grains of relatively pure alloy, a localized galvanic corrosion may exist between the crystals and the alloy in the grain boundaries. For example carbon depletes intergranular chromium concentration as it forms chromium carbide. A low chromium level may initiate intergranular corrosion leading to cracks between metal granules. This is why a low level of carbon is desirable in surgical stainless steel.

Ion Release

Implanted metal releases ions in the tissue. The tissue reaction to ion release decreases with time, and since tissue reaction is not a major clinical factor, internal fixation devices need not be removed routinely for reasons of metal ion concentration. Occasionally, patients may be sensitive to chromium or nickel found in stainless steel implants, requiring removal.

REFERENCES

1. McKibbin B. The biology of fracture healing in long bones. J Bone Joint Surg 1978;60-B:150–62.
2. Perren S. Physical and biological aspects of fracture healing with special reference to internal fixation. Clin Orthop 1979;138:175–96.
3. Wagner M, Frigg R. Internal fixators. Davos Platz, Switzerland: AO Publishing; 2006. p. 18.
4. Merloz P. Macroscopic and microscopic process of long bone fracture healing. Osteoporos Int 2011;22:1999–2001.
5. Chao EYS, Aro HT. Biomechanics of fracture fixation. In: Mow VC, Haves WC, editors. Basic orthopaedic biomechanics. New York: Raven Press; 1991. p. 303–9.
6. Giannoudis PV, Einhorn TA, Marsh D. Fracture healing: the diamond concept. Injury 2007;38(S4):S3–6.
7. Woo SLY, Lothringer KS, Akeson WH, Coutts RD, Woo YK, Simon BR, Gomez MA. Less rigid internal fixation plates: historical perspectives and new concepts. J Orthop Res 1984;1:431–49.
8. Borrelli J Jr, Pape C, Hak D, Hsu J, Lin S, Giannoudis P, Lane J. Physiological challenges of bone repair. J Orthop Trauma 2012;26:708–11.
9. Calori GM, Albisetti W, Agus A, Lori S, Tagliabue L. Risk factors contributing to fracture non-unions. Injury 2007;38S:S11–18.
10. Takahata M, Awad HA, O'Keefe RJ, Bukata SV, Schwarz EM. Endogenous tissue engineering: PTH therapy for skeletal repair. Cell Tissue Res 2012;347(3):545–52.
11. Toolan BC. Current concepts review: orthobiologics. Foot Ankle Int 2006;27(7):561–67.
12. Langer R, Vacanti JP. Tissue engineering. Science 1993;260:920–26.
13. Matthews SJ, Nikolaou VS, Giannoudis PV. Innovations in osteosynthesis and fracture care. Injury, Int. J. Care Injured 2008;39:827–38.
14. Synthes Medical (P) Ltd Plot no 118, sector-44 Gurgaon-122002, (Haryana) India.
15. Kolk A, Handschel J, Drescher W, Rothamel D, Kloss F, Blessmann M, Heiland M, Wolff KD, Smeets R. Current trends and future perspectives of bone substitute materials — From space holders to innovative biomaterials. J Craniomaxillofac Surg 2012;40:706–18.
16. Dimitriou R, Jones E, McGonagle D, Giannoudis PV. Bone regeneration: current concepts and future directions. BMC Med 2011;9:66.
17. Schmidmaier G, Schwabe P, Wildemann B, Haas NS. Use of bone morphogenetic proteins for treatment of non-unions and future perspectives. Injury 2007;38(S4):S35–41.
18. Pohler O, Strausmann F. Characteristics of the stainless steel ASIF/AO implants, In ASIF/AO basic course manual. Davos, Switzerland: Association for Study of Internal Fixation; 1975.
19. Litsky AS, Spector M. Biomaterials. In: Simon SR, editor. Orthopaedic basic science. Rosemont, IL: American Academy of Orthopedic Surgeons; 1994. p. 468.

20. An YH, Burgoyne CR, Crum MS, Glaser JA. Current methods and trends in fixation of osteoporotic bone. In: An YH, editor. Internal fixation in osteoporotic bone. Stuttgart: Thieme; 2002. p. 93–5
21. Petrini L, Migliavacca F. Biomedical applications of shape memory alloys. J Metallurgy 2011. Volume Article ID 501483. doi:10.1155/2011/501483.
22. Ciccone WJ, II, Motz C, Bentley C, Tasto JP. Bioabsorbable implants in orthopaedics: new developments and clinical applications. J Am Acad Orthop Surg 2001;9:280–8.
23. Woodruff MA, Hutmacher DW. The return of a forgotten polymer—Polycaprolactone in the 21st century. Prog Polym Sci 2010. doi:10.1016/j.progpolymsci.2010.04.002.
24. Doma S, Akdemir ZB, Özdiler F, Nacar OA, Köksal I, Kerman S. Innovative Materials and Technologies in Orthopedics. Republic of Turkey Ministry of Health Medicines and Medical Devices Agency. Ankara, Turkey: Department of Medical Devices; 2013. Accessed 7 Aug 2014. Available on http://www.who.int/medical_devices/global_forum/G08.pdf.
25. Roeder RK, Smith SM, Conrad TL, Yanchak NJ, Merrill CH, Converse GL. Porous and bioactive PEEK implants for interbody spinal fusion. Adv Mater Proc 2009;167(10);46–8. doi:10.1361/amp16710p37.
26. Mahamood RM, Akinlabi ET, Shukla M, Pityana S. Functionally graded material: an overview. In: Proceedings of the World Congress on Engineering, July 2012 Vol III. WCE 2012, July 4 - 6, 2012, London, U.K: International Association of Engineers, 2012. p.1593–7.
27. Baumgart F. Mixing of implants. Product information. Davos, Switzerland: AO/ASIF Foundation; 1990.

CHAPTER 3

BONE SCREWS

Anatomy of a Screw
   The Screw Head
   Recess
   Countersink
      Function
   The Shaft
      Run Out
   The Thread
      Core Diameter
      Pitch
      Lead
      Outside Diameter (Thread Design)
      Thread Design
   The Tip
      Self-Tapping Tip
      Non-Self-Tapping Tip
      Corkscrew Tip
      Trocar Tip
      Self-Drilling Self-Tapping Tip

Screw Types
   Machine Screws and Wood Screws
   Cortical and Cancellous Screws
   Self-Tapping Screw
   Non-Self-Tapping Screw
   Full and Partially Threaded Screws
   Cannulated Screw
   Locking Screw
   Locking Buttons
   The Herbert Screw

Screw Insertion
   Drill Bit
   Principles of Cutting Instruments
   Drill Size Nomenclature
   Heat Generation in Drilling
   Effects of Heat on the Bone
   Factors Affecting Heat Production
   Techniques to Minimize Heat Production
   Mechanics of Drilling
   Drill Bit Failure
   The Power Drill
   The Drill Sleeve
   Drilling Depth
   Pilot Hole
   Importance of Pilot Hole
   Measurement of Screw Length
   Tapping
   Countersink
   Washers
   Insertion
   Efficiency of Screw Insertion

Screw Removal
      Removal of Screw with Stripped Head
      Removal of the Broken Distal Screw Tip

Holding Power of the Screw
   Definition
   Modifying Factors
   Screw Failure

Clinical Considerations
   The Lag Screw
   Fixation of Spiral Fracture
   Good Practices for Locking Screw
   Screw vs Bolt

ANATOMY OF A SCREW

A bone screw is used for internal fixation more often than any other implant; it serves to hold two or more objects and to lag, i.e. compress two objects together. Though it appears a simple device, a great deal of complex engineering technology has contributed to its design.

A bone screw has four functional parts: head, shaft, thread and tip (Fig. 3.1).

The screw head serves as an attachment for the screwdriver. The countersink refers to the hemispherical or conical undersurface of the screw head. The shaft is the smooth part of the screw between the head and the thread. The 'run out' is the spot where the shaft ends and the thread begins. The thread is wrapped around the core, which provides the main support of the screw. Core (or root) diameter pertains to the minimum diameter of the screw across the base of the thread. The pitch defines the distance between the adjacent threads, while the lead of a screw refers to the distance the screw will advance with each turn; the lead is therefore equal to the pitch. The thread (or outside) diameter is the widest diameter of the screw. The thread design relates to its cross-sectional shape. The tip of the screw is the end opposite the head.

Each constituent of the screw has several special features and plays an important role in its function.

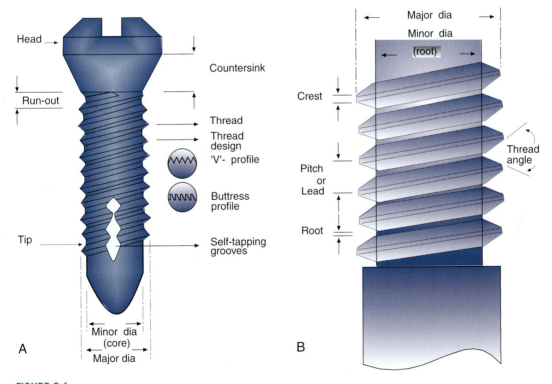

FIGURE 3.1

(**A**) Schematic details of the orthopaedic bone screw.[1,2] (**B**) Enlarged view of the thread.

The Screw Head

'Screw drive' is a system designed to turn a screw; it is a feature on the screw head that allows it to be turned; a matching screw driver is an essential implement. Firm purchase of the screwdriver on the screw head is all-important during insertion or removal of a screw. If the screwdriver suddenly disengages under load, it may cause considerable trauma to surrounding tissue and may distort the recesses in the screw head, making subsequent removal difficult.

Recess

Five designs of screw head recess are in common use (Fig. 3.2).

1. **Single slot head.** The single slot is an inefficient design. In this conventional design, a slot extends across the diameter of the head. A standard screwdriver is used to insert or remove this screw. Its tip is prone to slip whenever there is any disparity between the screwdriver tip and the screw slot. The torque transmission takes place only at two points and there is a danger of distortion of the slot. It is also difficult to align the screwdriver without visualization of the slot.
2. **Cruciate head.** Also known as Frearson screw head after its nineteenth-century English inventor, it has two slots at right angles provide a wider contact area than in the single slot design. An exact fit between the driver tip and slot is essential for secure hold. Cross-slot drives are more effective than single slot design for torque transmission but are sensitive to misalignment of the screwdriver.
3. **Phillips head.** Created by Henry F Phillips, its form resembles the cruciate head, but is so designed that the screw driver cams out if the screw stalls; this avoids damage to the screw head and to the material it is being inserted because the screw driver disengages. The slots stop short of the periphery and are recessed. The recessed cross-slot provides a secure grip on the screw head. On the negative side, the torque transmission is somewhat dependent of axial thrust and may compromise initially unstable reduction of the fracture fragments. Corrosion may commence in the depths of the head due to decreased oxygen concentration, escalating the chances of screw head breakage during removal. In the cruciate and Phillips heads, the torque transmission takes place at four points of contact.
4. **Recessed hexagonal head (Hex head).** This is currently the most popular design. The hexagonal head driver makes a strong and alignment-insensitive connection with the screw and offers a good lateral guidance that allows 'blind' insertion and removal. The driver tip snugly fits in the screw head and is unlikely to slip out or distort the head. Thus, the operator knows the inclination of hex screw of which only the head protrudes from the

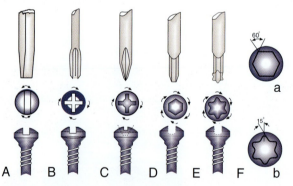

FIGURE 3.2

Five designs of screw heads and screw driver tips in common use: (**A**) Single slot; (**B**) Cruciate[1]; (**C**) Phillips; (**D**) Recessed hexagonal[2]; (**E**) Torx-6 Stardrive™. (**F-a**) The force is applied tangentially to the flats of the hexagonal screw drive during insertion and removal (**F-b**) in Stardrive™ the force is exerted nearly perpendicular to the flats of screw and the transmission of torque is superior than hexagonal drive.[3]

ANATOMY OF A SCREW

bone because the screwdriver by necessity aligns with screw axis. This alignment helps in avoiding collision of sequentially inserted plate or lag screws. The torque transmission is independent of axial thrust and thus does not compromise initially unstable reduction of the fracture fragments. On the negative side, hex is somewhat difficult to manufacture, especially considering the necessity for the close tolerance fit to the head of the screw. The flats of the hex screwdriver and hex-recess are oriented tangentially to the applied force (Fig 3.2F-a). Such torque transmission may strip resulting in expansion of the screw head with application of excessive torque. This happens when the screwdriver is worn out.

5. **The new socket and driver tip,** Stardrive™ (Synthes)[3] maintains the advantages of the hex but offers a better resistance to stripping, as the flats are orientated more perpendicularly to the applied force (Fig 3.2E and F.b). Furthermore, the size of the drive connection now conforms to general technical standards.

Several designs of screw heads and corresponding drivers exist in industry; a few are shown in Fig. 3.3.

Countersink

The countersink, or the undersurface of the head, is either conical or hemispherical. A screw with a conical undersurface should be inserted centred and perpendicular to the hole in a plate (Fig. 3.4). If set to any other angle, the undersurface does not adapt well to the plate hole and its wedge shape creates undesirably high forces. Uneven contact also predisposes to corrosion: both factors weaken the screw. However, a conical undersurface can be used to produce a compression effect (Fig. 3.4B).

In 1958 this principle was used by Bagby and Janes.[8] Earlier in 1948 Eggers employed similar screws to achieve compression.[9]

Since the 1980s a screw with a hemispherical undersurface has been in vogue. A hemispherical head allows the screw to be angulated in all directions within a washer or the screw hole of a plate while

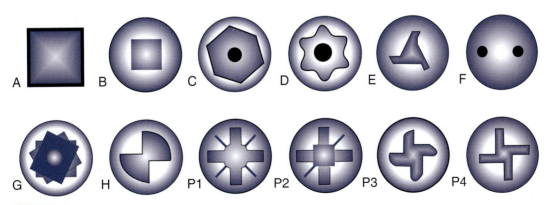

FIGURE 3.3

List of screw drives: **(A)** Square drive; **(B)** Robertson; **(C)** security hex socket; **(D)** security Trox socket; **(E)** Tri wing; **(F)** Spanner head; **(G)** Triple square; **(H)** One-way. Four variants of Phillips drive[4] are Posidriv (P1), Supadriv (P2), Mortorq (P3) and (P4)Torqset.

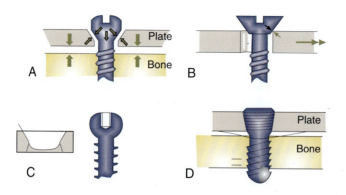

FIGURE 3.4

(A) A screw with conical undersurface should be centred in plate hole for close fit. (B) Such a screw may be inserted eccentrically in a plate hole to achieve compression since the head displaces the plate.[5] (C) A screw with hemispherical undersurface provides a congruent fit between screw head and plate hole or a washer.[6] (D) A screw with threaded conical undersurface: the threads engage in the plate hole that has matching threads.[7]

maintaining concentric contact between the screw and the side of the plate (Fig. 3.4C). The range of angulation varies with the shape and design of the hole in the plate. A hemispherical head allows for transmission of force to a plate and reduces the shearing forces when the screw is inserted at the angle other than a right angle; a frequent occurrence in surgery. Its only disadvantage is its prominence when used without a plate. The hemispherical shape is an integral part of the self-compressing plate design.

A new type of screw with conical threaded surface and very steep sidewall like a Morse cone is being used since 2000 (Fig. 3.4D). It is used only in a locked internal fixator plate hole. The pitch of the thread on the head is identical to thread on the shaft. The shape of the plate hole is same as the screw head with a misfit of 0.13 degree and has threads matching those on the screw head. The steep conical design of the screw-to-screw hole does not allow for much inclination of the screw or for compression of the fracture and locks efficiently, extending angular and axial stability to the screw. The design calls for minimum rotational force (torque) – less than one third of the usual torque. This screw locks even when minimal axial tension is produced during insertion. The formfit of this design locks efficiently against any tilting motion of the screw. An inadvertent benefit of these two properties is that the screw cannot pull-out during insertion. This property is valuable in minimally invasive surgery. However, the threaded design does permit inconsequential amount of inclination between screw and body, allowing locked misfit. A conical screw with shallow threads on the countersink is easier to remove than a similar screw with smooth walls because on over-tightening the later pattern easily welds with the plate.

Function

The screw head serves two functions (Fig. 3.5). Firstly and obviously, it provides the means of applying torque (twisting force) to the screw. Secondly, it acts as a stop. As the head comes in contact with the bone surface, the translational motion of the screw stops and the torque transforms to tension in the screw, which in turn induces compression between the two surfaces. Compression develops only after the translational motion of the screw stops.

ANATOMY OF A SCREW

The Shaft

The shaft or shank is the smooth link between the head and the thread. The shaft length is variable; in a standard cortical bone screw it is almost non-existent but in a cortical 'shaft screw' or in a cancellous screw it is significant (Fig. 3.5C–F). Screws with long shafts are used as lag screws. The smooth shaft has no purchase in the proximal hole and ensures compression by lagging.

Run Out

The 'run out', the transitional area between the shaft and the thread, represents a location of significant stress concentration (stress riser) because of abrupt changes in the diameter and presence of sharp corners (see Fig. 3.1). The screw may break at the run out during insertion if it is incorrectly centred over the hole or is not perpendicular to the plate. Typically, it breaks with a spiral configuration, indicating failure under torsional load. Under cyclic loading in an insufficiently tightened plate–screw construct, sufficient shear and bending forces may develop to break the screw at the run out. The run out of a fully threaded screw used to be of the same diameter as that of outside diameter of the screw thread. This caused significant expansion stresses as the screw was being forced into a bone hole (pilot hole) of smaller diameter. Undercutting or reducing the diameter of the run out has eliminated this unwitting over-sizing (Fig. 3.5G and H).

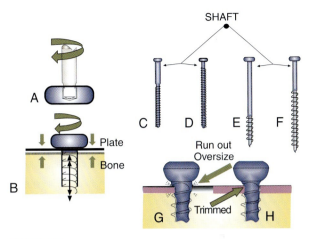

FIGURE 3.5

(**A**) Two functions of a screw head. A means of applying the torque to the screw. (**B**) It also acts as a stop and transforms torque to compression. The length of the shaft varies with type of the screw. (**C**) Partially threaded cortical screw. (**D**) Fully threaded cortical screw. (**E and F**) Partially threaded cancellous screws. (**G**) Run out segment of the same diameter as the screw's major diameter causes high expansion stresses when forced into the pilot hole. (**H**) Reducing the diameter of the run out sector by undercutting eliminates unsolicited stresses.

The Thread

A screw thread can be visualized as a long inclined plane or a wedge encircling core (root) (Fig. 3.6). A screw is as a simple machine that converts a small applied torque into a large internal tension along its axis while producing compression between the two surfaces being held together.

The standard orthopaedic screw has a single thread. A screw may, however, have two or more sets of threads; though a double-thread screw advances twice as fast as a single-thread screw, the former consumes more torsional energy than the latter to produce the same amount of compression and is deemed inefficient.

Core Diameter

The core diameter, also known as the inside or root diameter, represents the narrowest diameter of the screw across the base of the threads. This diameter determines the minimum solid cross-sectional area

CHAPTER 3 BONE SCREWS

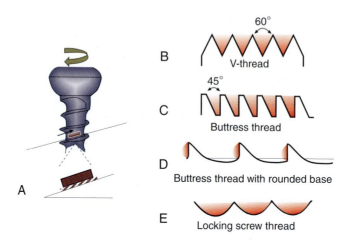

FIGURE 3.6
(A) A screw thread may be compared to an inclined plane on which a block of material is moving along its surface. The inclined plane being a simple machine, converts the torque to a force which moves the block upwards and along the surface. This moving force generates tension in the screw and the consequent compression that the screw applies to the fracture surface.[10] Six classical simple machines are lever, wheel and axle, pulley, inclined plane, wedge and screw; a simple machine is a mechanical device that changes the direction or magnitude of a force (B) 'V' thread (C) schematic buttress thread,[2] (D) buttress thread with rounded base[2] and (E) thread profile of a locking screw. Shaded areas represent the width of bone engaged in the screw threads.

of the screw (root area). It is also the weakest part of the screw. The smaller the root diameter, the greater the tendency to shear off during insertion and removal, or under various other loading conditions. The torsional strength of a screw varies with the cube of its root diameter. Doubling the root diameter of a screw increases the extent of torque that it can withstand by a factor of 8. Its tensile strength changes by the square of its diameter. The root diameter of the screw and its constituent material are the two factors which limit the torque that can be applied.

Pitch

The pitch is the distance between the adjacent threads (see Fig. 3.1B). A cortical screw with a fine thread has a small pitch whereas a cancellous screw with a coarse thread has a large pitch. The stronger the bone (cortex), the smaller the pitch; the weaker the bone (cancellous), the larger the pitch. The pitch also determines the rate of advance of the screw (lead) through a material. A fine-pitched screw moves a smaller distance linearly for a given angular rotation, offers greater mechanical advantage, produces greater compression, and has more leverage than a coarse-pitched screw. In a cortical bone screw the pitch typically measures 1.75 mm; this is also expressed as the number of threads per inch (tpi): AO cortical screw – 40.5 tpi; AO large fragment cancellous screw – 2.75 mm, or 9.2 tpi.

Lead

The lead of a screw means the distance it travels on a complete turn. For a screw with a single thread the lead equals the pitch; the smaller the lead, the greater the mechanical advantage of the screw. The

Outside Diameter (Thread Diameter)

Outside diameter of a screw refers to the diameter across the maximum thread width and affects its pull-out strength. The larger the outside diameter, the greater the resistance to pull-out. Up to a reasonable limit, the larger the size and surface area of the threads that are engaged, the greater the holding power. This explains why most 'cancellous' screws have a wide diameter thread.

Thread Design

The screw thread may be of a 'V' or a buttress profile (Fig. 3.6B). A 'V' thread has a slanted profile on both sides. A buttress thread widens at its base to form a buttress that resists bending of the thread under load. The rounded corners at the junction of the base of the thread and the screw shaft reduce the stress concentrators that are associated with sharp corners. A buttress thread is slanted only on the leading edge; the trailing edge is perpendicular and faces the screw head. This thread transfers forces between the bone and screw at right angles to the direction of the applied force. In principle, 'V' and buttress threads should have the same pull-out strength if each has identical outer diameter. This is disputed on the grounds that a 'V' thread produces compression and shear forces at the bone–thread junction, whereas a buttress thread mainly produces compressional forces. Shear forces promote bone resorption and result in lessened pull-out strength. It has been argued that a buttress thread is less likely to loosen as it produces very little shear component and offers greater pull-out strength in the long run. Thread profile of a locking screw is symmetrical, shallower and coarser (wider base) than that of a conventional screw. The screw does not produce compression, mainly resists shear loads. Its symmetrical thread is best suited in both cortical and cancellous bone.

The Tip

There are five common types of tips of bone screws.

Self-Tapping Tip

Included in the self-tapping (ST) tip is a thread cutting device called a 'flute' (Fig. 3.7). This mechanism cuts threads in the bone over which the screw advances. The flute has a cutting edge with a positive rake angle (see Fig. 3.16); three to four flutes ensure effective thread cutting. As the screw advances, the cutting flutes chisel into the bone and direct bone chips away from the root. These flutes also act as channels and transport the bone chips away from the bone face and place them in a position to be packed by the oncoming threads. The chip volume depends on the thickness of the bone, but the volume of the cutting flutes accommodates total chip production during insertion. The cutting flutes continue towards the head as the sizing flutes and give final shape to the bone thread. The conical tip of the screw assures that it self-centres in the axis of the pre-drilled hole.

The geometry of the cutting flutes in a bone screw has considerable effect on the insertion torque, on the axial force necessary for insertion and on the movement or clearing of bone debris. The sharpness of the cutting edge is an important parameter. Superior machining and advanced surface treatment procedures improve the cutting performance. However, the ST tip has no purchase on the distal cortex

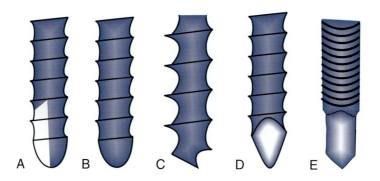

FIGURE 3.7

Five types of screw tips: **(A)** blunt tip of ST cortical screw; **(B)** blunt tip of NST cortical screw; **(C)** corkscrew tip of cancellous screw; **(D)** trocar tip[11]; **(E)** self-drilling, ST tip.

due to presence of flutes and a length of the screw should be so chosen to ensure that the entire fluted segment protrudes beyond the distal cortex.

The main advantage of this screw is simplicity, as it requires no pre-tapping of the bone before insertion. The number of steps and necessary instruments is reduced, thus decreasing the operation time. Furthermore, a very tight fit of screw thread to bone is ensured as the screw cuts its own thread. An ST screw can be removed and reinserted safely; its reinsertion should be manual as power insertion may inadvertently create a new track.

Non-Self-Tapping Tip

In a non-self-tapping (NST) screw the thread extends to the tip, which lacks a thread-cutting device (Fig. 3.7B). The threads must be pre-cut in the pilot hole before a screw may be inserted; a specialized tool – a tap – is used for this purpose. The conical tip self-centres in the axis of the pre-drilled hole and accurately guides the screw into the pre-tapped hole.

As the thread is tapped before the insertion of the NST screw, greater 'effective torque' can be produced when the screw is inserted and results in higher interfragmental compression (see Fig. 3.22). An NST screw can be removed and reinserted with a minimum of torque and without scarring the thread. Since there are no flutes in the screw tip, length for length, the NST screw offers greater resistance to pull-out than the fluted ST tip and provides better purchase on the distal cortex of diaphyseal bone. For the past few years, these screws have been extensively used in cortical bone.

Corkscrew Tip

A corkscrew tip is used in cancellous screws where the tip clears pre-drilled hole (Fig. 3.7C). The cancellous screw forms its own threads by compressing the thin-walled trabecular bone. Thread-forming tip is suitable only for use in a cancellous bone, and is inadequate for cortical bone.

Trocar Tip

A trocar tip functions somewhat like an ST screw (Fig. 3.7D). The trocar does not produce a true thread but rather displaces the bone as it advances.

The 'malleolar' screw has a trocar tip which is well suited for soft cancellous bone of the distal tibia and medial malleolus. Other screws with a trocar tip are Schanz screws, and locking bolts for intramedullary nails.

Self-Drilling Self-Tapping Tip

A screw tip similar to a conventional drill bit has been available since year 2000 (Fig. 3.7E). The screw compliments minimal invasive plate osteosynthesis (MIPO) and is used only in a locked internal fixator plate hole. The additionally sharpened tip of the screw drills a hole efficiently, reduces heat generation and the resistance as the drilling tip penetrates the bone. Similar to standard drilling procedure cooling by saline stream is essential. A tap is also crafted in the tip and trails the drill-bit section. A self-drilling ST screw is used exclusively for monocortical insertion because there is no possibility of measuring the exact screw length and a sharp, drill bit like tip may injure the structures 'outside' the bone. A screw with self-drilling ST tip is deployed mainly in the diaphyseal area where accurate length is not required. A self-drilling ST screw appears to have a better purchase than an ST screw, particularly in osteoporotic bone and in metaphyseal region.

SCREW TYPES

Machine Screws and Wood Screws

There are two major types of screw: the wood screw and the machine screw. To understand the difference between the types, one should recapitulate Newton's Third Law of Motion: 'Every force has an equal (in magnitude) and opposite (in direction) reaction force'. Once the screw is set, the force pulling the two components together must be generated by an elastic reaction somewhere within the screw or in the material into which it is inserted.

A wood screw has relatively large threads and is usually tapered; it is put into the material with a small pilot hole. The threads of the screw form their own mating threads by compressing the material. The screw is much stiffer than the wood into which it is inserted; the spring or elastic force therefore arises from the deformation of the surrounding material, not the screw. It is this force that draws together the two wooden surfaces held by the screw (Fig. 3.8A).

A machine screw differs from a wood screw in that it is intended to be placed into a hole in which threads have already been cut by a tool known as a tap. A pilot hole matching the size of the screw core is first drilled and then tapped by a tool that is twisted into the hole, cutting the threads with a sharp edge.

In the case of a machine screw placed in metal, the elastic reaction which lends the screw its compressive force comes primarily from the shank of the screw itself. The machine screw, rather than the much larger cross-section of the surrounding metal, deforms plastically (Fig. 3.8B).

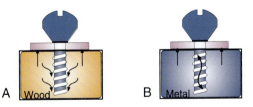

A Wood — Elastic force by the wood
B Metal — Elastic force by the screw

FIGURE 3.8

The different modes of action of (**A**) a wood screw and (**B**) a machine screw. The wood screw generates elastic force by deforming the softer wood to hold two pieces together. The machine screw placed in metal deforms plastically to generate desired elastic force necessary to hold two metal pieces together.[12]

Cortical and Cancellous Screws

A cancellous bone screw is a modified wood-type screw. Its tip is not tapered. It has larger threads and a higher pitch as compared to the cortical screw. The core diameter, which is smaller than that of the shaft, provides a greater surface area for purchase of the screw threads on bone. An increase in the thread diameter of a cancellous screw increases its pull-out strength. A cancellous screw is inserted into an untapped pilot hole; the size of the pilot hole equals the core diameter of the screw. Its large threads form companion threads in the bone by compression and by deforming the bone trabeculae. The spring reaction comes from the cancellous bone as it is deformed during the thread forming process.

The cortical bone screw is a machine-type screw. The threads are smaller (in diameter) and are closely placed (lower pitch). The core diameter is relatively large and provides the necessary strength. The smaller pitch increases the holding power of the screw. Threads are cut in the pilot hole before this screw is inserted; this is achieved either by a separate tool (tap) or by the ST tip of the screw. The elastic reaction, vital to hold the bone surfaces together, comes from elastic deformation of the bone and not the screw. This happens because the screw is stiffer than the cortical bone. The modulus of elasticity screw is more than 10 times that of bone; therefore, the elastic deformation occurs in the bone. Irrespective of the type of screw or the kind of bone, whenever a screw is inserted in the bone, the bone deforms and provides the elastic binding force (Fig. 3.9).

Self-Tapping Screw

The term 'self-tapping screw' refers to a screw which is inserted directly into a pre-drilled hole without first tapping a thread. ST screw may further be subdivided into thread-forming and thread-cutting screws. The thread-forming type moulds, i.e. forms threads by elastic–plastic deformation or by local destruction of the bone. The thread-cutting screw cuts its threads through the bone over which it advances.

The cancellous bone screw is a thread-forming, ST screw. The screw thread forms its own mating bone thread by compressing the soft cancellous bone. A tap should not be used to insert a cancellous screw – a cancellous screw inserted in a tapped hole has lower pull-out strength than one inserted in an untapped hole because tapping removes cancellous bone from the hole, and effectively enlarges it

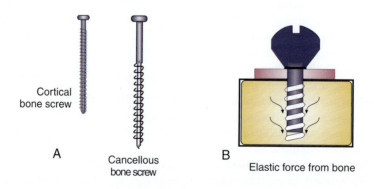

FIGURE 3.9

(A) Cortical and cancellous bone screws. **(B)** The bone always deforms to provide the elastic force.[12]

(Fig. 3.10). The amount of bone removed by tapping increases as the density of bone decreases; the mean volume increase is about 25%. When a cancellous screw is to be inserted first through hard cortical it is necessary to tap the cortical bone. Cancellous taps are provided for this reason alone. The smooth shaft of the cancellous bone screw provides the lag effect without the need for over-drilling. This becomes significant in the larger 6.5-mm screws, where a very large hole would need to be drilled in the near cortex to produce a lag effect. Varying lengths of partly threaded and fully threaded cancellous screws are used as indicated in different clinical situations.

A cortical bone screw may be ST or NST.

An ST cortical screw is a thread-cutting screw and has the cutting lip of a tap actually milled into its tip. This device cuts a thread in the dense cortical bone on which the screw advances. The ST screw was criticized for a long time since it was believed that an ST screw would provide a poor hold in the bone because it caused more damage at the time of insertion and became embedded in fibrous tissue rather than in the bone. Later research has shown this view to be incorrect. Size for size, an ST and an NST screw have almost the same holding power. The design of the cutting flutes of an ST screw is important. A poorly designed tip encounters considerable resistance, particularly in thick cortical bone. At times the resistance may be such that the torque required to drive-in the screw is greater than the tolerance of the screw, and the screw may break. The resistance to insertion may interfere with the accuracy of placement, particularly when a screw is being inserted obliquely to lag together two bone fragments.

ST screws are widely used in bone surgery as they may be inserted rapidly, decreasing the operation time for internal fixation. Furthermore, relatively fewer steps and instruments are required. The screw tip must protrude from the far cortex so that the flutes are clear and at least one complete thread engages the cortex. Reinsertion of an ST screw into the same threaded hole may not always be a cause for concern; reinsertion, however, should be manual and a drill machine should be avoided as power insertion may inadvertently create a new track.

The main advantage of this screw is simplicity, as pre-tapping is unnecessary. Additionally, a very tight fit of screw thread to bone is ensured as the screw cuts its own precise thread.

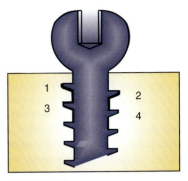

FIGURE 3.10

Tapping enlarges the drill hole. (1 and 2) The diagram shows loose fit in upper two threads inserted after tapping (3 and 4) The lower two threads show close contact with bone when a screw is inserted without tapping.[2]

Non-Self-Tapping Screw

An NST screw empowers precision placement in hard cortical bone, particularly when a screw is being inserted obliquely to lag together two bone fragments. The NST screw is incapable of cutting a bone thread. If it is inserted without tapping, the applied torque will be lost in overcoming friction at the bone–screw interface and only 5% of the applied torque may be utilized to develop the desired compression. Tapping the pilot hole prior to insertion improves this proportion to 40%. The bone tap, a special instrument for cutting threads in bone, is made of special steel and cuts high quality threads in the cortical bone. Minimal torque is then required to overcome the friction, and a higher percentage of the applied torque is converted to effective tensile force in the screw. After the use of a tap, a screw can be threaded into bone with minimal force, reducing the likelihood of loss of reduction of the fracture. The NST screw is incapable of cutting a channel in cortical bone but can be removed and reinserted without the fear of inadvertent damage.

Fully and Partially Threaded Screws

Cortical and cancellous screws are available as fully and partially threaded screws. A cortical bone screw is usually fully threaded. In plate fixation, a screw must purchase firmly on both the cortices. The purchase on the near cortex contributes 80% of the grip and the distal cortex contributes about 20%. A fully threaded cortical screw can function as lag screw only when the near cortex is over-drilled and thus does not offer any hold at near cortex. A fully threaded cortical screw may be ST or NST.

A partially threaded cortical screw is called a shaft screw. The shaft diameter corresponds to the outer diameter of the thread. This screw has better strength and stiffness than a fully threaded screw which is an advantage when it is used as a lag screw and as an axial compression screw (see Fig. 3.32).

A cancellous screw may be fully threaded or partially threaded. A fully threaded cancellous screw is used as a placement screw to fix a bone plate in metaphyseal and epiphyseal regions. A partially threaded cancellous screw is used as a lag screw.

Cannulated Screw

A cannulated screw is used over a guide wire for precise insertion in metaphyseal or epiphyseal site to eliminate the problem of having to remove and reposition an incorrectly placed screw. A guide wire accurately visualizes the path of the screw. In addition, the guide wire maintains the reduction and controls the fracture fragments. If guide wire position must be changed, it can be done without enlarging the hole and sacrificing holding strength of the bone. Final placement of the screw requires use of cannulated drill, a cannulated tap and a cannulated screwdriver. Cancellous cannulated screws come in large and small sizes. Large cannulated cancellous screws are used to fix fractures of the femoral neck, femoral condyle and tibial plateau. Small cannulated cancellous screws are employed for fixation of the distal radius, distal humerus, distal and proximal tibia and carpal scaphoid. A larger root diameter as compared to an equivalent non-cannulated screw is needed to accommodate the central bore of a cannulated screw. This effectively decreases the volume of bone between the screw threads and to some extent curtail its holding power.

The cannulated screw head has either an internal hexagonal recess to work with a cannulated screwdriver, or an external hexagonal or square head and a cannulated wrench (see Fig. 6.27) The internal recess design allows use of a slim screwdriver, and permits a spherical outer shape to the screw head. This can be important in screw removal. Bone growing around a screw head with an external hexagonal head makes removal difficult, since bone must be removed to allow engagement of a wrench. If two external hexagonal screw heads touch, they may lock. The advantage of using the external hexagonal head is the strength provided to the coupling with the driving wrench. The round head with an internal recess puts more demand on the screwdriver's tip. The screwdriver hexagonal tip must be small enough to fit within the recess in the screw head, yet itself must be cannulated, leaving little material in it. In addition, strength of the screw head–shaft junction is important. The internal hexagonal recess removes material from the head. If this recess is too deep, strength may be lost at the head–shaft junction.

To maintain the strength, the diameter of the shaft of a cannulated screw is often designed slightly larger than that of a solid screw of comparable size. Since the stiffness of a cylinder in bending is a function of the third power of its radius, a small increase in the outer radius of the shaft will compensate for the cannula. An example of medium-sized screw of comparable dimensions is shown in Fig. 3.28. Cannulation does not appear to be a problem in the larger screws, but in a smaller screw leaving a cannulation large enough for stiff guide wire, may require the shaft diameter to be significantly increased or the screw will be considerably weaker.

There is a mistaken belief that a solid screw is stronger than a cannulated screw of equivalent outer thread diameter. The 6.5-mm cannulated screw typically has a somewhat larger shaft (root) diameter than its solid 6.5-mm equivalent. A solid 6.5-mm screw has a 3.0-mm thread root diameter, while the 6.5-mm corresponding screw has a root diameter of 4.8-mm. When the cannulation for guide wire is 2 mm in diameter, the area and polar moments of inertia of the cannulated screw would be 102.6 mm^3 and 514.8 mm^4 compared with 27 mm^3 and 81 mm^4, i.e., 3.8 and 6.4 times greater respectively than those of the solid screw. A cannulated screw must have a larger root diameter than the solid screw to allow room for the cannula. However, this does decrease its holding power, because of smaller thread depth. Clinically cannulated screws appear to function well and have more than adequate holding power.

A cannulated screw for cancellous bone should be self-cutting and self–tapping. The screw tip cuts only when rotated clockwise and is blunt when turned counterclockwise (removal direction). Such a tip is advantageous in percutaneous procedures. After the guide pin is place, the screw is advanced through the soft tissue while turning it in a counterclockwise direction. The tip doesn't cut or wind the soft tissues. When cortex is reached, the rotation is reversed to clockwise, allowing it to cut into the bone.

Locking Screw

Locking screw is a bone screw with threads on the undersurface or countersink of the head, which on tightening, lock in the matching threads in the plate hole and the screw becomes axially and angularly stable. A locking screw popularized by AO is described here. The anatomy of locking screw is similar to a conventional bone screw with some differences. The head is conical and has either hexagonal or hexalobular recess (Fig. 3.11). Its conical countersink offers better distribution of forces between the screw head and the threaded holes and improves locking fixation in the screw hole. The conical threaded surface has steep sidewall like a Morse cone. There are two threads running side by side on the undersurface giving an illusion of compacted pitch (Fig. 3.12). The screws with single thread on the undersurface do not lock well; a single thread occasionally slips and screw may unlock. The pitch of each of the two threads on the head is identical to thread on the shaft. The shape of the thread in the plate hole is the same as the screw head with a misfit of 0.13°. The steep conical design of the screw-to-screw hole does not allow for much inclination of the screw and locks efficiently, extending angular and axial stability to the screw. The design calls for minimum insertional torque (rotational force) – less than one third of the usual. During insertion the screw locks even when minimal axial tension is produced; it also locks efficiently against any tilting motion of the screw. An unintended benefit of these two properties is that the screw cannot pull-out during insertion; a property valuable in minimally invasive surgery. However, the threaded design does permit inconsequential amount of inclination between screw and body, allowing locked misfit. A conical screw with shallow threads on the countersink is easier to remove than a similar screw with smooth walls because on over-tightening the latter

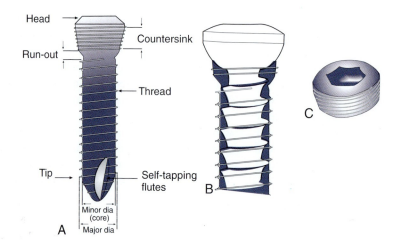

FIGURE 3.11

(A) Schematic details of a locking screw. The conical screw head has threads that lock in the plate hole with similar threads; other features of the screw are similar to a conventional bone screw. **(B)** Superimposition of silhouette of a conventional screw on a locked screw design. The major diameter of a locked screw is larger than that of a conventional cortical screw.[13] **(C)** A locking button or locking head insert installed to fill empty holes opposite a non-union or comminuted sector of a fracture; it increases plate's fatigue life without decreasing its flexibility.[14]

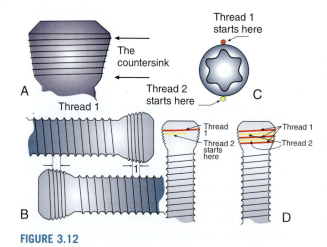

FIGURE 3.12

(A) Conical screw head with threads. **(B)** The screw head has two threads and running side by side. This gives an illusion of compacted pitch; the pitch each of the threads on the head is same as that of the thread on the shaft of the screw.[15] **(C)** The threads on the head start at two different points. **(D)** The subsequent turns give a false impression of compacted pitch. Double threads give more stability to the interface. At a given time only one thread engages.

pattern easily welds with the plate. A locking screw is used only in a locked internal fixator plate hole; it has no stand-alone application.

There is a single thread on the shaft of a locking screw. It is symmetrical in design and has a pitch coarser than that of a conventional screw. The thread is also shallower as compared to a conventional screw. A locking screw does not produce or maintain compression between the plate and the bone but resists only the pull-out forces. In a conventional plate–screw construct the force along the long axis of the screw is in the order of magnitude of several hundred kilograms. In Locking Internal Fixation Plate (LIFP), the locked screws produce only a few kilograms of static preload; this is so because the steep conical connection of the screw-to-screw hole locks upon minimal axial tension. The core diameter of the screw is 1.3 mm larger than a conventional cortical screw, which can resist the increased bending moment and higher shear force; likewise its outer diameter is also bigger. This difference in diameters enables the locking screw to withstand substantially larger bending moment and higher shear force. Increased projection area by 40% permits the distribution of the applied forces to a larger bone surface. Due to the larger core diameter the screw tolerates 100% more shear stress and 200% more bending load, whereby the incidence of screw failure is markedly reduced; this increased strength is an advantage, especially in the vicinity of the joint where cancellous bone is in abundance. The locking screw has a larger and coarser pitch when compared to a cortical screw. The pitch of a 3.5-mm locking screw measures 0.8 mm and 31.75 tpi. The pitch of the locking thread in the head of the screw is 0.4 mm but it is a double thread that equals 0.8 mm for one full turn of the screw, which is identical to the pitch of thread on the shaft. The locking screws are available with ST and self-drilling ST tips.

Locking Buttons[14]

Locking buttons or locking head inserts are screw heads with threads on its countersink but without the shaft. These are used in round hole locking plates to fill the empty holes opposite the fracture or non-union site. Filling up the empty holes increases the fatigue life of the plate. The tightly screwed in button eliminates the stress riser effect of the empty holes and prolongs the fatigue life of the plate as the plate then in this region acts more like a solid plate. Over-tightening these buttons further increase the fatigue life by 48–52% and prevents their early loosening. Presence of these inserts does not alter plate's stiffness.[16] Such insertion does not affect the flexibility of the plate and desired effect of decreasing the stiffness of the construct to attain higher levels of interfragmentary movements at the fracture site is achieved. Filling oval or oblong hole of integrated locking hole with a metal plug does not increase that plate's fatigue life because the oval plug cannot be screwed in the hole and does not eliminate the stress riser effect. Use of a locking plate with round holes and filling the screw holes nearest the defect or osteotomy with locking buttons may increase the fatigue life of plate in management of non-unions and bone defects.[17]

The Herbert Screw

The Herbert screw is a specialized implant to achieve interfragmentary compression. In this unique device there is no head and threads are present at both ends of the screw, with a pitch differential between the leading and trailing threads (Fig. 3.13). The intention is for the screw to be buried beneath a bony surface. Interfragmentary compression is achieved by the difference in thread pitch: the coarser pitch moves the screw a greater distance through bone with each turn than does the finer pitch. As the screw is turned, the leading thread penetrates the bone faster than the trailing threads, slowing penetration, reducing the surfaces to come together and creating compression during insertion. A screw head is therefore not required. In absence of a screw head it is possible to insert this screw through articular surfaces without the head being prominent. A cannulated Herbert screw is typically made of titanium and facilitates percutaneous scaphoid fracture fixation, avoids prolonged cast immobilization and allows a more rapid return to sport or work. Placing a guide wire first allows for accurate visualization of the path, position and length of the screw. The guide wire also helps in control and reduction of fractured fragments. Current indications include fractures of the carpal scaphoid, capitellar fractures,

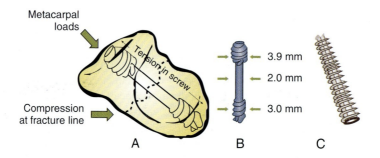

FIGURE 3.13

(A) The Herbert screw acts as a tension band to resist bending in the Scaphoid.[18] (B) Dimensions of a Herbert screw.[19] (C) Newer screw made on similar principles; the design is available in titanium and in biodegradable material. It is used in several locations for fracture fixation and joint fusion.

radial head fractures, osteochondral fractures, osteochondritis dissecans and small joint arthrodesis. The Herbert screw can be quite difficult to remove and is routinely left in place. Headless, variable pitch, cannulated screws are now available in many innovative modifications (Fig. 3.13C).

Headless compression screws with differential threading have found use in many situations like Greater tuberosity fractures, capitellum fractures, navicular fractures, fifth metatarsal fractures, radial head and styloid fractures, malleolar fractures, talus fractures, fusions of various small joints in the foot and wrist, osteotomies and OCD repair.

SCREW INSERTION

Successful insertion of a screw starts with the drilling of a pilot hole and ends with the screw achieving a firm purchase in the bone.

Drill Bit

Drilling is the most common single procedure performed in fracture surgery. A pilot hole can be drilled with a Kirschner wire, bur or drill bit. A drill bit (twist drill) is normally used. It has a smooth shank which is gripped in a chuck. The blunt end of the shank is sometimes modified for quick attachment to the drilling machine. The body of the drill bit contains spiral flutes (grooves) which carry bone chips out of the hole being drilled (Fig. 3.14). The cutting end is conical in shape and has two cutting edges or lips that are inclined away from the centre. The cutting edges act as wedges that shear bone from the surface being cut. Cutting is performed by the two lips at the end of the drill and not by the flutes along the side; likewise the drill bit is sharpened by grinding the two cutting edges, not the flutes. In fact, the hole will be truer if the flutes of a bone drill are dull, rather than sharp.

The face of the conical cutting end is usually slanted back slightly from the two cutting edges to allow clearance, since this facilitates cutting. The cutting edge angle determines the angle of the cutting surface with respect to the bone surface. The cutting edges meet at the dead centre of the drill bit. The angle

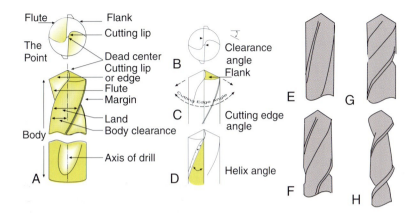

FIGURE 3.14

Parts of a bone drill bit.[2] (**A**) The three angles of the drill bit are clearance angle or angle at which the cutting surface is raked away from the bone surface (**B**), cutting angle (**C**) and the helix angle (**D**), which controls the rate of advance of the drill through bone. Type of helix determines the cutting speed of the drill bit. (**E**) Used for material that clears easily like dry bone, steel, a slow helix has smaller helix angle and fewer turns (**F**) than a quick helix which has larger helix angle and more turns on the shaft and is used for wet bone that is difficult to clear and must swiftly be removed to prevent blocking the flutes. (**G**) A bit with intermediate helix. (**H**) The most efficient design in terms of cleaning debris and contribute to enhance drilling efficiency is parabolic-shaped flute.[21]

between the dead centre and the cutting edge is the clearance angle. This angle defines how much of the cutting surface of the drill is actually engaged in bone. With no clearance angle, the whole cutting surface of the drill behind the cutting edge engages the bone surface, increasing its temperature. Too high a clearance angle encourages chipping. The helix angle affects the speed at which material is removed from the hole and the same time the speed at which the drill advances through bone (Fig. 3.13E–H). Table 3.1 presents a glossary of technical terms used in drilling technology and Table 3.2 details various parameters for drilling in different materials.

Principles of Cutting Instruments

The basic principles of cutting are similar for various types of cutting processes such as turning, shaping, plaining, milling. The underlying mechanism, which is common to all, is a wedge (the tool) progressing though a material in a direction parallel to its surface, with the edge of the wedge at a depth below the surface (Fig. 3.15). The cutting wedge is placed at certain angle to the material being progressed; this angle is known as the rake angle (Fig. 3.16). This basic relationship is the same for a rotating tool, as it is for a planer, if the direction of rotation is perpendicular to the cutting edge. The material which flows over the wedge forms the chip and that which flows under the wedge forms the machined surface. Osteotomes and chisels cut in a similar fashion.

The process of drilling results in deformation of bone. Elastic deformation occurs as the tool indents the bone surface, and plastic deformation to failure in shear results as the material is cut away and forms a chip.

Table 3.1 A Brief Explanation of Common Drilling Terms[21]

Term	Explanation
Body	Portion of the drill that extends from the shaft and couples with the driver
Chisel edge	Apex or tip of drill bit
Chisel point	Point of bit that drills into bone
Clearance angle	Angle by which the non-cutting flank clears the material
Cutting face	Portion of drill that functions as a blade; cutting edge or lip
Flank	Flat portion of the drill when viewed end-on
Flutes	Channels along the shaft that clear bone chips from the cutting surface
Helix angle	Angle that subtends the tangent of the lead and axis of the bit
Land	Peripheral edge of the flutes
Lead	Leading face of the land
Point angle	Angle between the two cutting lips in the sagittal plane
Rake angle	Angle at which the cutting face is presented to the material
Web	Inner portion of the drill separating the flutes
Wedge angle	Angle between the cutting face and the flank

Table 3.2 Effective Cutting and Helix Angles for Different Materials

Material	Cutting Edge Angle	Helix Angle	Progression in Material	
Wood	86	17.2	Fast	
Bone	90–110	24	Medium	Reduces chipping, allows rapid advance of the drill
Metal	113–118	13.5	Slow	

Drill Size Nomenclature

Drill size nomenclature is based on the diameter of the drilled hole. Several different systems were used in the past, designating the size by a fraction of an inch, a decimal of an inch, a number or a letter (Table 3.3). These are being discontinued and the system expressing the sizes in metric measurements is being gradually adopted.

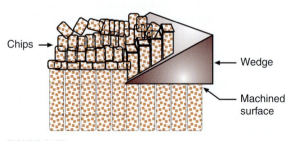

FIGURE 3.15
Schematic presentation of cutting process by a sharp tool.[22]

Heat Generation in Drilling

The energy input to a cutting tool is converted partly to heat as a result of friction between the cutting edge of the drill and the bone. About two thirds of the energy is

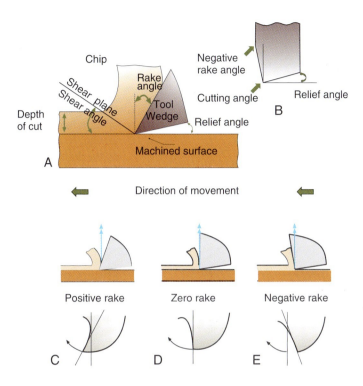

FIGURE 3.16
(**A**) Cutting terminology used in industry.[2] The angle between a vertical line and edge of the flute is known as rake angle. The cutting flutes of ST screws can have negative, neutral, or positive rakes. (**B**) Detail drawing of a negative rake. (**C**) Although slightly weaker mechanically a positive-rake cutting tip is very effective in bone. A positive rake is fabricated by removing minimal metal from the first couple of threads of a bone screw with very little change to the overall thread surface area. It cuts like a chisel with minimum force, generates very little heat and is only sharp when being turned in the clockwise direction.[11] (**D and E**) Zero and negative rakes are used in industry but have little use in orthopaedics.

absorbed by the action of cutting which disrupts the molecular and atomic bonds of the material. The rest of the energy is lost as heat, and a small fraction is converted to mechanical vibration and sound energy.

Infrared photographs of a drilling operation show the distribution of heat as the drill bit proceeds through the material. These indicate two areas of highest temperature; the bone chips immediately behind the drilling edges of the drill bit, and in the bit itself, just behind its leading edge. A large part of the heat generated by a sharp drill bit is either in the drill bit or in the bone chips, and very little heat is present in the bone itself. As the drill bit begins to dull, it no longer shears the material but rather gashes and fragments the particles from the bone. The amount of frictional heat increases, most of which is now located in the bone itself. With a dull drill bit, not only does the temperature of the bone surface increase but also the drilled hole is no longer clean; rather the bone is somewhat crushed, resulting in minute fractures on the bone surface.

A bur is sometimes used in bone surgery on small bones. Heat is rapidly generated with a bur, the temperature rising as the pressure and the speed (revolutions per minute or rpm) increase. Steel burs

Table 3.3 Frequently Used Drill Sizes in Millimetres and Their Equivalents in Fractions, Decimals and Numbers[23]

mm[2]	Inches[a]	Inches[a]	Number[a]
0.4	1/64	0.0156	79
0.8	1/32	0.0312	68
1.2	3/64	0.0468	56
1.5	1/16	0.0625	53
2.0	5/64	0.0787	47
2.5	3/32	0.0984	38
2.7	7/64	0.1063	36
3.2	1/8	0.1260	30
3.5	9/64	0.1378	28
4.0	5/32	0.1574	20
4.3	11/64	0.1778	18
4.7	3/16	0.1875	12

[a]Nearest equivalent

produce most heat. Tungsten carbide is superior material in this respect, and diamond tip burs produce least heat.

Pins (Kirachner wires) produce more heat than a drill bit. As the pin shaft is smooth, there is no way of eliminating the debris which is inevitably compressed against the wall of the hole leading to an increase in friction and higher temperatures. Heat production is directly related to speed and increases markedly above 500 rpm, which is the optimum recommended speed for a pin.

Effects of Heat on the Bone

After a bone is heated to 44.6°C, temperature elevation causes deactivation of alkaline phosphatase and the degradation of the collagen–hydroxyapatite bond resulting in permanent alterations in its mechanical properties. Necrosis of osteocytes can be produced in the long bones of rabbits by exposure to 47°C for one minute.

Factors Affecting Heat Production

Factors which increase the amount of heat include drill diameter, sharpness of the drill bit and the feed rate (cutting speed is expressed as metres/minute; feed rate as millimetres/minute; both are related to operating speed of the drill bit). The perfection of the cutting edge and the rate are related; the sharper the drill bit, the less pressure it takes to advance a given distance in a given amount of time. Time is also an important factor. As a drill bit drills at a specific point, heat radiates. The longer the drill bit remains at one point, the higher the temperature achieved. Bone density also influences heat generation; the denser the bone, the greater the heat produced.

Heat Production in Drilling

Increase
- Dull drill bit
- Time
- Thick bone
- Excessive thrust and speed

Decrease
- Sharp drill bits up to 3.2 mm at slow speed, with appropriate cutting angle
- Simultaneous saline irrigation
- Frequent drill bit cleaning
- Drilling large holes in stages

Techniques to Minimize Heat Production

Heat generated during drilling could be present in one of four places: the drill bit, the bone chips, the bone and the coolant. Under ideal conditions the majority of the generated heat should be in the coolant, with very little heat in the drill or in the bone chips and a negligible part in the bone itself. Irrigation with normal saline solution ('saline') is effective. This should commence simultaneously with drilling as the temperature increases almost instantaneously at the start of the act and much more slowly thereafter. A sharp drill bit of adequate tip angle (80–118°) cuts efficiently while producing minimal heat. The drill bit should be checked frequently to remove material lodged in the cutting face or flutes, particularly when working on dense cortex. When a large diameter hole is needed, the temperature as well as the accuracy of the placement will be easier to control if a smaller hole is drilled as a first step. The geometry of the drill bit tip is important. A smaller tip angle (60–70°), i.e. a sharper tip, produces more heat because it creates smaller axial forces and takes longer to achieve the objective. In essence, drill bits up to 3.2-mm diameter, at a speed of 750–1200 rpm, and higher feed rate with saline irrigation generate minimum heat.[24]

Recommending change in specifications of drill bits to reduce heat generation for orthopaedic use, Saha et al. and Natali et al. in separate studies demonstrated a 45% decrease in thrust load and 41% decrease in peak temperatures with shorter duration of sustained peak temperatures than a standard orthopaedic drill bits. Specifications of two commercially available drill bits are shown in the Table 3.4.[21]

Mechanics of Drilling

The drill point should be sharp; a blunt drill causes thermal necrosis of the bone. A bent drill bit wobbles, produces a hole larger than intended for the screw and thereby compromises the fixation. A drill bit should be replaced after making 12–15 holes. When commencing drilling, the drill may be rotated slowly to bite the bone. Once the drilling angle is established, it should be maintained during drilling, tapping and placing of the screw. A wobble during these procedures can damage the hole. A drill bit should be used with a close-fitting drill sleeve.

Table 3.4 Ideal and Available Drill Bits for Orthopaedic Use

Company	Drill Point	Flutes	Helix	Angle
Saha et al.	Split point	Parabolic flutes	Quick helix	118°
Natali et al.	Split point	Parabolic flutes	Quick helix	118°
Synthes	Standard point	Parabolic flutes	Slow helix	83°
Smith and Nephew	Standard point	Parabolic flutes	Slow helix	94°

Parabolic design has increased spacing between the flutes when compared to standard drill bits[21]

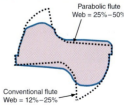

Drill Bit Failure

Drill bit failure is known to occur at a frequency of 3–25 drill bits per 1000 internal fixations. There are two possible causes of failure. The bit may touch an implant or may graze an instrument and fail; this is an avoidable cause. Rotational bending failure following contact with the far cortex at an unfavourable angle is an unavoidable cause of failure (Fig. 3.17).

Drill bit failure is more often seen during insertion of hip screws and in fixation of angled blade-plates in the hip region than in any other internal fixation procedure. When drilling, it is important to avoid bending the drill bit and to ensure that its tip does not contact an implant. A three-fluted drill bit is more stable than the two-fluted version; its use is likely to reduce the possibility of failure.

A broken drill bit in the vicinity of a joint should be removed. A drill bit fragment not in contact with an implant can be left indefinitely in the body. A broken drill bit in contact with an implant is well tolerated

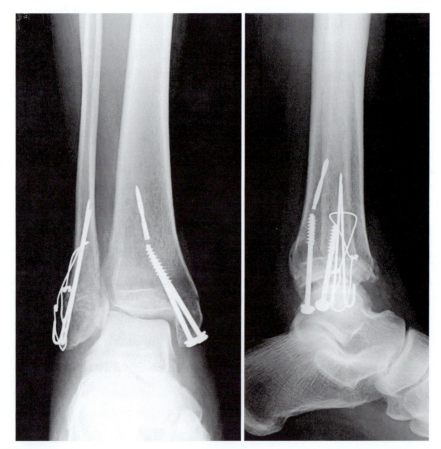

FIGURE 3.17
A drill bit is prone to breakage when it veers off a bone face; other common site is medial face of neck of femur. The drill bit bends under continued thrust and breaks is a possible explanation for frequent breakage.

by the body for months and years despite corrosion. Every effort should be made to remove a broken bit at the time of implant removal after bone healing; however, excessive surgical trauma is unjustified.

The Power Drill

Even under controlled conditions a drill hole is always significantly larger than the drill bit. Biomechanical and video analysis of power versus hand drilling shows a 'wobble factor' induced by hand drilling. A round drill hole turns to an oval shape. Less wobbling occurs if a drill sleeve and power drill are used. A power drill and abundant coolant are both necessary for good drilling.

Excessive speed and thrust on the drill machine may cause thermal necrosis of the bone. Excessive thrust may bend the drill bit and destroy the shape of the hole. In an extreme case, a drill bit may break. The thrust should be relieved as the drill emerges from the far cortex. This avoids micro-fracture of the bone and excessive penetration of the soft tissue.

The drill should be rotated in the same direction, even when it is withdrawn from the hole, and should not be reversed because it may then break. The drill fluting is designed to push the dust out of the hole. Trying to reverse the drill will only force dust back into the hole, making it difficult to remove. If the drill bit jams, the drilling machine should be taken away and the bit should be removed with the help of a T-handle.

Irrigation of the hole with saline should start simultaneously as saline reduces the friction and avoids thermal damage by cooling the tissue. A steady stream of saline on revolving shaft of the drill bit effective reaches the bone face (Fig. 3.18). The drill flutes should be cleaned periodically to remove the bone chips during a procedure. The optimal speed for drill machines is 750–1200 rpm.

A hand drill often wobbles, resulting in an eccentric hole. Pressure exerted by the surgeon on the hand drill may disrupt the fracture reduction, or the pointed drill may slip from the curved surface of bone to impale the adjacent soft tissues. Use of the power instrument helps to position the hole in the mid-axis of the bone.

The Drill Sleeve

A drill sleeve (drill guide) is an instrument used to direct the placement of a drill hole and simultaneously protect the surrounding soft tissues. The sleeve and the drill should have a close fit without play (Fig. 3.18B and C); the sleeve increases the accuracy of drilling and prevents the drill point from wandering across the bone. The drill sleeve also protects a bone plate from accidental scratching by the rotating drill bit.

Drilling Depth

As a drill point begins to exit a cortical bone surface it slows slightly and the pitch of the drilling sound changes. This should be used as a signal to ease pressure on the drill machine and to arrest the forward motion of the drill bit to avoid over-penetration. Accurate drilling depth is established through practice.

Good Drilling Practice
- Use a straight, sharp drill bit of recommended size
- Clean the tip and the flutes frequently.
- Start slowly, establish and maintain the drilling angle.
- Use a drill sleeve.
- Use the power drill; drill with simultaneous saline irrigation.
- Achieve proper drilling depth; avoid over-penetration.

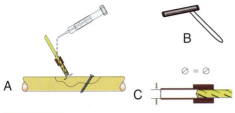

FIGURE 3.18

(**A**) A stream of normal saline on revolving drill bit shaft reaches bone face in sufficient volume. Normal saline directly lowers bone temperature by conduction, eliminates bone chips that cause increased friction, lowers friction by lubricating the drill bit.[24] (**B**) A common drill sleeve. (**C**) The inside diameter of the sleeve matches the diameter of the drill bit.

Pilot Hole

A pilot hole is the first step in inserting a bone screw. The diameter of the drill bit should be the same as the core of the screw.

Importance of a Pilot Hole

A screw may break during insertion if the pilot hole is too small, while it will have no hold in a hole that is as large as its thread diameter. The holding power of a screw increases in progressively smaller holes. A hole with a diameter that is 90% of the thread diameter of the screw provides optimal hold. Holes smaller than 90% do not offer any advantage; the smaller the hole, the higher the resistance, with inevitable higher insertion torque. The pilot hole size should therefore be large enough to minimize the torque needed to drive the screw, but be well below the critical diameter for optimal pull-out strength. The manufacturer's recommendations on drill bit size for a screw should be meticulously followed (Table 3.5).

Tapping

Cutting an internal thread by means of a multiple-point cutting tool is known as tapping. Tapping is necessary to allow the penetration of screws into hard cortical bone. The tool necessary to cut threads in a drill hole is called a tap (Fig. 3.20). The tap is essentially the inverse geometry of the internal thread to be cut where the threads consists of sharp cutting edges. To ease tapping process, the threads on the tap increase gradually in height up to the desired thread depth. A pilot hole is hand-tapped for better quality of bone thread. The tap centre line should coincide with the hole centre line. This is facilitated by a long taper on the bone tap. Such centring produces maximal thread strength. Any movement away from the centre line will cut an uneven thread. The tap is gently twisted and should progress at the rate governed by the helix angle of the thread. Any thrust distorts the thread; excessive thrust may bend or break the tap.

When a hole is tapped, bone is cut away and forms a thread chip. The amount of bone removed with every revolution of the tap is the difference in heights between two successive rows of thread cutters. As the tap is reversed, the chips break off and accumulate within the flutes that run along the side of the tap. The flutes act as channels for transport of bone chips. The length of the flutes is in general the same as the threaded part of the tap. It is a good practice to make a half back-turn after every two forward turns (Fig. 3.20B). Excessive torque may break the tap inside the bone. Tapping is continued until two threads of the tap emerge from the far cortex. A tap is removed by twisting gently in the reverse direction. Pulling on the tap may damage the threads.

Table 3.5 Different Drill Bits for Pilot and Gliding Holes for Varying Screw Sizes

Screw Size	Drill Bit For	
	Thread Hole	Gliding Hole
4.5	3.2	4.5
3.5	2.5	3.5
2.7	2.0	2.7
1.5	1.0	1.5

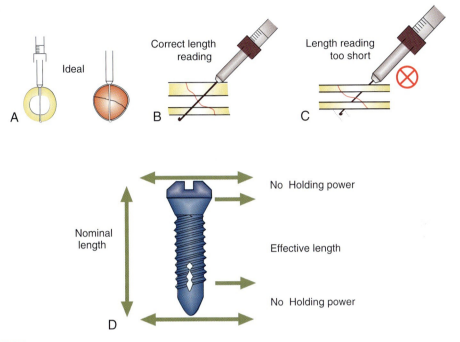

FIGURE 3.19

(**A**) Depth gauge is used for correct estimation of the screw length. (**B**) In an oblique hole, the small hook of the depth gauge tends to slip off the obtuse angled tip of the thread hole, yet this is the correct site for making an accurate measurement. (**C**) The acute-angled lip of the thread hole is easily engaged with the hook, but provides inaccurate measurements.[26] (**D**) The nominal length of a screw is its total length including the head. Effective holding length of a screw is less than the nominal length.[27]

The tapped hole is irrigated and the debris is cleared by suction. The debris, if left behind in the hole, jams the screw and destroys the threads. The tap should be cleaned before each use. The removed bone chippings make a ready source of bone graft for small bone gaps often encountered at the end of a fixation procedure.

Taps are engineered to minimize heat production (by distributing the cutting area over many small surfaces) and to reduce micro-fracturing of the cortical bone. The use of a sharp tap results in a stronger and better constructed thread in the bone. Tapping reduces the incidence of cortical screw failure during insertion and allows a greater percentage of the applied torque to be converted into compressive force between the fracture surfaces across which the screw is placed.

In lower-density material such as cancellous bone the resistance to penetration of a screw into a non-tapped hole is lower and shear failure of the screw becomes less of a concern. The cancellous screw forms its own matching threads by compressing soft cancellous bone; tapping is thus limited only to the hard proximal cortical bone. The far cortex need not be tapped. A separate tapping operation to insert an ST cortical screw is unnecessary, but the precautions suggested for tapping are applicable here and ensure satisfactory screw insertion.

Countersink

The screw undersurface exerts high wedging pressure on the bone. To disperse this high pressure over a wider area a hemispherical or conical hole is gouged into the bone; this hole as well as the cutter used to gouge the hole is called 'countersink' (Fig. 3.21). When a screw is used without a plate, a countersink hole is created to reduce the risk of fracture as the screw is tightened. Besides, countersinking reduces the prominence of the screw head over the malleolar area. The risk of bone splitting is also reduced by undercutting or reducing the diameter of the 'run out' of a screw (see Fig. 3.5G and H).

Washers

A washer is often used with a cancellous screw to prevent the screw head from burying into the thin cortex overlying the cancellous bone (Fig. 3.20C). The flat side of the washer rests on bone while its countersunk side matches the underside of the screw head.

Insertion

The insertion torque is an important parameter controlled by the surgeon. The insertion torque is equal to the applied force times the length of the lever arm (centre of the screw head to the tip of the handle of the screw driver). It is determined mainly by the design of the screw and strength of the bone. The surgeon feels the insertion torque in two different ways while turning the screwdriver. The first mechanism is by the contact forces felt at the finger tips; this feeling depends on the screwdriver handle diameter—larger the diameter, lesser the feeling. The second process is by the direct feeling of the torque in the forearm; this feeling does not depend on the diameter of the screwdriver handle. Insertion torque and axial force should be kept as low as possible to avoid additional load on the bone threads, excessive heat generation and fatigue of the surgeon who may at a time be inserting numerous screws.

In the initial phase of insertion the bone threads in the near cortex may easily get distorted as the moment arm of the torque is large and the screw is largely unsupported. Likewise, in osteoporotic bone a substantial torque produced by a large screwdriver handle also can easily destroy the bone threads produced by an ST or cancellous screw. If excessive torque is required to insert an ST screw, it should be removed and its flutes be cleaned before reinsertion. An ST screw may be inserted with a powered or hand-operated drill machine. The accuracy of power insertion is better than that of manual insertion. In very hard bone, a STS may be handled similar to a tap during insertion. The heat generated during insertion is independent of the machine speed.

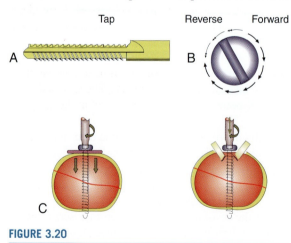

FIGURE 3.20

(A) A tap cuts high quality threads in a hole.[28] **(B)** Doing frequent back-turns is a good tapping practice.[12] **(C)** A washer prevents a screw head from sinking into cancellous bone or from cracking thin cortical bone.[26]

The screw is centred and inserted perpendicular to the hole in a plate. When a screw is driven-in off-centre it may jam or bone threads may get damaged. Besides, bending moments may be created which may damage the bone threads and perhaps weaken the screw.

A wedge-shaped countersink of a screw creates higher forces, while a rounded one permits compensation for small degrees of error. It is recommended that the selected ST screw should be 2 mm longer than the measurement to ensure that the cutting flutes extend beyond the far cortex. This is important when the screws are inserted obliquely in relation to the axis of the plate.

Once the screw enters the medullary canal, it is possible to miss drill hole on the opposite cortex. Less experienced surgeons must always drive screws by hand; hand-driving is also necessary when the bone quality is poor. A power driver with matching screwdriver tip is useful when multiple screws are being inserted into hard cortical bone, but this technique requires practice.

The screw is then made snug but over-tightening should be avoided as it can result in fracture of the bone or failure of the screws. Over-tightening also predisposes the screw to premature failure. In healthy young cortical bone, it is generally recommended that torque of about 2.824 N·m be applied to the screw. This can be learned by practising with a torque screwdriver.

Efficiency of Screw Insertion

To insert a screw, torque (rotational force) is applied to the screw head. Of the total applied torque, part is utilized to cut the threads, part to overcome the thread friction and another portion is consumed at the countersink interface. When the undersurface of the screw meets the surface of a bone, a tensile stress is induced in the screw, resulting in compression of the opposing bone surfaces. In practice, a very small portion of the applied torque is put to use to induce tension in the screw (Fig. 3.22).

The efficiency of insertion is the percentage of applied torque which is finally converted into tension in the screw. For maximum efficiency and least risk of premature failure of the screw, this tensile stress should be generated with the lowest possible applied torque. Under the most adverse circumstances only about 5% of applied torque is used to induce tension, but under ideal conditions about 65% can be usefully employed.

To improve the efficiency of insertion, the thread friction can be reduced by increasing the size of the pilot hole. The standard hole should be slightly larger than the minor diameter of the screw. The average diameter of commonly used drill bit from standard manufacturers is 200 μm larger than the minor diameter of the corresponding surgical screw. When a screw is inserted by a continuous rotatory movement, as opposed to intermittent movement of the screwdriver, it further reduces the torque. The torque lost at the screw–bone interface and that lost through thread friction can be reduced by lubrication; saline is a satisfactory agent.

MEASUREMENT OF SCREW LENGTH

A depth gauge is used to measure the required screw length (Fig. 3.19). In cortical bone this should be measured after countersinking but before tapping the thread, since the depth gauge may damage the thread by tearing the bone. Care is required to avoid an erroneous reading arising either from engaging only the near cortex or the soft tissues on the far side. It is a safe practice to palpate the screw tip on the other side or to view it under fluoroscopy intensification.

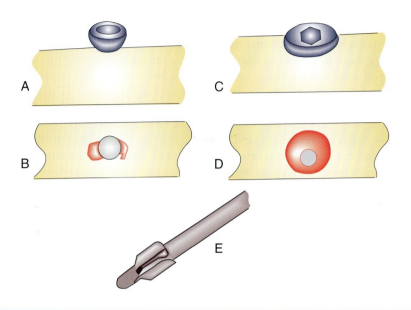

FIGURE 3.21

Countersink. **(A and B)** A screw head remains prominent and exerts uneven pressure on the bone. **(C and D)** A countersink hole reduces the screw prominence, helps it to sit flush with or below the surface of the bone, and evenly distributes pressure. **(E)** The tool to gouge out a countersink hole is also called countersink.

The nominal length of a screw equals its total length including the head (Fig. 3.19D). In cortical bone, the appropriate screw length is such that one full thread exits the far cortex. When inserting an ST cortical screw, the screw tip must protrude further from the far cortex so that the flutes are clear and at least one complete thread engages the cortex. This is unnecessary with a cancellous screw and is inadvisable where the sharp tip of the screw threatens soft tissues on the opposite side of the bone. In cancellous bone the depth gauge is used without the use of countersink.

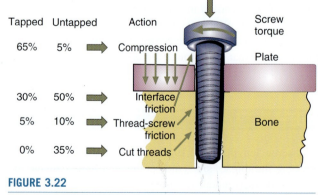

FIGURE 3.22

The efficiency of screw insertion. Utilization of applied torque at important interfaces in tapped and untapped pilot hole.[29]

SCREW REMOVAL

An isolated screw may be left in place for good. However, a single screw in cancellous bone without autologous cancellous grafts may be removed only after 3–6 months. The fibular positioning screw used for malleolar fractures should be removed after 6–8 weeks, as it serves little purpose after that time and, if left in place, may become loose or break. An ST screw is more difficult to remove than an NST screw because bone may grow into the cutting flute of the screw and block the rotation. Unless the new bone is removed, the screw cannot turn. The recommended procedure is first to tighten the screw by one turn to break the bone growth in the cutting flute and then to remove it by anti-clockwise rotation of the screwdriver. An oversized screwdriver is useful to remove a screw with single slot head.

Bone may also grow in the screw head recess. A sharp-pointed instrument is used to remove the new bone so that the screwdriver can get a firm purchase.

Removal of Screw with Stripped Head

Stripping of the screw heads is a common occurrence. It is most commonly caused by slippage of a screw driver that is incorrectly aligned with the screw axis. This can occur during either insertion or attempted percutaneous removal. It is important to ensure that the screwdriver is aligned co-linearly with the screw axis to obtain complete engagement in the screw head. Even after one event of slippage, the maximal torque values in both clockwise and counterclockwise directions can be reduced to one half the pre-slippage values.[30] The hexalobular sockets offer better resistance to stripping and are superior to 'hex' sockets in this respect (see Fig. 3.2).

When slippage and stripping occurs, various techniques may aid removal of screws with damaged heads. One technique is to interpose the foil from a suture pack between the screwdriver and the screw head in an attempt to improve the connection. Placing gauze between the screw head and screwdriver creates an interference fit and provides additional torque necessary for removal. Additional folds may be required to increase the gauze swab thickness. However, these techniques are successful only with minimal screw head stripping.

Whenever the screwdriver fails to firmly engage in the screw socket, a conical extraction screw with left-handed threads is inserted firmly into the screw head and is turned in anti-clockwise direction to engage the head (Fig. 3.23). Lightly tapping the appropriately sized extractor with a mallet is successful when purchase is not initially obtained with manual pressure. Conical extraction devices are available in sizes for screws ranging from 1.5 to 7.3 mm.

At times even this method fails. The use of a carbide drill bit or diamond-impregnated metal cutting disk will be required to remove a cold-welded screw. The cold-welded screw head is then drilled out through the use of the carbide drill. The conical extraction screw is jammed in with power drill at slow speed or by a T-handle. Once it engages in the screw head, it becomes easier to remove the screw.

Removal of the Broken Distal Screw Tip

The removal of the distal screw tip portion is not always necessary. However, it may be required to eliminate a potential infective nidus or to insert an intramedullary nail. When a portion of the screw shaft protrudes above the bone, a vise grip-type plier is useful to grasp and turn the screw (Fig. 3.24).

A broken distal screw tip also can be removed by impacting the screw and driving it through the far cortex. A well-fixed distal screw tip in cortical bone may be tough to remove. It can be removed by using hollow reamer to enlarge the near cortical hole and gouging out area around the broken screw. An extraction bolt is passed to engage the broken screw bit and removed by counterclockwise moment. If the extraction bolt fails to create purchase on the remaining screw tip, the far cortex is drilled with the hollow reamer to dislodge the screw; this method causes greater bone loss. A Kirschner wire is useful to judge the correct screw trajectory of a broken cannulated screw. At times, a spade-tipped Kirschner wire is impacted to create an interference fit and the screw is twisted out. Routinely a reverse-threaded conical extraction device is used to remove a broken cannulated screw.

CHAPTER 3 BONE SCREWS

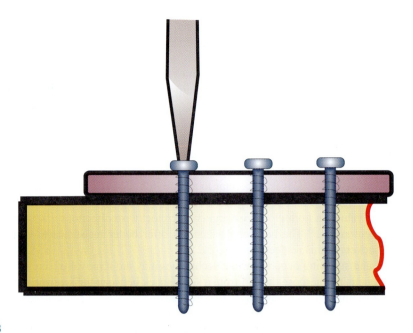

FIGURE 3.23

Removal of a stripped screw using a conical extraction device.[31]

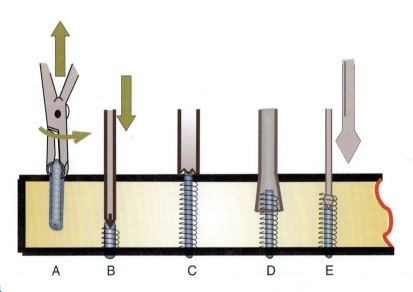

FIGURE 3.24

(A) Vise-grip pliers can grasp and twist out a broken screw. **(B)** Broken bit is driven out from the far cortex.[31] **(C)** A hollow reamer is used to remove bone and tissue around the broken half of the screw. **(D)** A reverse threaded extraction bolt is threaded on to the broken screw. **(E)** A spade-tipped Kirschner wire when impacted in a cannulated screw creates an interference fit and the screw may be twisted out.

HOLDING POWER OF THE SCREW

Definition

The so-called holding power of the screw is difficult to define because it largely depends on how it is measured. Two common tests are the measurement of the pull-out strength and the measurement of maximum axial tension that a screw can develop as it is being tightened. To determine its pull-out strength, a screw is pulled along its longitudinal axis and the force required to rip the threads is measured. The pull-out strength, a function of both the size of the screw and number of threads engaged, is usually specified in units of Newtons per millimetre (of screw length). For this reason, a bicortical screw will hold better than a unicortical screw in the same bone.

Estimation of the maximum axial tension that a screw can produce may be more useful than pull-out strength since it is a measurement of how tightly a screw can compress when lagged across a fracture site, or how tightly a screw can fasten a plate to the bone. This measurement is somewhat more difficult to obtain, as specialized instrumentation is required. In any test of holding power, the conditions must be identical when comparing different types of screw.

Modifying Factors

Holding strength is dependent upon the screw and the material in which the hole is situated. The screw holding strength increases as the threads become deeper and are placed closer. The thread shape factor (TSF) is defined as 0.5 plus the ratio of thread depth to pitch multiplied by a constant. The TSF (and screw holding strength) increases whenever the thread depth becomes larger (larger threads and smaller root diameter) and the distance between the threads (pitch) becomes smaller, with either factor changing in isolation or in tandem. The thread angle decides the shape of the thread. If a constant angle is maintained, the pitch increases as the thread depth is increased: conversely, decreasing the pitch decreases the thread depth (Fig. 3.25).

In reality, there is a limit to which the holding strength of a screw (TSF) could be increased. For a given thread shape, to increase its TSF, a smaller thread angle is required, which in effect makes the thread thinner and weaker. There is a practical upper limit of altering screw thread geometry, and TSF values up to 1.0 are considered optimal. If the threads cut by a screw in the bone become very narrow and too long, they are easily broken by bending loads that are substantially smaller than shearing pull-out loads. Holding strength or pull-out resistance is, in general, proportional to the bone volume between threads, the length of the screw and its triangulation with the plate (Fig. 3.26).

Other factors that modify holding strength are the number of threads engaged (bone thickness),

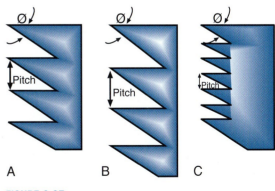

FIGURE 3.25

Effect of change in thread depth and pitch. (**A**) Example of a thread angle; the same angle is used in all the examples. (**B**) Increased thread depth increases the pitch. (**C**) Decreased thread pitch results in decreased thread depth.

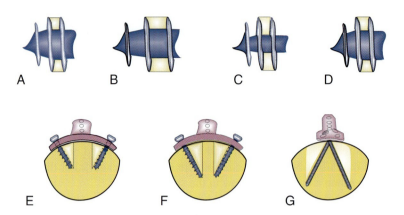

FIGURE 3.26

Holding strength of a screw. **(A)** Screw holding strength or pull-out resistance is proportional to bone volume (yellow shaded area) between screw threads. **(B)** Increasing the pitch (the distance between threads) increases the volume of bone between the threads. **(C)** Increasing the thread depth reduces the thread width. **(D)** Another method of altering the volume of bone between threads is by changing the thread shape. Position of the screws affect their pull-out resistance. For example, increased screw penetration and the use of triangulation increase the pull-out resistance. **(E)** Pull-out resistance is proportional to the triangular area defined by the screw, the perpendicular and the bone surface abutting the plate depicted by the shaded area. **(F)** The triangular area increases with longer screws or with increase in the screw angle. However, this triangulation effect requires that the screws be inserted through plate holes.[32] **(G)** The effective overlapping triangles enhance the screw hold in the porotic bone. Application of triangulation principle is seen in deployment of crossed screws in locked internal fixator plates for head of the humerus and radius (see Fig. 4.70 and Fig. 4.72).

the size of the hole and the shear strength of bone. In addition, when the screw is implanted in the bone, the tissue reactions and the bone growth also affect the holding strength.

When a machine screw is placed in a metal, it is the core area of the screw that is the most critical factor in determining how far the screw can be tightened before it fails. In bone, the threaded hole plays a more important role since the bone threads will fail well before the screw snaps. Up to a reasonable limit, the larger the hole in the bone, the larger the size and the surface area of the threads that are engaged and the greater the holding power. This rule assumes a pitch which allows engagement of at least three intact threads in a cortical bone in which they are being used. Nevertheless, when placing a screw in a bone, the goal should be to engage an aggregate of five to six threads in the cortical bone in order to achieve maximal holding power; this takes care of the eventuality that threads may break or be defective.

Screw Failure

Screw fixation may fail in several ways. A screw may break during insertion if the applied torsional load exceeds its torsional strength. This can occur when pilot hole is too small, is not tapped in a hard bone, or there is a lack of lubrication. High stresses develop in the screw when there is significant resistance to insertion causing the screw to shear at a cross-section and leave a part lodged in bone (Fig. 3.27).

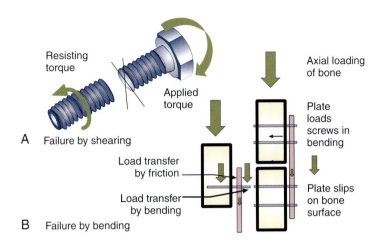

FIGURE 3.27

Modes of screw failure. (**A**) Failure by shearing due to excessive torque. (**B**) Bending failure due to loading of the plate against the screw.

Such a situation may also arise during removal if bone grows intimately to the threads of the screw and in the flutes of an ST screw. The coefficient of friction between metal and bone is approximately 0.4. When axial force is produced in tightening a screw, friction results from the screw threads sliding against bone and a part of torque is lost in overcoming friction. Increased resistance provokes the surgeon to increase the torque, which increases the shear stress in the screw. This shear force develops due to twisting of one cross-section against another. The stress magnitude depends directly on the applied torque and inversely on the cube root of the diameter of its cross-section, given by the formula:

$$\tau = 16T / (\pi d \times 3)$$

where, τ – shear stress, T – applied torque, d – root (minor) diameter of the thread

The load exerted on the screw is governed by the maximum torque that the surgeon can apply and the resistance of the screw to insertion, while the stress generated is a result of the torque applied and its root diameter. The root diameter changes with the screw under consideration. A cortical screw has threads that are shallower than cancellous screw; therefore, cortical screw has a larger root diameter than a cancellous screw that has deeper threads but smaller root diameter. Cannulation of a screw shaft also affects its torsional strength. A cannulated screw has less material in the cross-section of the body, as it has a bore for the guide wire.

Fig. 3.28 shows the cross-sectional dimensions of a standard cortical, cancellous and cancellous cannulated screw of nearly equal size. A solid cancellous screw of nearly equal size to a cortical screw can support about 25% of the peak shear stress that the cortical screw can sustain. In comparison, the cannulated screw, which has a larger minor diameter to compensate for the central bore, can sustain 58% of the shear stress of the cortical screw and 227% of that of the solid cancellous screw. An orthopaedic surgeon, who typically can apply a torque ranging from 26 to 52 inch-pounds, is capable of shearing a screw with a minor diameter as large as 2.92 mm during insertion if the screw jams. The actual torsional strength of a screw differs due to manufacturing tolerances (variations). All reputed

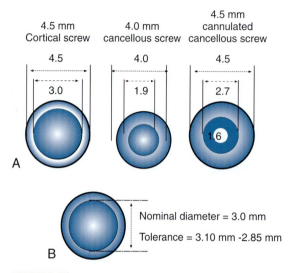

FIGURE 3.28

(A) Root, cannulation and outside diameters of bone screws in common orthopaedic use. (B) Variations permitted by standards institutions in root diameter of a 4.5-mm cortical bone screw.

manufactures follow standards that dictate the allowable tolerances in screw dimensions. For cortical screws of 4.5-mm outer diameter, the allowable dimensional tolerances are shown in Fig. 3.20B. This results in a variation of ±10 to 14% in the cube root of the cross-sectional area, and ultimate torsional strength. For a cannulated screw, using the same dimensional tolerances (±0.10 mm) for the root diameter and the bore of the cannula of the screw shown in figure result in an estimated variability in the torsional strength of ± 24%. These larger variations are the result of the tolerances on both the root diameter and the cannula itself.

Assuming that a bone screw is inserted properly, screw failure by fatigue has still been found to occur in up to 6% of implanted fixation plates. The failure occurs if the screws are tightened below the optimal level. A loose screw is unable to stand high cyclic loading for a long time. This mode of failure is usually seen several months after screw insertion and occurs when fracture fixation has not been rigid and bone healing has not occurred. Compressive force generated between a plate and a bone surface has an important effect on the strength of the screw itself. If the plate slips, load is applied directly to the screws in a direction transverse to their long axis, producing cantilever bending of the screws and the fatigue life of the screws is significantly reduced, resulting in early breakage (see Fig. 3.19B). The tensile stresses at the surface of the root of the screw are inversely proportional to the moment of inertia of the cross-section (i.e. to the diameter) raised to the power 4. Cortical screws of 4.5 mm diameter have been tested by cyclic loading. Based only on cross-sectional dimension, a solid cortical screw can support 6.2 times the maximum bending stress of a solid cancellous screw of equivalent diameter and 1.7 times the stress of a cannulated cancellous screw. It is important therefore to apply as much torque as possible to a screw to generate the frictional force that holds a plate against bone and prevents slipping of the plate so that the screws become loaded in bending. Cyclic bending load significantly decreases the fatigue life of a screw.

Another cause of delayed screw failure is corrosion. Old-style bone screws frequently fail as they get weakened by corrosion which is initiated and perpetuated because of the saline environment of the body. The stainless steel screws used today are more resistant to corrosion because they form a protective oxide or passivation layer on the surface. This layer prevents interaction between the underlying metal and corrosive environment. In addition, polishing reduces the surface exposed to the corrosive environment. Anything that damages the surface allows corrosion to occur until a new passivation layer can form. Repeated damage, such as a loose screw rubbing against a plate, prevents regeneration of the passivation layer and favours progression of corrosion, increasing the possibility of screw failure.

The bone into which a screw is placed may also fail. Usually, this failure occurs in the threaded portion of the bone. A large enough force along the longitudinal axis of the screw will cause the bone thread to fail as the screw is ripped free. If a screw is over-tightened, the threads may strip and a screw may lose its holding power. Cortical thinning reduces the length of engagement of bone screw that in turn reduces the maximum screw torque that can be applied, and the frictional force between plate and bone, thus increasing the potential for fatigue failure. Similarly if the density of trabecular bone decreases to half that of normal bone, its shear strength decreases to nearly one quarter; and therefore a screw of four times the diameter would be required to produce holding power equivalent to that of normal bone. This is impractical.

CLINICAL CONSIDERATIONS

A screw is used to compress fracture fragments together (lag screw), to hold a plate against bone (placement screw) or to buttress a fracture.

The screw, being an elementary machine, converts a small torque to a large axial force and creates this requisite elastic force in the bone. In attachment of a plate to bone, the screw creates a perpendicular (normal) force between bone and plate, increasing friction between them. The screw itself depends on the friction around the threads to hold its place.

The Lag Screw

The lag screw is a technique of insertion and not a screw. It is the most effective way to achieve compression between two bone fragments; it pulls the fragments together producing pressure across the fracture line. It achieves this by providing purchase on the distal fragment while being able to turn freely in the proximal. If the screw threads engage both cortices, the fragments remain apart like two nuts on the same bolt. The fracture gap remains open and uncompressed, as no compression is generated (Fig. 3.29).

Lagging is an excellent technique with any screw because the threads in the proximal cortex do little to improve the purchase and tend to hold fracture fragments apart. Compression between fragments increases the friction force so that inter fragmentary motion is less likely and therefore strengthens the structure. Additional stability between the two bone fragments is created by interlocking of the bone surfaces, hence the need for accurate reduction.

The lagging technique can be applied to virtually all types of screws. In diaphyseal fractures a cortical screw is applied as a lag screw. As the screw is threaded over its entire length it can act as a lag screw only if it passes freely through the near cortex. A 'gliding hole' is drilled through the near cortex with a drill bit equal to or larger than the outside diameter of the screw thread. The distal hole is precisely tapped. The screw thus has no hold on the near cortex but has a firm purchase on the far cortex (Fig. 3.29B). Alternatively, a cortical shaft screw may be used.

In the cancellous bone of epiphyseal or metaphyseal fractures, cancellous screws are employed. Cancellous screws and cortical shaft screws are lag screws with a long shaft. A gliding hole is not required. The unthreaded portion of the shaft, however, must be long enough so that the threaded portion will engage only the far fragment (Fig. 3.30). The shaft diameter of these screws corresponds to their outer diameter.

Lag Screw Practice

A lag screw must glide freely through the near fragment and engage only the far fragment
- Whenever a screw crosses a fracture line, it should be inserted as a lag screw
- Two small screws produce a more stable fixation than one large screw

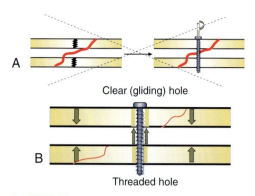

FIGURE 3.29

(A) The fracture gap remains open if the screw has purchase on both the cortices. (B) Clear gliding hole in near-cortex and firm purchase of the screw on the far-cortex produces requisite lag effect.[12]

To effect maximal interfragmental compression, lag screws must be inserted into the centre of fragments and at right angles to the fracture plane (Fig. 3.31). A single lag screw is insufficient to achieve stable fixation of diaphyseal fragments. Two screws distribute the interfragmental compression uniformly over the fracture interface and restrain rotation of the fragments around the screw axis (Fig. 3.31B). At least two, and preferably three, screws are required.

Lag principle does not obtain when applying a plate over a segment of bone without fracture lines, since both cortices are part of the same intact structure and so are active in drawing the plate tight against the bone. A plate fixation screw that crosses a fracture line should be applied as a lag screw (Fig. 3.32). A gliding hole in the proximal cortex is essential if a fully threaded screw is used. Use of an inclined fully threaded screw within a plate as a lag screw results in 50% loss in compression effect because of indentation of the screw threads within the cortical bone of the gliding hole (Fig. 3.32B). A shaft screw, when used as a lag screw, does not engage the near cortex and its use significantly improves the static compression force exerted by the lag screw (Fig. 3.32C and D). As the screw is tightened, the sliding fit of the shank screw in the gliding hole avoids the locking effect secondary to movement of the screw in a direction other than along its longitudinal axis.

Fractures can be fixed successfully with screws alone in situations where high bending loads are not anticipated or can be protected against. The goal is to create a composite structure that will bear a load. The more perfect a reduction that can be achieved, the more the fragments will be locked

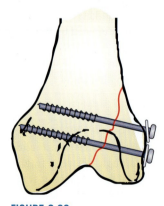

FIGURE 3.30

Bone screws with long shaft do not require clear hole. The threads must engage only the far-fragment.

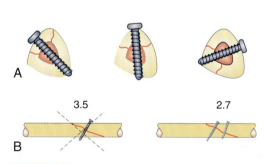

FIGURE 3.31

(A) A lag screw should be inserted into the centre of the fragment and at right angles to the fracture plane. (B) Two small screws produce more stable fixation than one large screw.[26]

together, and the lesser the loads that will be placed on the fixation. Without a plate it is difficult to achieve an integrated structure. The addition of a plate to the structure simply adds mechanical support and generates forces that resist bending.

Screw fixation alone can provide adequate stability only if the fracture length is at least 2–3 times the diameter of the bone, thus permitting fixation with a minimum of two screws. It follows that only long oblique and long spiral fractures can be stabilized with lag screws alone, and this is possible only in short tubular bones such as phalanges, metacarpals and metatarsals (Fig. 3.33). The third use of a screw is to buttress a fracture: a lateral wedge fracture is buttressed at its tip with a cortical screw and a washer (Fig. 3.33B). Lag screws by themselves are sufficient to fix a few fracture types. If lag screws alone are used for the fixation of long bones, such as the femur and the humerus,

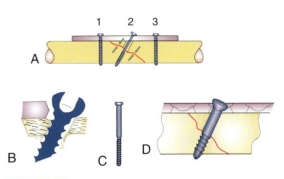

FIGURE 3.32

Lag screw nuances; a lag screw can produces force of 2500–3000 N magnitude and achieve absolute stability. (**A**) Screws 1 and 3 must take purchase on both cortices. The near-cortex of screw 2 is over-drilled to the size of the shaft of the screw only to accommodate the wider diameter of the shaft screw. (**B**) An inclined fully threaded screw within a plate as a lag screw digs in cortical bone of the gliding hole and hampers free gliding. (**C**) Detailed view of a 'Shaft' screw. (**D**) A lagged shaft screw does not engage the near cortex and precludes its secondary movement during tightening.[6]

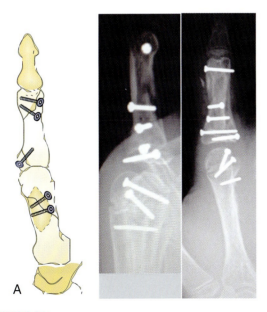
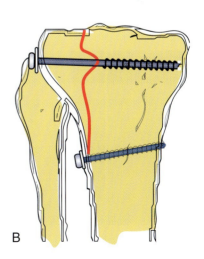

FIGURE 3.33

(**A**) Short tubular bones could be fixed with the screws only.[26] (**B**) A lateral wedge fracture fixed under compression with the proximal cancellous lag screw and buttressed at its tip with the lower cortex screw.[33]

they almost always end in early failure because of mechanical overload. Occasionally they may be successful (Fig. 3.34).

Fixation of a Spiral Fracture

In the matter of the fixation of a spiral fracture, there is an unresolved controversy whether a screw placed to fix an oblique fracture should be perpendicular to the bone or perpendicular to the fracture line. No single screw insertion angle provides satisfactory rigidity against all load configurations. The screw placed at right angles to the fracture plane produces stability against tension load but is weak in neutralizing compression loads (Fig. 3.35). When the screws are placed at right angles to the shaft, they do ensure stability against compression load but are unsatisfactory against the tension loads. Most long bones in the lower limb are intermittently subjected to compression and tension forces and therefore neither of the mentioned insertion angles is satisfactory (Fig. 3.36).

The direction of each screw is critical. In a spiral or lengthy oblique fracture, at least one screw should be inserted at right angles to the shaft of the bone to prevent overriding of the fragments. Another screw should be positioned at right angles to the fracture surfaces to provide maximal compression of the fragments. Other screws may be aligned as a compromise between these two angles (see Fig. 3.35D).

Good Practices for Locking Screw

Lag before you lock.[35] Locking screw does not bring the plate and bone together, but maintains the distance. This is why all the conventional screws placed as lag or placement screw should be installed before any locked screw is inserted; no conventional screw should be placed after a locked screw anywhere in the construct. A locked screw is stable in porotic bone because it achieves its stability by its hold in the plate and like conventional screw does not depend on quality of bone. As a rule locking screw insertion should be the last step in osteosynthesis.

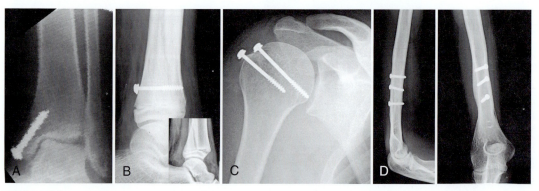

FIGURE 3.34

Lag screws alone are sufficient to fix a few fracture types. **(A)** Malleolar fracture **(B)** Triplane fracture of distal tibia. **(C)** Avulsion fracture of humeral tuberosity. **(D)** Four-year follow-up radiograph of a long spiral fracture of humerus fixed only with screws in 13–year-old girl; parents forestalled second surgery of plate removal; the arm was supported in a cast for 4 weeks.

CLINICAL CONSIDERATIONS

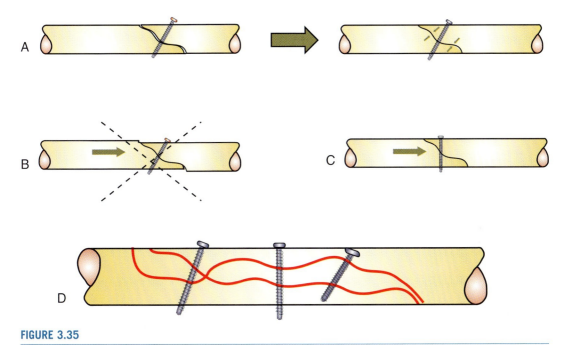

FIGURE 3.35

A lag screw inserted at right angles to the fracture plane provides maximum interfragmental compression but minimal axial stability. (**A**) Under axial load, one fragment tends to glide on the other with loss of reduction and fixation (**B**) If a screw is inserted at right angles to the long axis of the bone, it provides maximum axial stability. (**C**) It is best to have one screw at right angles to the long axis of the bone and the other at right angles to the fracture line. In a spiral fracture which is often fixed with more than two screws, the central screw is usually set at right angles to the long axis of the bone and is thus able to prevent axial displacement. (**D**) The other two screws should be at right angles to the spiral fracture plane to ensure maximal compression.[34]

Screw vs Bolt

A screw is an externally threaded headed fastener which is tightened by applying torque to the head, causing it to be threaded into the material it will hold. A bolt is also an externally threaded headed fastener, which is used in conjuction with a nut and is tightened or released only by twisting a nut (Fig. 3.37). To obtain reliable and repeatable fastener torque the bolt/nut combination should always be tightened by holding the bolt head stationary and turning the nut.[36] A further clarification aimed at disambiguation is available.[37] Bolts are headed fasteners having external threads that meet an exacting, uniform bolt thread specification such that they can accept a non-tapered nut. Screws are headed, externally threaded fasteners that do not meet the above definition of bolts.

A screw is designed to cut its own thread; it has no need for access from or exposure to the opposite side of the component being fastened to. A bolt is the male part of fastener system designed to be accepted by a pre-equipped nut of exactly the same thread design; it needs access from or exposure to the far side of bone being fixed. Cancellous and cortical screws are unsuitable to be used as bolts; a specific implant is mandatory.

CHAPTER 3 BONE SCREWS

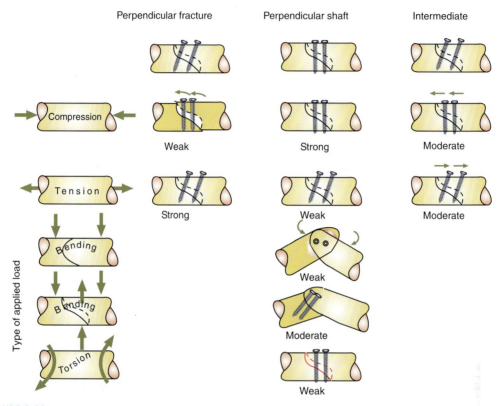

FIGURE 3.36

Screw fixation of oblique fractures. The degree of stability of fracture fixation changes with the angle of screw insertion (perpendicular to the fracture line, perpendicular to the long axis of the bone or angle between these two positions) and type of applied load.[1]

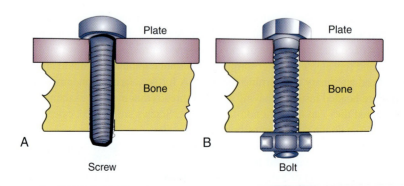

FIGURE 3.37

Bolt and screw both are threaded fasteners with similar function but different in detail: **(A)** screw; **(B)** bolt.

REFERENCES

1. Gozna ER, Harrington IJ, Evans DC. Biomechanics of musculoskeletal injury. Baltimore: Williams & Wilkins; 1982.
2. Albright JA, Johnson TR, Saha S. Principles of internal fixation. In: Ghista DN, Roaf R, editors. Orthopaedics mechanics: procedures and devices. London: Academic Press; 1978. p. 124–222.
3. Haas NP, editor. New products from AO development. Davos Platz: AOTK; 2002. p. 10.
4. Phillips screw heads. Available at: http://screwsnutsbolts.wix.com/screwsnutsbolts#!credits/c1j4q. [Accessed 2014 October 12].
5. Mears DC. Materials and orthopaedic surgery. Baltimore: Williams & Wilkins; 1979.
6. Perren SM, Allgöwer M, Burch HB, et al. The concept of biological plating using the limited contact-dynamic compression plate (LC-DCP). Injury 1991;22(Suppl. 1):1–41.
7. Frigg R. Locking compression plate (LCP). An osteosynthesis plate based on the Dynamic Compression Plate and the Point Contact Fixator (PC-Fix). Injury 2001;32:S-B-63–66.
8. Bagby GW; Janes JM. The effect of compression on the rate of fracture healing using a special plate in acute diaphyseal fractures of the radius and ulna. Am J Surg 1958;95:761.
9. Eggers GWN. The contact splint. Rep Biol Med 1946;4:42.
10. Tencer AF, Johnson KD. Biomechanics in orthopaedic trauma: bone fracture and fixation. London: Martin Dunitz; 1994.
11. Perren SM, Cordey J, Baumgart F, Rahn BA, Schatzker J. Technical and biomechanical aspects of screws used for bone surgery. Injury Int J Orthop Trauma 1992;2:31–48.
12. Cochran GVB. A primer of orthopaedic biomechanics. New York: Churchill Livingstone; 1982.
13. Wagner M, Frigg R. Internal fixators concepts and cases using LCP and LISS. Davos Platz: AO Publishing; 2006. P. 34, Fig. 1-20a–c.
14. Smith & Nephew Healthcare Pvt. Ltd., Andheri East, Mumbai - 400 059.
15. Frigg R. Locking plate- Principles and Design. Presented at Advance course on fracture management November 20-23. Phuket, Thailand; 2007.
16. Cartner J, Messina A, Baker C, Russell TA, Tornetta P, III, Ricci WM. Does insertion torque affect the mechanics of locking hole inserts and fatigue performance of bridge plate constructs? Bone Joint Sci 2011;02(03):1–3.
17. Tompkins M, Paller DJ, Moore DC, Crisco JJ, Terek RM. Locking buttons increase fatigue life of locking plates in a segmental bone defect model. Clin Orthop Relat Res 2013;471:1039–44.
18. Herbert TJ, Fisher WE. Management of the fractured scaphoid using a new bone screw. J Bone Joint Surg 1984;66B:114–23.
19. Zimmer India Pvt Ltd, Gurgaon 122001
20. Accumed LLC, Hillsboro, Oregon, USA
21. Fincham BM, Jaeblon T. The effect of drill bit, pin, and wire tip design on drilling. J Am Acad Orthop Surg 2011;19:574–79.
22. Jacobs CH, Pope MH, Berry JT, Hoaglund F. A study of the bone machining process - orthogonal cutting. J Biomech 1974;7:131–6.
23. List of drill and tap sizes. Available at: http://en.wikipedia.org/wiki/List_of_drill_and_tap_sizes. [Accessed 2014 October 12].
24. Augustin G, Davila S, Mihoci K, Udiljak T, Vedrina DS, Antabak A. Thermal osteonecrosis and bone drilling parameters revisited. Arch Orthop Trauma Surg 2008;128:71–7.
25. Parabolic drills. Available at: http://www.guhring.com/documents/catalog/drills/GT.pdf. [Accessed 2014 October 11].
26. Heim U, Pfeiffer KM, Brenwald J. Internal fixation of small fractures: technique recommended by the AO-ASIF group. 3rd ed. Berlin: Springer-Verlag; 1988.

27. Bechtol CO, Ferguson AL, Laing PG. Metals and engineering in bone and joint surgery. Baltimore: Williams & Wilkins; 1959.
28. Sequin F, Texhammar R. AO/ASIF instrumentation. Bern: Springer-Verlag; 1981.
29. Perren SM, Cordey J, Baumgart, F, Rahn GA, Schatzker J. Technical and biomechanical aspects of screws used for bone surgery. Nt J Orthop Trauma 1992;2:31–48.
30. Behring JK, Gjerdet NR, Mølster A. Slippage between screwdriver and bone screw. Clin Orthop Relat Res 2002;404:368–72.
31. Hak DJ, McElvany M. Removal of broken hardware. J Am Acad Orthop Surg 2008;16:113–20.
32. Lastra JJ, Benzel EC. Biomechanics of internal fixation. In: Vaccaro AR, Betz RR, Zeidman SM, editors. Principles and practice of spine surgery. St. Louis: Mosby; 2003. p. 43–65.
33. Müller ME, Allgower M, Schneider R, Willenegger H. Manual of internal fixation. 2nd ed. Berlin: Springer-Verlag; 1979.
34. Müller ME, AIlgower M, Schneider R, Willenegger H. Manual of internal fixation. 3rd ed. Berlin: Springer-Verlag; 1991.
35. Kulkarni GS. Plate fixation of fractures. In: Kulkarni GS. editor. Textbook of orthopedics and Trauma, Vol. 2. New Delhi: JP Brothers Publishers; 2008. p. 1447.
36. Screw vs Bolts – The engineer explains. Available at: http://engineerexplains.com. [Accessed 2014 October 8].
37. Bolts vs screws. Available at: http://en.wikipedia.org/wiki/Bolt_(fastener)#Bolts_vs_screws. [Accessed 2014 October 9].

CHAPTER 4

BONE PLATES

Introduction
Classification
  Protection (neutralization) Plates
  Compression Plate
    Role of Compression
    Static and Dynamic Compression
    Methods of Achieving Compression
  Tension Band Plate
  Buttress Plate
  Bridge Plate
  Condylar Plate
General Principles of Plate Fixation
  Plate-Related Factors
  Screw-Related Factors
  Bone-Related Factors
  Construct-Related Factors
  Effect of Compression
Additional Principles of Plate Fixation
  Tension Band Plate
  Prebending of Plate
  Plate Fixation of Oblique Long Bone Fractures
  Double Plating
  Plate Bending
  Biomechanics of a Conventional Bone Plate
    Effect of Forces on a Conventional Plate–
      Screw Construct
      Bending and Axial Load
      Torsional Load
    Load-Sharing and Load Bearing Constructs
  Plate Length and Screw Density
    Forces Acting on the Plate-Screw Interface
    Length of a Plate
    Plate Length and Plate Working Length
    Screw Type and Placement
  Conventional Plate and Bone Vascularity
  Insufficiencies of Compression Plate
  Relative Stability and Bone Plate
    Accomplishing Relative Stability with
      Conventional Self-Compression Plate
  Minimal Invasive Plate Osteosynthesis
Locked Internal Fixator Plate
  Fixed Angle Plates
  Variable Angle Plates
    Pros and Cons of Fixed and Variable Angle
      Locking Systems
  The Undersurface of a Locked Hole
  Biomechanics of the Locked Bone Plate
    External Fixator vs Locked Internal Fixator Plate
    Effect of Differing Forces on a Locked
      Screw-Plate Construct
      Bending and Axial Load
  Optimized Plate Anchorage with Divergent or
    Convergent Locked Screws
  Unicortical Screw
    Hazards in Unicortical Insertion
  Indications for Use of LIFP
    LIFP in Compression Mode in Accordance
      with the Principle of Absolute Stability
    Lag Screw and Protection Plate
    LIFP in Splinting Mode in Agreement with
      Principle of Relative Stability
    LIFP in Combination of Two Methods
    Combinations of Different Screws
  Contraindications

Advantages
    Limitations
Disadvantages
Far Cortex Locking
    Flexible Fixation
    Load Distribution
    Progressive Stiffness
    Parallel Interfragmentary Motion
Plate Removal
    Removal of LIFP
        Fan Blade Effect
Regional Considerations
    Preshaped Plates
    The Femur
        Subtrochanteric Fracture
        Femoral Shaft
        Distal Femur
        The Condylar Plate
    The Tibia
        Proximal Tibia
        Tibial Locked Internal Fixator Plate
        The Calcaneus
    The Humerus
        The Proximal Humerus
        Shaft of Humerus
        Distal Humerus
            Orthogonal Plating
            Parallel Plating
    The Radius and Ulna
        Fractures of Radial Head
        The Proximal Ulna
        Fractures of Diaphysis of the Radius and the Ulna
        Distal Radius
        Fragment-Specific Implants
        Fluoroscopic Evaluation of Locked Screw Placement
        Distraction Plating for Distal Radius Fracture
    The Hand
    The Clavicle
    The Rib
    Paediatric Applications
        Limb Lengthening and Bone Transport
        Epiphysiodesis

INTRODUCTION

The goal of plate fixation is to restore anatomy and impart mechanical limb stability, ultimately allowing uneventful fracture healing, thereby promoting early joint mobility and return of function.[1]

Bone plates are like internal splints holding together the fractured ends of a bone. These plates are a popular splinting device and are available in all sizes, thicknesses and shapes. The evolution of the shapes and sizes of the plates has taken place over many years, reflecting clinical usage and developments in engineering and material science.

Early in the twentieth century, surgeons such as Lane and Lambote applied plates merely to fix two bone fragments in an approximate alignment. Mechanical failures were frequent owing to the metal reaction as well as to the inadequate design of screws and plates. In 1949, Danis of Belgium was the first surgeon to report the use of interfragmentary compression by applying plates under tension along the longitudinal axis of the bone. The concept was further explored and perfected by Müller and the AO group.

A bone plate has two mechanical functions. It transmits forces from one end of a bone to the other, bypassing and thus protecting the area of fractures. It also holds the fracture ends together while maintaining the proper alignment of the fragments throughout the healing process.

CLASSIFICATION

The names given to bone plates can often be confusing. At times, these refer to the shape of the plate (semitubular or one third tubular plate), or sometimes to the width of the plate (broad or narrow plate). A name may be derived from the shape of the screw holes (round hole plate), from the surface contact characteristics of the plate (low contact) or from the intended site of application (condylar plate).

Regardless of their length, thickness, geometry, configuration or type of holes, all plates may be classified in six groups according to their function.

1. Protection (neutralization) plates
2. Compression plates
3. Buttress plates
4. Tension band plates
5. Bridge plates
6. Condylar plates

Protection (neutralization) Plates

A plate used in combination with a lag screw is a protection (neutralization) plate (Fig. 4.1A), counteracting the torsional, bending and shearing forces that tend to disrupt the screw. The lag screw contributes the interfragmentary compression and the stability. The plate merely protects the lag screw, allowing mobilization of the extremity. In exceptional circumstances, if the geometry of the fracture permits, a neutralization plate can produce compression at the fracture site. The most common clinical application of the protection plate is to shield the screw fixation of an oblique fracture, a long spiral fracture and a butterfly fragment; shelter a mildly comminuted fracture of a long bone, and for the fixation of a segmental bone defect in combination with bone grafting (Fig. 4.1B).

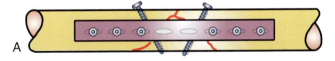

A

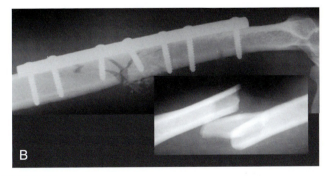

B

FIGURE 4.1

(A) The plate protects the lag screws which contribute the stability.[2]
(B) Radiograph showing protection plate shielding the interfragmentary screw; inset illustrates the butterfly fragment.

Compression Plate

A compression plate produces a locking force across a fracture site to which it is applied. The effect occurs according to Newton's Third Law (action and reaction are equal and opposite). The plate is attached to a bone fragment. It is then pulled across the fracture site by a device, producing tension in the plate. As a reaction to this tension, compression is produced at the fracture site across which the plate is fixed with the screws. The direction of the compression force is parallel to the plate.

Role of Compression

What does a compression plate achieve? Any one or all of the following effects may result:

a. Compaction of the fracture to force together the interdigitating spicules of bone and increase the stability of the construct. It achieves superior fracture immobilization to that obtained with a protection plate alone because it generates axial interfragmental compression
b. Reduction of the space between the bone fragments to decrease the gap to be bridged by the new bone.
c. Protection of the blood supply through enhanced fracture stability.
d. Generate friction, which at the fracture surfaces resists the tendency of the fragments to slide under torsion or shear. This is advantageous as plates are not particularly effective in resisting torsion.
e. Accomplish absolute stability to facilitate primary osteonal contact healing without periosteal new bone formation.

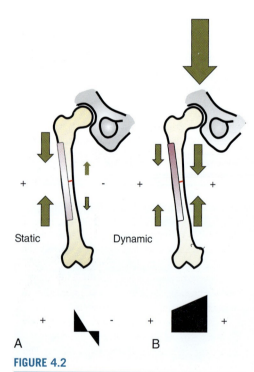

FIGURE 4.2

(A) Compression plating produces static high pressure only on the near cortex. (B) Tension band principle induces higher levels of dynamic compression on the far cortex.[3]

Static and Dynamic Compression

Compression may be static or dynamic. A plate applied under tension produces static compression at a fracture site; this compression constantly exists when the limb is at rest or is functioning. Dynamic compression is a phenomenon by which a plate can transfer or modify functional physiological forces into compressive forces at the fracture site. Fig. 4.2 shows a compression plate on the lateral side of the shaft of the femur exerting static compression both when the limb is at rest and when it is functioning. When functional activity begins, the physiological forces, which are normally destabilizing for a fracture, are converted to a stabilizing and active force by the same plate, which now acts as a tension band. A dynamic compression is thus exerted at the fracture site. With cessation of physiological activity, this dynamic compression force will cease but the static compression force will continue to act.

Methods of Achieving Compression

Compression may be produced by one of following techniques:
1. Self-compressing plate. This is a device that converts the torque (turning force) applied to the

screw head to a longitudinal force that compresses the fractured bone ends. The screws and plates are designed to facilitate this conversion.

As the screw advances in a self-compressing plate it slides down on an inclined plane that is part of the plate's screw hole (Fig. 4.3). The effect is to create a tension force in the plate and compression force across the fracture fragments. One or both ends of a screw hole may be sloped, thus making it possible for compression to be produced in either direction.

2. **Tensioning device.** A special tensioning device can be attached between the bone plate and the adjacent bone cortex (Fig. 4.4A). A bolt is then tightened to pull the plate across the fracture site. This produces tension in the plate and large compressive forces across the fracture. The attachment of the device to the bone necessitates a larger surgical exposure.

Compressor/expander tool is a new device used to compress small fractures; it does not need additional exposure for application (Fig. 4.4B).[6]

In certain situations, for example in a smaller bone, a Verbrugge forceps may be used as a tensioning device. One jaw of the forceps is fixed in the terminal hole of the plate and the other jaw abuts against the specially inserted screw. Closing the jaws produces tension in the plate and compression across the fracture site (Fig. 4.5).

3. **Eccentric screw placement.** Eccentric placement of a screw in a plate hole creates considerable shear stress in the screw. The same force is transmitted to the plate and can occasionally be used to produce interfragmental compression. To achieve this, a semitubular plate is fixed to one fragment by a placement screw. On the opposite side of the fracture, another screw is eccentrically placed in a plate hole (Fig. 4.5B and C). The technique of eccentric screw placement, however, is mechanically inefficient. The screw head is at risk and may break. Eccentric screw placement can be used to simulate a self-compressing plate, but the technique has definite limitations and should not be used as a planned procedure.

4. **Lag screw.** Lag screw efficiently executes compression across a fracture (see page 99).

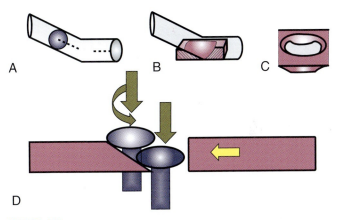

FIGURE 4.3

(A) A ball confined to an inclined cylindrical path slides down and horizontally. **(B)** The screw hole resembles two half cylinders placed at an angle. **(C)** The spherical gliding principle is implemented at both ends of the plate hole, which enables compression in either direction along its longitudinal axis. This geometry of the hole adds more flexibility to the plating technique and eases handling of interfragmental compression of multifragmentary fractures.[4] **(D)** The undersurface of the screw resembles the ball, and sloping wall of the screw hole is analogous to the inclined path. The screw descends as it is inserted by twisting. The slope of the screw hole causes the plate to move at right angles to the direction of descend; the horizontal cylinder (path) facilitates this movement. The plate, which is fixed by placement screws to opposite bone fragment glides and brings the fracture gap under compression.[5]

CHAPTER 4 BONE PLATES

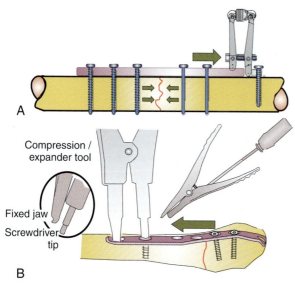

FIGURE 4.4

(**A**) Articulated tension device can produce compression force up to 120 kp.[1] (**B**) Compressor/expander tool.[6] The plate is secured to distal fragment. An eccentrically placed screw, farthest from the fracture is partially inserted in the slotted hole; the driver tip engages the screw hole and jaw of the tool is inserted in the last hole away from the fracture. The tool is squeezed to apply compression; the screw is firmly tightened to maintain the compression.

Tension Band Plate

The function of a tension band is to convert tensile force into compressive force. After fracture reduction the opposite cortex must provide a bony buttress to prevent cyclic bending and failure of fixation.

Buttress Plate

The mechanical function of this plate, as the name suggests, is to strengthen (buttress) a weakened area of cortex. The plate prevents the bone from collapsing during the healing process. It is usually designed with a large surface area to facilitate wider distribution of the load.

A cancellous lag screw has conventionally been used to produce compression forces across the cancellous surfaces of fractures passing through the wide metaphyseal–epiphyseal ends of the long bones. This fixation, however, is insufficient to resist the axial loading forces that are applied to joint surfaces during weight bearing and other muscular activities. To prevent shearing at the fracture site, or displacement of the fracture fragments bringing about widening of the articular surface, it is necessary to apply a plate that extends from the diaphysis across the outer surface of the metaphyseal–epiphyseal fragment. Such a plate acts as a buttress or retaining wall. A buttress plate applies a force to the bone which is perpendicular (normal) to the flat surface of the plate.

A buttress plate must be firmly anchored to the main fragment. It must fit the underlying bone cortex snugly, or the deformity could recur. A buttress plate should first be contoured accurately to the segment of bone. The fixation to the bone should begin in the middle of the plate, i.e. closest to the fracture site on the shaft. The screws should then be applied in an orderly fashion; screw insertion in buttress mode implants begins in the area of greatest potential motion and moves away in both directions towards both ends of the plate.

A buttress plate is used to maintain the bone length or to support the depressed fracture fragments. It is commonly used in fixing epiphyseal and metaphyseal fractures. A representative clinical example of a buttress plate is the T-plate used for the fixation of fractures of the distal radius and the tibial plateau (Fig. 4.6). A buttress plate is also used to fix fractures of the tibial pilon and the distal humerus. A special application of the buttress plate is termed 'anti-glide plating' (Fig. 4.7).

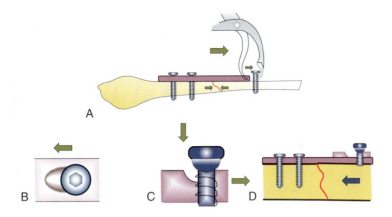

FIGURE 4.5

Other methods of producing compression across the fracture. (**A**) Verbruge clamp used to tension a small bone plate.[7] (**B**) Eccentric screw placement in an oval hole of semitubular plate. (**C**) The hemispherical geometry of the undersurface of the screw helps plate movement and induces compression of the fracture.[8] (**D**) Application of the technique to generate compression across the fracture line.

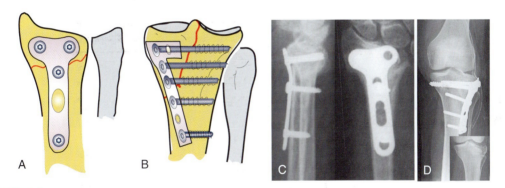

FIGURE 4.6

(**A**) Buttress plate for the distal radius fracture or (**B**) tibial plateau fracture.[9] Radiographs illustrating buttress plate application. (**C**) Lateral and anteroposterior view of distal radius. A locking plate is applied to support the fracture. (**D**) A conventional T plate buttresses the fracture against the vertical shear forces; Inset: Injury radiograph showing the fracture of the lateral condyle before treatment.

In this mode a one-third tubular plate is so applied as to prevent the displacement of the tip of an oblique fracture of the distal fibula (Fig. 4.7E–H). In tibial injuries bone void is often encountered which needs to be filled with bone graft and bone substitutes to prevent secondary loss of fixation.

Bridge Plate

A neutralization plate acts as a 'bridge'. It transmits various forces from one end of the bone to the other, bypassing the area of the fracture. Its main function is to act as a mechanical link between the

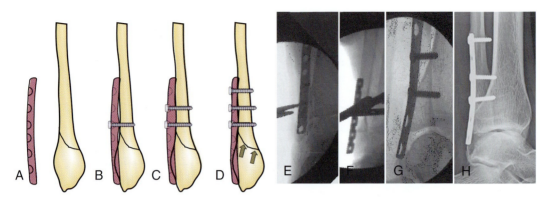

FIGURE 4.7

Anti-glide plate. **(A–C)** One-third tubular plate is placed on posterior surface and fixed only to the proximal main stable fragment of fibula. **(D)** The plate supports the distal fragment and prevents its displacement. Note that there is no screw inserted in the distal fragment.[10] Illustrative radiographs for application of one-third tubular plate on the posterior surface to buttress the fracture of lateral malleolus **(E)** posterior placement of the plate. **(F)** Application of the first screw just proximal to fracture line applies reductive pressure on the distal fragment. **(G)** More screws applied on the proximal fragment. **(H)** Screw in the distal fragment is unnecessary.

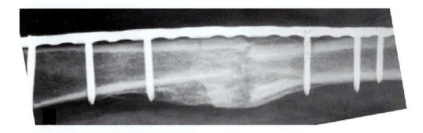

FIGURE 4.8

Radiograph illustrating a bridge plate application. Forces are transmitted from one end to other; there is no compression at the fracture site.

healthy segments of bone above and below the fracture. Such a plate does not produce any compression at the fracture site (Fig. 4.8).

Condylar Plate

The condylar plate differs from the plates described above because of its distinct mechanical function. As shown in Fig. 4.9, its main application has been in the treatment of intra-articular distal femoral fractures. It has two mechanical functions. It maintains the reduction of the major intra-articular fragments, hence restoring the anatomy of the joint surface. It also rigidly fixes the metaphyseal components to the diaphyseal shaft, permitting early movement of the extremity. This plate functions both as a neutralization plate and as a buttress plate. Since the plate can be attached to a tensioning device and has specially designed screw holes, it also functions as a compression plate.

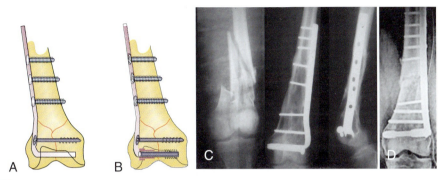

FIGURE 4.9

(**A**) The condylar plate (95° angled blade plate) maintains the reduction of intra-articular fragments and fixes the metaphysis to the shaft assisting early joint movement.[9] (**B**) A condylar compression screw (CCS) works on the same principles and is regarded as a superior innovation both technically and mechanically even in porotic bones.[11] Radiographs showing fixation of distal third of femur by (**C**) 95° condylar plate (**D**) condylar compression screw.

A 95° condylar plate is used to fix a proximal femoral osteotomy, four-fragment proximal femur fracture and an intercondylar fracture of the femur. It is also used for fixation of trochanteric fractures with lateral wall explosion, in subtrochanteric fractures and in those events where the fracture lines are going into the piriform fossa, because both sliding hip screw and cephalomedullary nail are then contraindicated.

In biomechanical terms these fractures frequently have short periarticular segments and long working length because of frequent metaphyseal comminution as well as absence of bony support on the medial side. The fixed angle of the plate overcomes the coronal plane instability and prevents consequent collapse. Special instrumentation is required for the application of a condylar plate. Its use is diminishing with the advent of the 'condylar screw', which is relatively easy to apply (Fig. 4.9C and D).

GENERAL PRINCIPLES OF PLATE FIXATION

Successful use of a bone plate depends on the properties of the plate, the screws, the bone and on the correct application of biomechanical principles.

Plate-Related Factors

The strength of a plate depends on its cross-section; thickness is the most important contributing factor. The strength varies with the cube of the thickness. The plate should be made from a material of adequate strength and its stiffness should be close to that of the bone. The stiffness of titanium is closer to that of bone, whereas stainless steel is stiffer than titanium. Very stiff plates can weaken the bone after fracture healing is complete. The contact surface of the plate is also a significant factor. The surface like the first generation of compression plate causes reduction of blood supply under the plate, leading to immediate post-fixation osteoporosis.

In the current design featuring reduced contact self-compressing plate to minimize bone-plate contact surface, substantial material is removed between the holes from the undersurface of the plate, giving it an arched appearance (Fig. 4.10). A conventional bone plate is weak at the screw holes. The excavation reduces the stiffness of the plate to the same level as of the screw hole area. The plate with this design now has uniform stiffness in both the areas. Such a plate can be bent in a continuous curvature with a good fit of the screw head in the plate hole and yet preserve the mechanical features that evenly distribute bending and torsional stresses over a long distance along the plate. The plate's fatigue life is prolonged as its holes are protected from localized high stresses. The plate holes are symmetrical, are evenly distributed along the plate and have oblique undercuts on the lower side of the plate. This undercut allows unhindered inclination of a lag screw up to 40° longitudinally, and 7° in the transverse plane, in both directions through the plate (Fig. 4.10E–G).

Use of a shaft screw as a lag screw through the plate in place of a fully threaded cortical screw gives superior static compression force. Plate holes are evenly dispersed along the plate length. This arrangement facilitates late shifting of the plate's position or using a longer one and still be able to use the same drill holes for fixation.

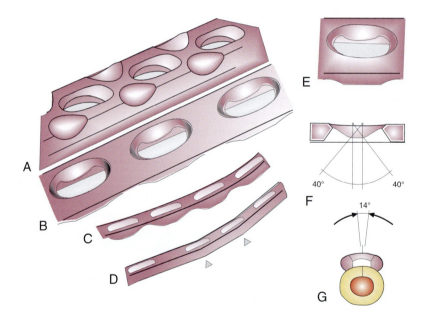

FIGURE 4.10

(A) The scalloped undersurface reduces the bone contact surface of the reduced contact self-compressing plate. (B) The surface of plate has evenly spaced holes. (C) When contoured to fit the bone surface, it forms smooth bends in contrasts to (D) a conventional self-compressing plate that tends to deform within the plate holes and bends producing kinks (arrows).[12] (E) Modified screw hole has contours on either side that allow gliding of the screw head and inclination of the screw in two directions and compression can be achieved in either longitudinal direction. (F) The oblique undercuts on the lower side of the plate as seen in the longitudinal section ensure that the screw threads have no contact with plate. The lag screw can be inclined up to 40° in longitudinal plane and (G) 7° in the transverse plane in both directions without impinging on the plate.[12]

The length of the plate is another important factor that affects the pattern of fracture healing. Too short a plate may make a construct unstable, while application of a very long plate may cause unnecessary damage to the soft tissue, when principles of minimal invasive plate osteosynthesis (MIPO) are deserted.

Screw-Related Factors

The screws fasten a plate to the bone. The effectiveness of a screw greatly depends on the design of its threads and its head. Well-designed threads are easy to insert and hold well in all circumstances. A well-designed slot for the placement of a screwdriver ensures ease of screw insertion. An adequate number of screws is essential to hold the plate. A minimum of two in each fragment are necessary to prevent rotation. The total number of screws needed for a fixation depends on the site and type of fracture. The ratio of the pilot hole to depth of the screw thread is crucial; the holding power of the screw depends on this ratio. Strength of the plate fixation depends in turn on the holding power of the screws. The screws should be made of strong material that can withstand heavy loads. Screws and plate should be of the same material to minimize corrosion.

The success of bone-plate fixation depends on the following:

- Plate thickness, dimensions, geometry, material used
- Screw design, material, number and hold in the bone
- Bone – mechanical properties and the health of the bone
- Construct – placement of plate and direction of load
- Compression between the fragments.

Bone-Related Factors

The health of the bone is a factor, which is usually overlooked while fixing a fracture. A young bone is dense in consistency and a screw holds well in such a bone. As the holding power of a screw is dependent on the elastic force provided by the bone, it is obvious that the denser the bone, the stronger the hold. In the elderly, the bone is porotic, being less dense than in the young. The holding elasticity of porotic bone is of a lower magnitude and leads to inferior screw hold. Thus, the health and mechanical properties of the bone are of importance in this context.

The interaction of the bone and the plate is important, since the two are combined in a composite structure that becomes a crucial entity in the strength of a fixation. The strength of a plate-bone construct is its ability to withstand load without structural failure. This entity can be described as a bending strength or a torsional strength, depending on the load application. A bone plate is a load-sharing device. Loads can be transmitted between plate and bone through the screws and through friction-type forces between the plate surface and the bone. Some of the load is supported by the plate and some load passes between the bone fragments. The reconstructed bone must support a certain load.

Construct-Related Factors

A plate may be applied to a bone in various positions. The strength of the construct will depend on the direction of the load and the position of the plate (see Fig. 4.15).

118   CHAPTER 4   BONE PLATES

The plate is applied on the side of the bone which is under compression during bending (Fig. 4.11A). The bending forces are acting in the direction of the plate. The effect of loading is to open up the fracture; this situation is also referred to as the 'bending open' configuration. This is an example of a weak construct. Let us assume its strength to be 1, and compare it with another construct in the Fig. 4.11B, which shows a satisfactory situation.

Here the plate is applied on the side of the bone that would come under tension during bending. The bending forces are active in the opposite direction of the plate. The fracture surfaces are closely apposed. This is a strong construct; 200 times stronger than the previous construct, and represents a 'bending close' configuration.

In another variation, the plate may be applied at right angles to that in the above situation (Fig. 4.11C). The construct is weaker than that in Fig. 4.11B but it is still 60 times stronger than that in Fig. 4.11A.

The plate-bone construct becomes strongest when two plates are applied at right angles to each other (Fig. 4.11D). The ensuing construct is 235 times stronger than the example in Fig. 4.11A. Such an arrangement works well when the bone apposition is poor or a gap is present.

Effect of Compression

Compression will increase rigidity in all these cases by ensuring closer contact and increase in friction between the bone ends. An attempt should always be made to apply a plate on the tension side of the bone and under compression to achieve good bone apposition.

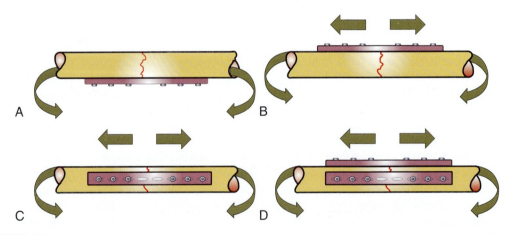

FIGURE 4.11

Plate application to well apposed transverse fracture. (**A**) This is a weak construct. The plate is located on the compression side of the bone.[8] (**B**) The plate is located on tension side and load is shared by the plate-bone construct. The fracture is compressed during physiological activities.[8] (**C**) The screws here are subjected to bending and rotational forces and may fail under the load.[13] (**D**) Double plating provides the strongest fixation regardless of the direction of applied force.[8]

GENERAL PRINCIPLES OF PLATE FIXATION

The strength of the reconstructed bone depends on the following:

1. Strength of the plate and screw – design, dimension, material and purchase
2. Configuration of the fracture – comminution and placement of the plate
3. Properties of the plate-bone construct – working length and load sharing

In a bone-plate construct, each component plays its part. A broken bone needs to be held together if it has to support the load of the limb. The plate holds the ends together, but on its own cannot support the load of the limb indefinitely. If it does so, it may break due to repeated overloading. The plate will endure only if the bone shares some of the load of physiological activity. Thus, a plate is a load-sharing device and not a load-bearing device.

Despite the strength and rigidity of a plate-bone construct, problems remain, and some may crop up. Whenever a gap exists between the bone ends (Fig. 4.12A), a plate will first bend under the load

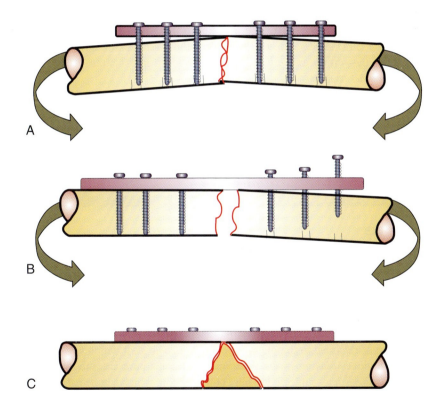

FIGURE 4.12

Plate application when bone contact is less than perfect. **(A)** If there is a gap between the bone ends the plate may bend or the screw may loosen till the bone fragments make a contact. Occasionally, if bone resorption occurs, such a situation may develop following a perfect reduction.[14] **(B)** If the plate is not tightly fastened to the bone, bending stresses occur on the screws.[13] **(C)** The plate will fail! The ruinous event may be averted either by reconstructing the bone cross-section to create an integrated bone-plate unit or by providing an external support.

until the bone fragments make contact. The load would be shared by the plate and the bone once the contact is made, but until that time it is the plate that bears all the load.

When a plate is not tightly set against the bone by the screws (Fig. 4.12B), the screws are subjected to bending forces.

The presence of a butterfly fragment or a more extensive comminution in the bone provides the worst instance (Fig. 4.12C). The bone does not support any load. All the load falls on the plate, resulting in high bending forces on the metal. The plate or the screws may break: this eventuality can be salvaged by achieving a near-perfect reduction of the butterfly fragment to create a unified plate-bone unit. Such a unit will then share the load. Another way to reduce the forces in a plate is to deploy a longer plate or provide an additional external support.

In fixation of spiral fractures, bending and rotational forces should be considered (Fig. 4.13). These fractures occur as a result of torsional forces; the fracture line follows a helical path. A plate placed at right angles to the fracture line counteracts the rotational forces effectively but fails to resist the bending forces (Fig. 4.13A and B).

When a plate is placed along the shaft, i.e. parallel to the bone, it efficiently resists bending but not the torsional force (Fig. 4.13C and D). In practice, the torsional strength of a plate depends on the holding power of the screws as well as on the frictional forces acting between the bone ends; compression increases the friction.

A spiral fracture can be stabilized by two methods (Fig. 4.13E and F). The first necessitates the use of a long plate to hold the bone beyond the fracture line. The second method utilizes a lag screw to achieve interfragmentary compression and a plate to protect this fixation from the disruptive forces. This method is more effective and is therefore preferred.

ADDITIONAL PRINCIPLES OF PLATE FIXATION

Tension Band Plate

The engineering principle of the tension band is widely used in fracture fixation. It applies to the conversion of tensile forces to compression forces on the convex side of an eccentrically loaded bone. In a femoral mid-diaphyseal fracture, axial load opens up the lateral cortex and angulates the distal fragment into varus (Fig. 4.14). This unstable fracture can be stabilized by the application of a plate as a tension band.

When a plate is applied as a tension band on the lateral (tension) side of the bone the neutral axis shifts from the centre of the bone to the plate-bone junction. The shift denotes restoration of stability. Any axial loading produces tension in the plate and distributes pure compression forces across the fracture line. The fracture is now subjected to pure compression, which can be called a stable situation. The plate and the bone share the load.

When a plate is applied on the medial side (i.e. compression side) of the femur, the axial load tends to open up the fracture, leaving the load to be borne by the plate alone. This is a considerably less stable plan of fixation. The plate is likely to fatigue, bend and fail.

Another argument for placing a plate on the tension side of a bone is its effect on the working length of the plate. The working length is the distance between the two points on either side of the fracture where the plate is firmly fixed to the bone. Working length does not necessarily correspond to the total

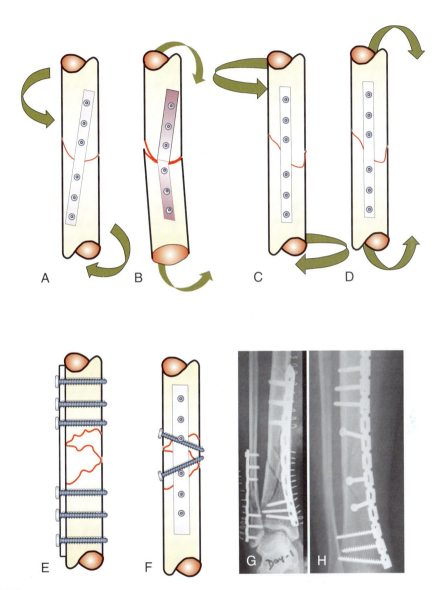

FIGURE 4.13

When a plate is placed at right angle to the fracture line it (**A**) resists torsion adequately (**B**) but bends poorly. When the plate is placed parallel to the bone it resists (**C**) bending reasonably well (**D**) but counteracts torsion poorly. (**E**) A long plate or (**F**) interfragmentary screw and neutralization plate can effectively stabilize a spiral fracture.[13] Radiographs showing stabilization of a spiral fracture of the tibia with (**G**) only A long plate (**H**) by interfragmentary screws and a protection plate.

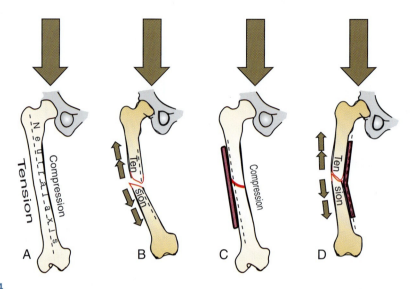

FIGURE 4.14

Tension band principle. **(A)** Forces on intact bone. **(B)** No fixation – unstable. **(C)** Tension band plate – stable. **(D)** Plate on compression side of bone – less stable.[9]

length of the plate but rather is a portion of the total length. Short working length increases the rigidity and strength of a construct and is ideal. The greater the working length of a plate, the lesser is its resistance to bending.

When a plate is applied as a tension band in the bending close construct, the working length (for bending) of the plate is minimal, since it is in contact with bone on either side of the fracture (Fig. 4.15).

The plated bone is particularly weak under loads that tend to bend open the fracture. The working length of a plate is greater in the bending open construct. The outer screws bear the highest stresses as the direction of the load is towards the plate.

When applying a tension band plate, it is important that the cortices on the opposite side should be intact. If there is any gap or defect in the opposite cortex, the plate may be subjected to bending rather than pure tension loads and may rapidly fatigue and break. A plate applied on the tension side of a bone produces a fixation, which is 200 times stronger than one on the compression side.

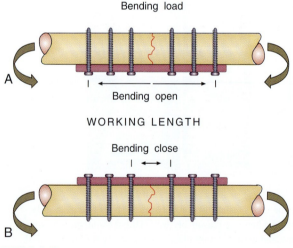

FIGURE 4.15

The relationship of working length with bending configurations for a plated fracture.[14] **(A)** Bending open construct is weak as it has a long working length. **(B)** Bending close construct is strong due its shorter working length.

ADDITIONAL PRINCIPLES OF PLATE FIXATION

The recommended site for placing a bone plate in the femur is anterolateral. In the tibia the 'tension' side varies from fracture to fracture. The subcutaneous surface of the tibia is a highly accessible and suitable site for a plate in many fractures, even though it is not the tension side of the bone under normal weight-bearing conditions. A plate can also be applied to the lateral surface of the tibia; in the humerus dorsal surface is the tension side and is choice location for plating. Deltoid insertion limits its proximal placement; often it is then applied on the anterolateral side. In the forearm, plates are usually applied on the subcutaneous borders of the ulna and the dorsal surface of the radius.

Prebending of Plate

When a straight bone plate is applied to a straight bone surface under static compression, the near cortex is brought under compression but the far cortex opens up (Fig. 4.16). This gap may result in micro movements with subsequent bone resorption and loss of fixation. If a plate is bent sharply opposite the fracture site before application, it first brings the far cortex under compression and then the near cortex. The prebent plate results in more uniform compressive contact across the fracture site without gaping than is achievable with a straight plate (Fig. 4.17). Radiographs in the figure illustrate this observable fact. Incidentally, Bagby and Janes had proposed plate over-bending as early as 1958.

When a prebent plate is applied to a bone, the screws closest to the fracture should be fixed first and then the next one farther away from the fracture site. When the farthermost screws are applied first, the near-cortex opens up as the inner screws are inserted; the plate is then comparatively longer than the bone to be fixed.

Prebending can be used only when dealing with a simple, two-fragment fracture. In a comminuted fracture, prebending will often jeopardize the reduction.

When fixing a straight plate to a curved surface, the outer screws should be applied first. This limits the length of the bone. Tightening of the screws from outside towards the fracture bends the plate, shortens the distance between the outer screws and thereby compresses the fracture (Fig. 4.18).

Application of a lag screw to an over-bent or contoured plate reduces strain on the plate surface. A straight plate is subjected to higher degrees of bending and torsional forces when it is applied without a lag screw or without following tenets of tension banding. The stability is best with the contoured plate and interfragmentary lag screw, followed by an over-bent plate and a lag screw (Fig. 4.19A and B). Moreover,

Prerequisites of tension band fixation

- Bone which is eccentrically loaded and is able to withstand compression
- An intact buttress of the opposite cortex
- A strong plate to withstand the tensile forces
- Plate placement on the tension side of the bone

'A bone plate will act as a tension band only if it is applied to the tension side of a bone'

Prebending plates

- Contour to fit the bone surface snugly
- Make a sharp bend opposite the fracture site; midsection is elevated
- Fix to the bone, starting on either side of the fracture and then moving outwards
- Plate then compresses the far cortex also
- Apply this technique only to two-fragment fractures

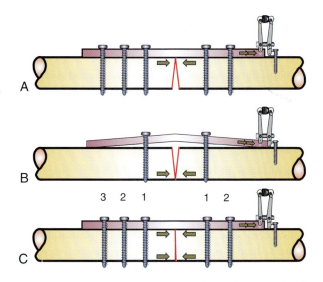

FIGURE 4.16

Application of static compression using a plate. **(A)** Application of tension to a straight plate results in compression only at the cortex immediately under the plate. A small gap appears at the opposite cortex. Cyclical closure of this gap under loading will result in repetitive bending stress to the plate. **(B)** Prebending of the plate results in initial compression at the cortex opposite the plate when the tension device is applied. **(C)** Continued tightening of the tension device on this prebent plate results in uniform compression across the fracture site without a gap.[2]

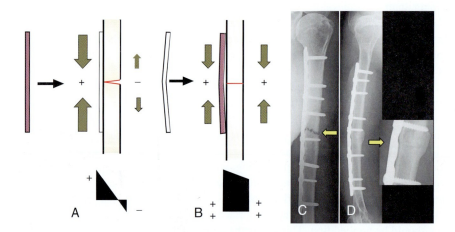

FIGURE 4.17

Pressure distribution in the fracture gap. **(A)** Application of a straight plate to a straight bone. The compression develops only over the near cortex and the far cortex opens up. **(B)** A prebent plate under compression produces high compressive force on both the cortices and firmly apposes them.[3] Radiographs presenting the effect of plate bending on fixation. **(C)** Application of a straight plate to compress a fracture; a gap is develops at the opposite cortex. **(D)** Bending of the plate before application results in uniform compression at the cortex opposite the plate. Inset shows abundant callus formation.

interfragmentary lag screw clearly reduces corrosion. Corrosion is proportional to the gliding distance in the contact zone and more marked with over-bent plate than for the contoured plate.

Plate Fixation of Oblique Long Bone Fractures

The bone fragments of an oblique fracture have a tendency to slip over each other. The greater the obliquity, the higher the shear forces and the greater the tendency of the fragments to slide over one another. The plate should be applied to function as a buttress plate and a compression plate. If a plate is fixed to the fragment that forms an acute angle with the fracture, then, as axial compression is generated the fragment is displaced and the reduction is lost. On the other hand, if the plate is fixed to the fragment that forms an obtuse angle with the fracture, then, as axial compression is generated, the spike of the opposite fragment is driven against the plate. As a result, displacement is prevented and axial compression is achieved. This is illustrated in Fig. 4.19C and D.

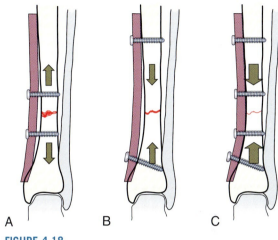

FIGURE 4.18

Application of a straight plate to a curved bone. **(A)** If the middle screws are applied first, the fracture gap opens up as the plate bends to come close to the bone. **(B)** Insertion of end screws effectively shortens the plate. **(C)** As the middle screws are applied, the fracture is compressed.[15]

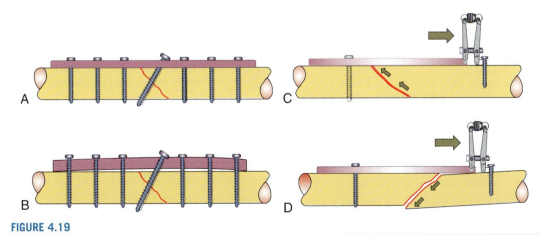

FIGURE 4.19

(A) Contoured plate and interfragmentary lag screw provides best stability, **(B)** followed by over-bent plate and lag screw.[16] **(C)** Placement of the plate over the tip of an oblique fragment before compressing prevents sliding of the fragments. **(D)** Failure to do so may cause overriding of the fragments.[9]

Double Plating

Double plating of a bone is usually not required. Exceptions include difficult non-union, a situation when the bone quality is less than optimal. Double plating may also be called for in a fracture configuration where solid bone contact on the cortex opposite the plate is impossible. The second plate should always be smaller, both in size and length, than the major fixation plate, as two plates of a similar length act as severe stress risers at their ends. Typically, double plating is used to fix subtrochanteric and supracondylar fractures of the femur.

Plate Bending

Plate bending and twisting is a skill that is often required. Special instruments such as a bending press, bending pliers and bending irons are needed to contour the plate to the curves of a bone. Malleable aluminium templates are useful aids. These are easy to mould to copy the bone curves and serve as a model for plate bending and checking the outcome.

Bending is more accurate and effective if an assistant holds the plate while the surgeon bends the plate. A plate should be bent between the screw holes. Bending in small increments avoids over-bending. Reverse bending of a plate substantially weakens it and is not recommended. Kinking of the plate is to be avoided.

Biomechanics of a Conventional Bone Plate

The stability and mechanical strength of the intact limb rely on stresses shared by muscle and bone. Applied to a fractured bone, a plate acts as a load carrier from one fragment to the other and assists the bone in mechanical function. The mechanical loads on the plate recede as bone healing proceeds. To achieve fracture stability, the axial, torsional and three-point bending forces must be neutralized (Fig. 4.20).

Conventional plating techniques are designed to provide absolute stability. Absolute stability requires anatomic reduction and compression of the fracture. Precise anatomic reduction and interfragmentary compression using a plate in compression mode is an established and leading method of fracture management. The fracture area is approached though extensive incisions to ensure good exposure necessary for accurate reduction and plate stabilization. The plate is contoured to snugly fit the anatomy and is secured to the bone with screws that achieve both, interfragmentary compression and firm fixation. In a bone fixed in compression, the structural function of the bone is maintained, i.e. the major part of the biomechanical load is taken over by the bone. The plate is not the main load-carrying element. The function of a compression plate in this situation is to maintain the reduction and to apply the interfragmentary compression.

Indications for compression plating
- Simple fractures of the diaphysis and metaphysis
- simple transverse or oblique fractures (compression plating or protection plating
- In combination with a lag screw or tension-band plate)
- Intra-articular fractures (buttress plate)
- Delayed union or nonunion
- Closed-wedge osteotomies

ADDITIONAL PRINCIPLES OF PLATE FIXATION

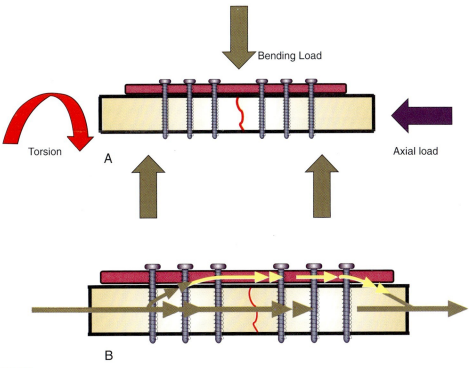

FIGURE 4.20

(A) The three forces that must be overcome by a plate and every other method of fracture fixation: axial, torsional and bending loads.[17] **(B)** Load transfer from bone to conventional plate and cortex screw construct (splint). Bone bears the load to greater extent than the plate.

Effect of Forces on a Conventional Plate Screw Construct
Bending and Axial Load

A conventional plate is fastened to a bone by inserting screws. As a screw is tightened against the plate, it generates a compressive force between the plate and the bone. A reactionary friction force develops that is equal to the compressive force and acts in the opposite direction. These opposing forces bestow stability on the plate. The stabilized bone-plate complex serves to bear load from one fragment to other helping bone carry on its mechanical function. Mechanically every plate works as a splint. Load transfer from bone to conventional plate occurs by friction. The bone and the conventional plate share the load though not in equal measure (Fig. 4.20B).

A well-fixed conventional plate resists external forces such as axial, torsional and bending loads. When loaded axially, either in compression or in tension, the applied force is converted to a shear stress at the plate-bone interface. This external axial force is countered by frictional force between the plate and bone (Fig 4.21A).

In fastening a plate to a bone, the screw with the greatest torque contributes the most amount of force perpendicular (normal) to the plate and therefore bears the utmost load. When axial load is higher

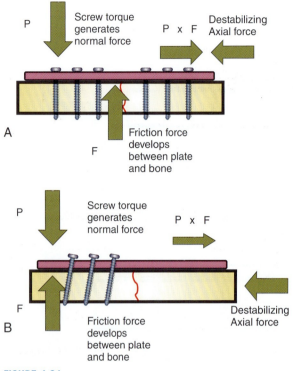

FIGURE 4.21

(A) Compression of the conventional plate to the bone creates a friction fit to hold them together. The construct requires bicortical screws to stabilize the fragment to the plate. A plate can resist an axial force that is equal to a force perpendicular to the plate generated by screw torque marked 'P' times the coefficient of friction between the plate and the bone marked 'F'. (B) Conventional plating is unable to prevent the screws from orienting parallel to the direction of a larger applied force within the plate. Fixation strength is equal to holding power of the screws; holding power is defined as bone shear stress times the area of bone within the screw threads.

than frictional force between the bone and the plate, the strength of fixation depends on the axial stiffness of a single screw; depending on the site of load application this screw may be the one closest to or farthest away from the fracture site. The conventional screws orient themselves parallel to the direction of the destabilizing axial force (Fig. 4.21B).

A conventional plate applied to a normal cortical bone with 3.5-mm cortical screws can resist a load greater than 1200 N. Normal cortical bone has a compressive strength of higher than 1200 N but diminishes in presence of comminution and osteoporosis. A plate-bone construct is strong enough to support the bone and its healing process when the frictional force between the plate and bone and the axial stiffness of the screw and that of the bone is superior to the destabilizing axial loads on the construct. A plate applied in compression mode is contoured to fit the local anatomy. Screws fix the plate and bone fragments together to eliminate any movement between them. When there is no movement between the bone, the plate and the screws, a fixed angle construct is created. If the construct loosens the axial stiffness offered by the screw and the plate is lost, then the bone provides the required axial screw control. If the cortical bone in the screw holes fails to resist the axial loads, the bone may either fail in compression or get absorbed leading to screw loosening (Fig. 4.22). The construct may loose its strength, causing instability at the fracture site and interruption of bone healing process.

In a plate-screw construct fixed on the tension side of a bone and subjected to bending loads, maximum stresses are generated at the screws placed farthest from the fracture (Fig. 4.23).

State of affairs takes a turnaround when the plate is applied on the compression side of the bone; shear stresses are highest on the screws that are closest to the fracture line. In this situation the fixation strength of a conventional plate is equivalent to the resistance to shear stress offered by the bone trapped in the screw threads; the site of maximum hold changes with site of load application; depending on the loading site it may vary between the screws closest to the fracture line to the ones farthest

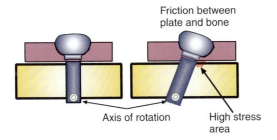

FIGURE 4.22

When axial load exceeds friction force, the conventional screw rotates about the far cortex, generating high stresses at the cortex nearest the plate.

from it. A conventional plate fails because it is unable to check the screws from aligning with the direction of the applied load. The shear resistance at bone-screw interface is the feeble link in conventional plating. The product of stress resistance of the bone times the contact area between the bone and the screw is the magnitude of force necessary to move a screw through a bone. Likewise, the force to failure is the product of force required to surmount the shear stress of bone multiplied by the surface area between a single screw and the bone. The screws show a domino effect in failure, one following other (Fig. 4.24).

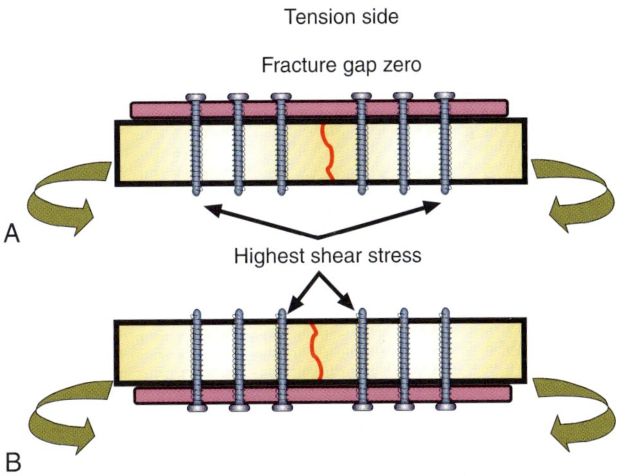

Under bending forces the screw-plate assembly loosens and ultimately fails when loads increase. A failure in bending is due to damaging action of the shear force larger than the strength of the cortical bone which causes bone absorption and screw loosening; the fracture site becomes mobile, leads to instability, disruption of healing process and ultimate failure. The susceptible link 'screw-bone interface' fails under severe shear stresses.

FIGURE 4.23

Location of highest shear stresses changes with position of the plate. **(A)** The screws farthest from the fracture line face the highest shear stresses when the plate is placed on the tension side of the bone. **(B)** The screws closest to the fracture site bear the highest shear stresses when the plate is located on the compression side.

Torsional Load

The torsional stability of a construct is more dependent on the number of screws rather than type of the screw – conventional or locked (Fig. 4.25). Four or more screws in each fragment offer optimum stability as long as the holes closest and farthest to the fracture line are filled. The positions of third and subsequent screws are inconsequential. Given this, a slight motion is possible between the screw head and the plate in the conventional plating. The range of motion depends on the torque used to place the screw, the size of the screw head, the design of the plate, and material the conventional screw is made of.

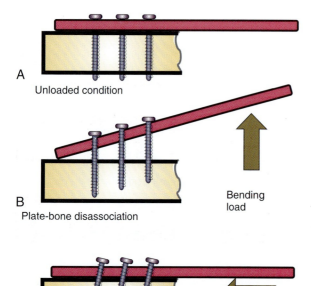

FIGURE 4.24

Effects of bending and axial loads on conventional plate screw construct. **(A)** plate-screw-bone construct of conventional screw and plate. **(B)** Bending load applied to construct. The plate on the compression side stresses the screw closest to the fracture site first with sequential screw toggle, pull-out and subsequent failure of the other screws. **(C)** A conventional screw rotates orienting parallel to the applied load. Fixation strength of a conventional screw is equal to bone shear stress times the area of bone within the screw threads.[18]

Load-Sharing and Load Bearing Constructs

Conventional screw-plate construct is a 'load-sharing beam construct'. Load-sharing construct is one where motion takes place between individual components of the beam. Smith-Peterson pin-plate (S-P Pin) is a load-sharing beam construct (Fig. 4.26).

In a 'single-beam construct', there is no motion between the components of the beam. It is also known as angle stable implant; 95° condylar blade plate and a Jewett nail for hip fracture are examples of angle stable implants (see Fig. 4.44). Single-beam construct is four times stronger than load-sharing construct. A conventional plate performs as single-beam construct only in ideal circumstances, such as good bone that permits screw torques greater than 3 Nm; sufficient coefficient of friction between the plate and physiological loads less than 200 N.

Plate Length and Screw Density

A plate must be sufficiently long and strong, and should be fixed with screws engaging an adequate number of cortices to provide rigid fixation for successful treatment of a fracture. This number of cortices to be engaged depends on the individual bone, the degree of stability, i.e. relative or absolute, desired, the type of plating, bone quality, fracture comminution, length of the plate and the anticipated forces exerting on the fixation. Fig. 4.27 exemplifies the method of numbering the cortices.

What is an appropriate length of a plate? Optimal conditions of splinting depend on the length of the lever provided by the plate on each side of the fracture site. Plate length is determined by the mechanical requirement of a particular fracture. In principle, low loading of the plate and screws avoids fatigue failure of the plate due to cyclic loading, or screw pull-out due to excessive single overloading.

Forces Acting on the Plate-Screw Interface

The placement and number of screws affect the function of a plate construct. More screws do not necessarily equate to more stability. When fewer screws are inserted at select site, the plate leverage increases, which in turn decreases the load on each screw. A plate is often subjected to bending moment, which is a product of a force and the distance. The force can be altered by changing the length or leverage; the longer the plate, the smaller the pull-out force acting on the screws (Fig. 4.28). The change is purely due to improvement of the plate leverage acting on the screws.

Longer plates reduce the stress in the plate as well as to the screws (Fig. 4.29). From the mechanical point of view, it is therefore better to use very long plates. Long plates inserted under MIPO guidelines cause minimal damage to soft tissues.

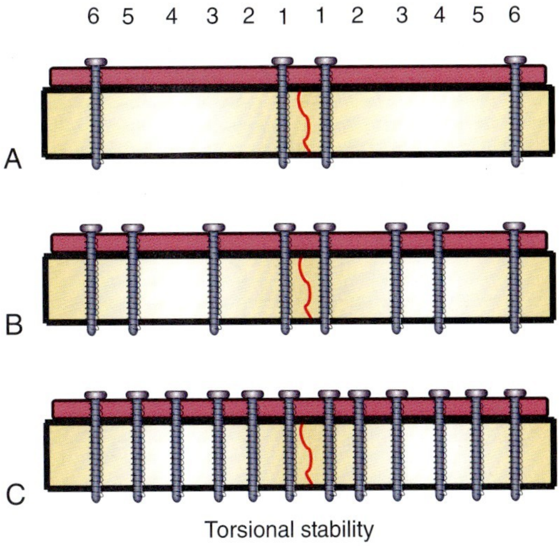

Length of a Plate

The choice of length of a plate is the key element in the fracture fixation stability provided by the construct and varies according to fracture pattern. The plate size, plate alignment and screw placement are important concerns for success of fixation, and the correct application of plating depends on many variables such as bone quality, bone geometry and soft-tissue damage.

Plate Length and Plate Working Length

In initial days of compression plating, it was a common practice to keep the plate length short to prevent soft-tissue damage from a large incision; however, the opposite is true in current practice as a long plate is usually applied by the smallest possible surgical incision to preserve the blood supply to the bone and adjacent soft tissues. The actual plate length depends upon the fracture pattern and the treatment principle to be made use of for a particular fracture. To treat a multiple fragment fracture, relative stability is desirable and a flexible splinting without compression is the method of choice. This situation needs a plate 2 or 3 times longer than the fracture length. The same calculation will apply to treat a simple fracture without compression. A simple transverse fracture is of short length and is treated with compression. The plate length should be 8–10 times longer than the fracture length. Thus, the plate length is based on the intended biomechanical behaviour at the fracture site. Plate span ratio and plate screw density influence level of stability at the fracture site.[20] Plate span width is determined by the quotient of plate length and fracture length (Fig. 4.30). It is recommended that the plate span width- the length of a bone plate should be 2–3 times the length of a comminuted fracture and more than 8–10 times the length of a simple fracture (Fig. 4.31).

It is known that a shorter plate with an equal number of screws caused a reduction in axial stiffness but not in torsional rigidity[22]; therefore, long plates should be used to optimize axial stability. The torsional rigidity of a construct is not compromised by change in the plate length.

Removal of screws nearest to the fracture site increases plate's working length, reduces its plastic deformation and its enhanced flexibility is tolerated by the construct (Fig. 4.32). The working length, i.e. the distance between the two screws closest to the fracture on either side of the fracture determines the elasticity of the fracture fixation and distribution of induced deformation caused by external load, a factor more important for durability of the plate.

FIGURE 4.25

(A) Screw insertion in the hole closest to and farthest from the fracture is important for torsional stability. (B) Four screws are essential for optimum torsional stability; locations of third and fourth screw are irrelevant. (C) More than four screws are inconsequential for torsional stability.

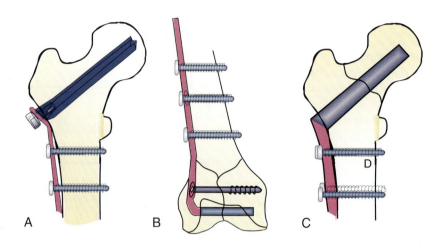

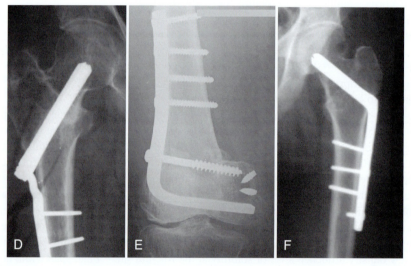

FIGURE 4.26

(**A**) Smith Peterson pin plate is a load-sharing implant. Its components are mobile and not fixed. (**B**) 95° angled blade plate and (**C**) Jewett hip nail are examples of angle stable implants; there are no movable components of these implants. Radiographs showing clinical use of these implants (**D**) S-P pin plate has moveable parts (**E**) 95° condylar blade plate and (**F**) Jewett Nail have no movable parts.

FIGURE 4.27

A method of counting the number of engaged cortices for plate fixation.[19]

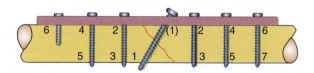

ADDITIONAL PRINCIPLES OF PLATE FIXATION

Longer working length, i.e. a larger distance between the two screws near to the fracture line, is beneficial, as it reduces plate's plastic deformation, distributes deforming forces over its longer section and prevents its breakage. A spanning distance of three empty screw holes over the fracture line ensures an elastic construct which distributes the induced stress over an adequate plate length; this schedule has been validated in clinical practice. Additional screws placed between the two most lateral screws and two screws close to the fracture improve the axial and torsional stability.

The most effective working length such that the plate does not break down easily by fatigue is dependent on the fracture gap size. As working length increases over a gap size of 6 mm or more, the plate fatigues earlier; the trend is not seen when the gap size is 1 mm or less.[22]

Screw Type and Placement

There are two factors to consider when inserting bone screws. First, it is important that they do not interfere with each other. Second, the quality of the bone; conventional screws have poor hold in osteoporotic bone and are prone to loosen.

The absolute minimal arrangement of screws is two unicortical screws placed in each main fragment of bone; however, this scheme works only in a bone of exceptional quality and when the screws are inserted with great accuracy. The screws can be either unicortical in that they only penetrate one cortex of the bone, or bicortical in that they penetrate both the cortices; unicortical screw has only 40% holding power when compared to the hold of a bicortical screw. Two bicortical screws have better hold than the two unicortical screws. To increase the safety factor of a plate-bone construct, the recommendation is for insertion of a

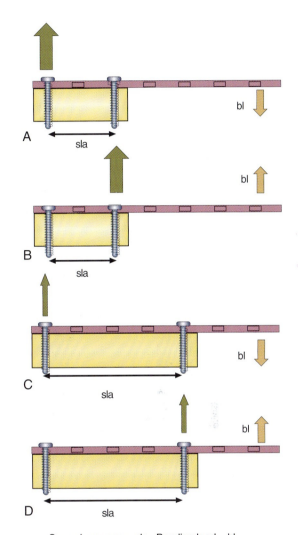

Screw lever arm = sla   Bending load = bl
Change in plate lever arm alters the pull-out force on the screw

FIGURE 4.28

Change in plate lever arm alters the pull-out force on the screws. **(A and B)** When a relatively short plate is used, the screw loading is relatively high due to the short lever arm of the screws in both directions of a bending moment. A line with two arrowheads shows the size of the lever arm of the screw. **(C and D)** Using a longer plate increases the lever arm of each screw. Under a given bending moment, the pull-out force of the screws is therefore reduced. This applies both to conventional and locking screws.

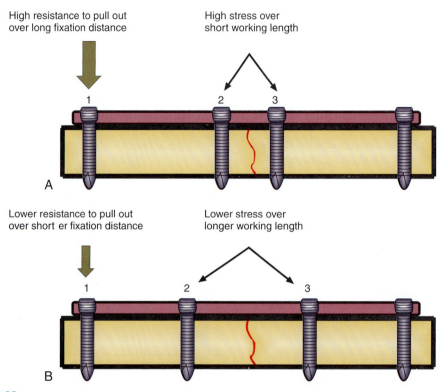

FIGURE 4.29

Pull-out force on screws changes with the fixation length i.e. distance between screws 1 and 2. **(A)** The greater the distance the higher the resistance to pull-out forces and vice versa. High stress concentration occurs when working length is short i.e. distance between screws 2 and 3. **(B)** Stress concentration eases over longer working distance.

minimum of three screws in each main fragment. Stoffel et al.[22] even suggest at least 3–4 screws on each side of the fracture in humerus and forearm because of the high rotational loads.

The axial stiffness of the construct remains steady once the plate has more than three screws in each fragment as long as two of the three screws are placed in the holes closest and farthest to the fracture line (Fig. 4.33). The placement of screws at each plate end ensures that the full plate length contributes to the fracture fixation. The position of the third screw does affect the axial stiffness; as the third screw moves away from the fracture line the axial stiffness decreases.

The torsional rigidity remains steady once the plate has four or more screws in each fragment and as long as the holes closest and farthest to the fracture line are filled. The positions of third and subsequent screws are inconsequential.

If the induced implant deformation is defined by closing and opening of a fracture gap (strain dependent), a longer distance between the two screws close to the fracture line distributes the given deformation over a longer distance and avoids the danger of plastic deformation of a overstressed short

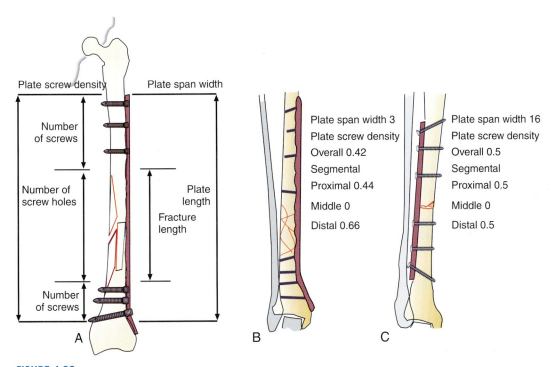

FIGURE 4.30

Estimation of length of a plate, number and positions of screws for fracture fixation (**A**) A schematic for calculating plate span width and plate screw density for a mechanically sound fixation of a multifragmentary diaphyseal fracture in the lower leg. Plate span width is shown on the right and is given by the plate length divided by fracture length. Plate screw density is shown on the left and is defined by the number of screws divided by the number of screw holes. The screw density is given for each bone segment as well as for the entire bone.[21] (**B**) A line sketch of fracture of tibia fixed with a plate. In this case, the plate span width ratio is high enough, that is, approximately 3 indicating that the plate is 3 times longer than the overall fracture area. The plate-screw density is shown for all the three bone segments. The proximal main fragment has a plate-screw density of 0.44 (four out of nine holes occupied); the segment over the fracture has a density of 0 (none out of three holes occupied) The higher plate-screw density 0.66 (four out of six) in the distal main fragment has to be accepted, because for anatomic reasons there is no way of reducing it. The overall plate-screw density for the construct in this example is 0.42 (6 screws in a 14-hole plate). (**C**) In the next example of a transverse fracture of a short fracture length and treated on compression principle, the plate span ratio is 16:1 and plate screw density is 0.5 (6 out of 12).

plate segment.[24] When bridging a large gap the screws should be kept close to the fracture line because such a placement decreases Von Mises stresses on the plate and protects it from fatigue failure. Conversely, when bridging a small gap the screws should be moved away leaving two to three screw holes. This shift decreases Von Mises stresses on the plate and protects it from failure by fatigue. When the fracture gap is small, e.g. 1 mm, a stainless steel implant is under higher stress than a titanium implant, but their stress levels are similar when they support a large gap. This singularity occurs because the two metals have differing mechanical stiffness of the two metals in combination with the motion at the fracture site and is dependent on elastic modulus of the material, cross-sectional area and

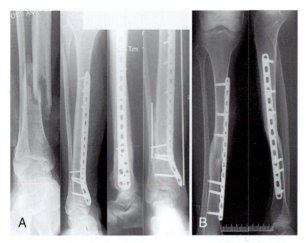

FIGURE 4.31

Radiographs of tibia (**A**). Plate length is 3 times longer than the fracture length. Plate-span ratio is 3:1. Out of 18 holes only 8 are occupied by the screws; plate-screw density is 0.4. In patient (**B**), plate span ratio is 9:1 and screw density is 0.4.

length of the implant. The Von Mises stresses of the screw show minimal change for a large fracture gap and they exceed the stresses for a small gap size. When the fracture gap is small the Von Mises stresses in the screw will decrease with increasing working length of the plate.

Plate screw density is determined by the quotient of the number of screws inserted and the number of screw holes. The optimum screw ratio (the number of screws used for fixation divided by the number of available screw holes) – for example, the screw ratio for a 10-hole plate with five screws is 0.5 – and the appropriate use of bicortical fixation when locked plates are utilized have not been well researched in the clinical setting. However, there is good biomechanical data to guide the achievement of the appropriate screw ratio. The recommended screw ratio is 0.4 to 0.5 (Fig. 4.34) for bridging fixation with three or four screws on either side of the fracture gap. The number of screws is far less important than their position within the plate. The placement of screws at each plate end ensures that the full plate length contributes to the fracture fixation. The distance between the two screws closest to the fracture on each fragment determines the elasticity of the fracture fixation, and, more important for the implant, the distribution of the induced deformation by applying load to the construct. An elastic spanning distance of three empty screw holes over the fracture line helps to distribute the induced stress over an adequate plate length.[25]

Conventional Plate and Bone Vascularity

Although mechanical stability is essential, bone vitality is paramount in fracture healing because a dead bone cannot heal. In initial days of plate fixation, primary bone healing, also known as direct or osteonal healing, was the golden aim and this was achieved only under an absolutely stable fixation. Wide exposure of the bone was necessary to gain access and to provide good visibility of the fracture zone to permit reduction and plate fixation. The bone fragments were extensively handled to accomplish perfect anatomical reduction and heavy implants were used. The screws had to be tightened to fix and compresses the plate onto the bone. Relative movement between fragments was eliminated by compression load and friction. Intramembranous bone formation, direct cortical remodelling and absence of external callus are characteristics of primary bone healing. In presence of absolute stability the blood vessels crossed the fracture line without disturbance and faster revascularization occurred. As there is no increase in bone diameter under direct osteonal healing, its load-bearing capacity does not increase and implant must be retained for longer time. Tightly fixed implants, as well as extensive bone and soft tissue handling, lead to a change in the bone which can be noted as porosis beneath the plate on early postoperative X-rays. Subsequent research has proved that the radiographic changes are

ADDITIONAL PRINCIPLES OF PLATE FIXATION

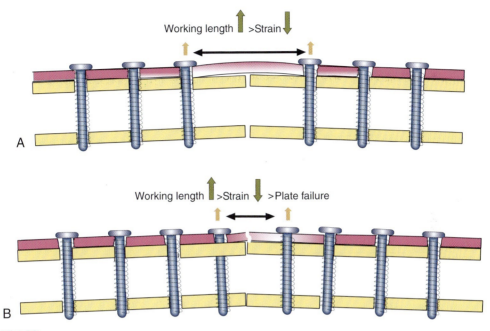

FIGURE 4.32
Relationship of working length and strain at the level of the fracture for LIFP. **(A)** When a fracture is bridged with a locked plate, three or four plate holes should be left empty at the level of the fracture to increase the working length and decrease the strain and stress concentration on the plate. **(B)** In contrast, if a locking construct is made too stiff with too many screws at the level of the fracture, the short working length will lead to an increased strain and stress concentration with loading and torsional forces, causing the plate to break.[23]

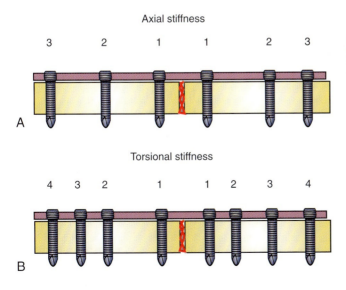

FIGURE 4.33
Effect of screw position on axial and torsional stiffness. **(A)** Axial stiffness of a construct. Holes closest (1) and farthest (3) to the fracture line must be filled. Position of the third screw is less significant; however, construct stiffness decreases as the third (2) screw moves away from the fracture site. **(B)** Torsional stiffness is optimal when four screws are inserted in each fragment. Holes closest (1) and farthest (4) to the fracture line must be filled. Positions of the third (2) and fourth (3) do not alter the magnitude of torsional stiffness. More than four screws are inconsequential for torsional stability.

$$\text{Plate span ratio} = \frac{\text{Plate length}}{\text{Fracture width}}$$

Simple fractures

$$\text{in compression} = \frac{8\text{-}10}{1}$$

$$\text{in splinting} = \frac{2\text{-}3}{1}$$

Multi fragmentary fractures

$$\text{in splinting} = \frac{2\text{-}3}{1}$$

$$\text{Plate screw density} = \frac{\text{Number of screws}}{\text{Number of plate holes}}$$

Simple fractures
0.3 to 0.4

Multi fragmentary fractures
0.4 - 0.5

FIGURE 4.34

Quick guide for plate length and number of screws for a variety of fracture patterns.

due to avascularity of the bone under the plate (Fig. 4.35). It was revealed that the compressive force under the plate prevents periosteal perfusion, resulting in periosteum as well as bone necrosis deep to the plate and adjacent to the fracture site. Such episodes may occasionally lead to localized bone resorption at the screw threads and result in implant loosening.

It is also noted that the loss of vascularity is directly proportional to the contact area of the plate; the smaller the contact area of the plate, the lesser the vascular damage (Fig. 4.36). It is further postulated that by preserving the blood supply to bone it would be possible to minimize or avoid delayed union, non-union and refracture after hardware removal as well as prevent development of infection in to a sequestrum under the deep surface of the plate.

An undesirable consequence of the use of rigid compression plates is post-union osteopaenia. This can translate into porotic transformation of the cortex beneath the plate with a net decrease of bone mass and with impaired mechanical properties of the healed bone. It has been related to the occurrence of refractures after plate removal. Most investigators believe that the structural change is secondary to the overprotection of the underlying bone from normal stresses – stress protection. The prevalence of post-union osteopenia in plated human fractures is unknown and there is uncertainty about the mechanism causing post-union osteopenia. The bone density at the fracture site is marginally reduced but this bone loss is offset by an increase in the total area of the bone. There are three potential solutions, to overcome these disadvantages (a) continue to use rigid plates but modify the timing of plate removal, (b) the use of biologically degradable materials for internal fixation.

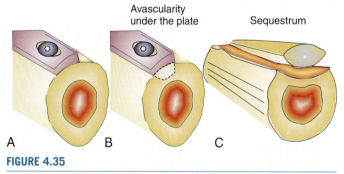

A B C

FIGURE 4.35

Observed patterns of bone loss beneath a plate did not correspond to the stress patterns of the corresponding bone segment.

Insufficiencies of Compression Plate

The concept of direct bone healing was introduced in the early 1960s. It professed perfect anatomical reduction and rigid internal fixation to achieve immediate mobility in the postoperative period; extensive handling of bone fragments was required to accomplish fixation with heavy implants. Wide exposure of

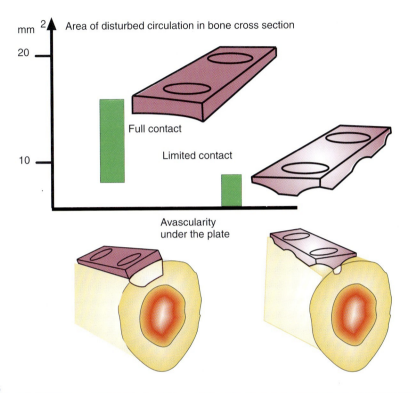

FIGURE 4.36

Loss of vascularity is proportional to the contact area of the plate. Smaller the contact area of the plate, the lesser the vascular damage.

the bone provided spacious access and good visibility of the fracture zone to achieve the objective. The rigid fixation doctrine set the stage for modern era of plate fixation; compression became the buzzword. Over the years many shortcomings of the self-compression plate came to light (Table 4.1).

Relative Stability and Bone Plate

Accomplishing Relative Stability with Conventional Self-Compression Plate

Conventional compression plate is designed to produce absolute stability at the fracture site. In 1960s, the goal for fracture stabilization of long bones was to achieve an exact reduction of all fracture fragments in combination with a rigid osteosynthesis, and the compression plate was the tool to achieve it; lag screws were used to obtain compression at the fracture site. This approach of osteosynthesis resulted in lack of callus formation. Moreover, it was tricky to scrutinize radiographs for signs of fracture healing. Delayed fracture healing and implant failures were frequent.

The goal for plate osteosynthesis in twenty-first century is to restore the length, axis and rotation of the bone by indirect reduction; small fracture fragments are left in place. It is now accepted that callus

Table 4.1 Inadequacies of Compression Plate

Designed for absolute stability; creates mechanical environment that favours primary bone healing Unnatural healing pattern – worthless soudure primer
Creates an environment where lack of stability is conducive to delayed or non-union
Components tend to move under loading/bicortical hold essential/load-sharing implant
Anatomical reduction is essential which requires large and direct exposure of the fracture thus disturbing the vascularity
Mismatch distorts reduction; plate must be shaped to bone curve
Extensive plate-bone contact under enormous pressure
Damage to bone vascularity; leads to necrosis induced bone loss, which is a potential nidus for infections
Delayed load bearing
Delayed return to normalcy
Inadequate fixation in osteopaenic or pathologic bone
Implant removal leaves bone in weakened state; needs protection for up to 16 weeks

formation is a normal and essential process in fracture healing and not a sign of instability. Micromotion at the fracture gap is needed to get callus formation.

Accomplishing plate fixation that allows micromotion using an implant designed to produce absolute stability is a challenge but can be addressed by applying mechanical principles to advantage. Axial stiffness and torsional rigidity are influenced mainly by the bridging length, i.e. the distance of the first screws on either side from the fracture site. Micromotion increases exponentially with increase in bridging length (Fig. 4.37).

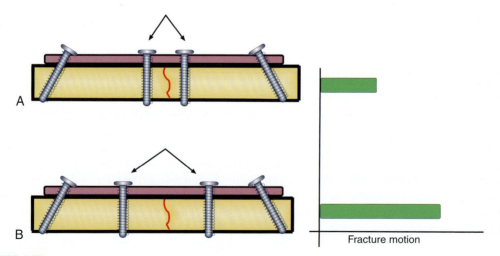

FIGURE 4.37

(**A**) Effect of bridging length on fracture motion: micromotion at the fracture gap increases rapidly with increasing distance of the screws from the fracture site. (**B**) Oblique placement of end screws improves pull-out strength of the screw.[26]

Omitting two or three plate holes at the fracture gap allows sufficient micromotion and therefore faster bone healing. Lag screw through the plate produces absolute stability; it should be avoided. The most important factor to improve pull-out strength of the screws in long bones is the length of the plate; longer the plate the stronger the pull-out strength. A surgeon can influence fracture healing by the number of screws used. Screws should not fill all holes in a long plate; three to five few screws per fracture segment are optimum for fixation. Oblique screws at the plate ends also increase pull-out strength.

Minimal Invasive Plate Osteosynthesis

MIPO means that a plate is placed through small incisions with as little dissection and stripping of the soft-tissue envelope as possible. It is also known as percutaneous (MIPPO), submuscular, minimal incisional and less invasive plating. Both conventional and locking plates can be inserted through these surgical techniques (see Chapter 10 for greater coverage of the technique).

LOCKED INTERNAL FIXATOR PLATE

Locked internal fixation plate (LIFP) is a screw and plate system where the screws can be locked in the plate and form one stable system. Locking the screw into the plate guarantees angular and axial stability, abolish the possibility for the screw to toggle, slide or be dislodged and eliminates the risk of postoperative loss of reduction. The plate needs not be pressed against the bone, thus the blood supply is preserved and there is no risk of loss of primary reduction.

Round holes with threads make the basis of a locked plate; threaded hole receives the threaded conical head of the screw; the shape of the hole and the head match. As the screw is tightened in the plate hole, the threads lock and a fixed angle construct is formed. Once secured, the locked screw does not toggle. Initial designs of locked plate had only threaded holes and every screw had to be locked in (Fig. 4.38A). Such a construct caused practical difficulties and adversely affected bone healing as extremely rigid constructs got created. Besides it was not possible to compress the fragments as and when required; subsequently the plates with alternate locking and compressing holes were produced.

In an improved plate design, the self-compression and the locking mechanisms have been combined to impart dual ability to compress and lock (Fig. 4.38B and C). This integrated hole makes it possible to exploit and combine the advantages of both, the conventional plate and screws and LIFP. The traditional self-compressing unit permits dynamic compression by eccentric placement of a standard screw as well as by lag screw technique to obtain maximal interface compression. The threaded screw head and an appropriately threaded plate hole offer angular stability, provide better anchorage, eliminate toggling and minimize the risk of reduction loss. A plate with integrated hole offers three alternatives: (i) fixation with conventional bone screws; (ii) fixation with threaded-head screws and (iii) fixation with combination of conventional and threaded-head screws. The plate with integrated holes is useful in all those situations where a traditional compression plate is used.

Types of Locking Plate

There are two kinds of locking plates: fixed-angle locking plates as described above and variable-angle locking plates where in the screw can be locked with a certain clearance within a cone with an angle

FIGURE 4.38

(A) Plate with threaded round holes and screw with threaded head – LISS plate. (B) A smooth sloping oval hole and a threaded round hole are integrated to form a new design, 'Combi hole'.[27] Integrated screw hole has a contoured slope of the conventional compression hole at one end that facilitates gliding and tilting of the screw head. The other end of the integrated hole has threads that match the ones on the head of the locking screw. (C) A threaded as well as a conventional screw may be inserted to achieve different objectives.

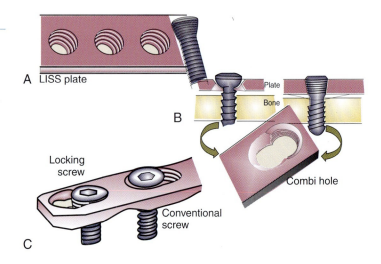

of 1–15°. Two locking mechanisms are prevalent: in the first the screw head is itself threaded and screws into the plate or into an adapted lip. In the second the screw head is locked in its chamber by a threaded locknut.

Fixed Angle Plates

In the first-generation locked plates screw insertion is unidirectional; the screw head is conical and equipped with a double threaded screw thread that locks within the threaded hole. The pitch of the screw head is identical to the pitch of the screw body to prevent compression. Best locking effect is achieved by inserting the screw at a predetermined angle to the hole. This is achieved by drilling a pilot hole through a sleeve that is screwed in the plate hole (Fig. 4.39). The predetermined angle of the threaded hole is often adequate, but difficulty arises in metaphyseal regions and in periarticular fixations. In these situations a shorter locked screw or conventional screw has to be placed through the hole; both procedures are undesirable when periarticular fixation needs to be maximized.

The above description is of AO system. Other fixed angle systems also are in use. In the Surfix® system[28] (developed nearly simultaneously with AO system but totally independently by Patrick Sürer, unchanged since its beginnings) locking is obtained with a locknut (Fig. 4.39D). The screw has a flat head that is locked into the chamber by the locking nut screwed through the plate thickness. Tornier®,[29] the third fixed angle system has used this concept with variation for the distal radial epiphyseal plates. A screwed-in cover that simultaneously locks several screws replaces the locking nut; there is a separate cover for radial and ulnar side (Fig. 4.39E). The system offers a choice of threaded screws, pegs that are partially threaded on the volar side and lag screws, partially threaded on the dorsal side. In this fixed angle system before locking it is possible to compress a bone fragment by a lag screw. There are two anatomically aligned screws for radial styloid. The distal lip of the plate has a low profile that prevents tendon impingement and overstuffing.

LOCKED INTERNAL FIXATOR PLATE

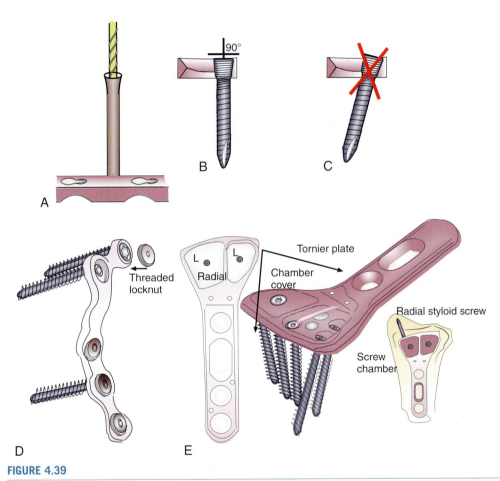

FIGURE 4.39

Fixed angle (unidirectional) systems. **(A)** A sleeve is screwed in the plate hole to guarantee precise screw positioning for matching the screw head threads into plate hole.[27] **(B)** Well-placed locked screw; optimal angular stability at 90° to plate axis. **(C)** Any angulation generates reduced angular stability. **(D)** Surfix® system uses a threaded locknut to prevent any change in its direction. The design has remained almost unchanged since its introduction.[28] **(E)** CoverLoc® by Tornier® has a snug fitting lid that simultaneously locks several screws. The side specific distal radius plate has radial and ulnar compartment. The design has a distinctive styloid screw.[29]

Variable Angle Plates

Current multidirectional systems permit screw angulation of up to 30° using several devices like special shape of the plate thread and the screw head, innovative mechanisms, synthetic material for washer and metals with dissimilar hardness. A few of these designs rely on some sort of hoop stress and an additional interface between the screw head and the plate. Most systems now offer the surgeon a choice of inserting a locked or conventional screw through the same hole; often traditional screws can be used to compress fractures and 'pull' the plate down to bone, facilitating reduction. Locked screws may then be used to further stabilize the construct. This 'hybridization' of the locked and conventional technologies is available with second-generation locked plates, which helps in achieving proper compression, plate positioning and fracture alignment.

One of the new designs has an expanding ring (arrow) that allows a screw to be put in chosen direction before locking[30] (Fig. 4.40A). When the screw is threaded into the mechanism its conical head engages with the matching threads in the expandable ring, which then locks into the plate; this maintains the screw's position at the chosen angle and direction. Before locking, it is possible to adjust the position of the bone with respect to the plate or to pull a bone segment closer to the plate, by using a 'special turning device'. Similar mechanism used by Newclip™ that has a washer and an additional clip in the assembly.[31] The screw head can be screwed into lock inside a cone with up to 10° clearance.

The variable-axis or so-called polyaxial screw system has a bushing in the threaded plate hole, and as the threaded conical screw head engages the bushing, the bushing expands, placing hoop stresses

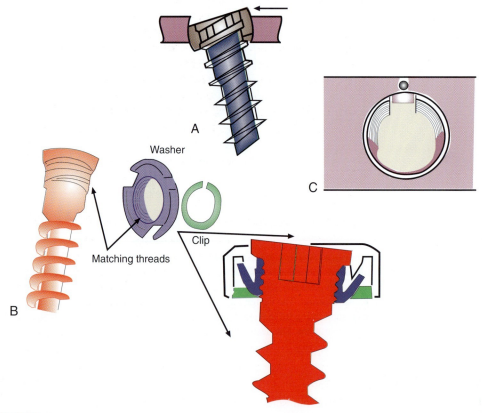

FIGURE 4.40

Multidirectional angular stability allows screws to be locked in the plate hole at a desired angle. **(A)** An expanding washer (arrow) allows a screw to be put in preferred direction.[30] **(B)** A locking washer and an additional clip is used in another system.[31] **(C)** POLYAX® variable-axis screw placement plate has a bushing in the threaded plate hole and as the conical threaded screw head engages the bushing, it expands and locks the screw to the plate.[32]

on the surrounding hole and locking the screw to the plate by a frictional interface between the bushing and the plate[32] (Fig. 4.40C). This device allows an approximately 40° cone of angulation prior to end-point locking.

Biotech International uses a synthetic material in the plate hole to lock in the self-tapping conical head (Fig. 4.41A) AO system has modified the system where in screws with round undersurface are used. The plates have four columns of threads in the variable angle-locking hole that provide four points of locking (Fig. 4.41B).

Another system locks the screw at a desired angle by placing a cap over the screw head that builds up friction (Fig. 4.41C). The NCB® system permits a screw to lag a bone fragment before locking it; the surgeon can feel the bone quality while tightening the screw. These features permit fracture reduction and interfragmental compression before locking, an element unique to this technique.[34] In laboratory testing the system showed high stability under load and no slip was detected. Cold welding or wear has not been reported in this system and removal is easy.

In another newer design the locking mechanism is located in the screw head and must be activated by a special key. In locked position it protrudes (arrow) beyond the head boundary[35] (Fig. 4.41D).

A further option for locking consists of reshaping the material in the plate hole (Fig. 4.41E). The implants are made of titanium of differing hardness and the screw head has a conical thread. The screw may be positioned in an arc of 15°. Screw insertion at greater angle may be carried out by using of a thread forming device. In Wolter system,[36] plate bending and use of conventional screw to draw the plate close to the cortex is possible and is recommended; the contact between the plate and the bone surface is considered an advantage. This technology allows insertion of threaded screw into a deformed hole, e.g. an oval plate hole; as the screw head is tightened, reshaping process occurs, radial compression widens the hole and its round outline is restored. It is postulated that Wolter's angular stable method reduces micro-movements, promotes unhindered in-growth of vessels and guarantees bone healing. A wide fracture gap is closed by compression but without placing the fracture surface under compression; fracture gap closure is expected to reduce consolidation time.

Pros and Cons of Fixed and Variable Angle Locking Systems

Unidirectional locking system has advantages. It avoids joint penetration as well as screw crossing, because the directions are predetermined in the designing process. It can also help in gaining correct alignment in the lower femoral metaphyseal comminuted fracture; inserting the juxta-articular screws parallel to the femoro-tibial joint space prevents malalignment in the frontal plane. The theoretical advantage of multidirectional locking is the ability to circumvent obstacles to fixation that would not be avoidable with the insertion of screws at a predetermined angle. This is at times true in vicinity of a joint. A variable-axis screw is weaker in resisting a bending load than a fixed angle locking screw because it depends on friction and not on the locked threads for stability; thus, there is compromise in strength between the fixation strength and ability to insert a screw at desired angle. However, clinical experience has shown that the variable-axis technology is effective in achieving high rates of union without varus collapse or mechanical failure of well-reduced complex fractures.[37]

Some surgeons question the need for variable angle devices. Implants in a variable–angle-locking system are thicker and are undesirable near a joint like wrist where several tendons, vessels and nerves are crowded in a compact space. Common argument in support of a variable angle system is its ability to adapt to different fracture types and to fix a particular fragment. However, only in conventional plating, it is absolutely necessary to engage all the fragments and multidirectional screw placement

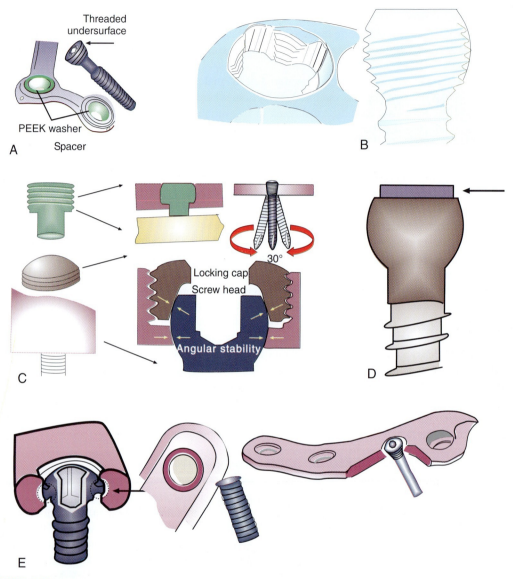

FIGURE 4.41

(A) This design uses a liner of synthetic material, polyaryletherketone (PEEK) to obtain the locking effort.[33] The conical and self-tapping screw head locks at the selected angulation in the PEEK insert set in the plate. (B) Four columns of threads in the variable angle locking hole provide four points of threaded locking between a plate and a variable angle locking screw, forming a fixed angle construct at the surgeon desired screw angle; screws can be angled anywhere within a 30° cone around the central axis of the plate hole. The head of the variable angle locking screw is round in shape to facilitate locking mechanism.[27] (C) Locking cap mechanism permits unique facility first to lag and then lock the screw at a desired angle in an arc of 30°; spacers maintain a gap between the bone and the plate, minimize the plate-bone contact area and protect the periosteal vascularity.[34] (D) The locking mechanism is located in the screw head and a special key is used to activate locking; in locked position it protrudes (arrow) beyond the head boundary.[35] (E) Locking is accomplished by reshaping the material in the plate hole (arrow); the screw and plate are made of titanium of differing hardness and the screw head has a conical thread. By mounting the screw head into the hole, its material-lip transforms to a part of the thread and solidifies by cold welding. The system permits insertion up to 15° variation of angle and easy removal.[36] To tilt the screw more than 15° one needs to use a special device to mould the lip of the plate.

becomes essential. A locking screw is stable because it is screwed in the plate hole; it need not a have bite in the bone fragment to support it; a grid of locked screws supports the reduced fragments. The directions of fixed-angle screws are so designed as to provide maximum support to the joint surface.

The Undersurface of a Locked Hole

Substantial material is removed between the holes from the undersurface of a locked internal fixator. This arrangement limits the contact area between the plate and the bone and minimizes vascular insult (Fig. 4.42).

Apart from this vital benefit, the excavation also reduces the stiffness of the plate to the same level as of the screw hole area. Thus, LIFP has uniform stiffness in all the segments; it can be bent in a continuous curve and yet preserve the mechanical features that evenly distribute bending and torsional stresses over a long distance along the plate (Fig. 4.42C). The LIFP fatigue life is also prolonged as there are no areas of high stresses. The undercuts allow unhindered inclination of a lag screw up to 40° longitudinally, and 7° in the transverse plane, in both directions through the plate (Fig. 4.42D and E). The plate holes are evenly distributed along the plate. This distribution pattern allows the plate's position to be adjusted or exchanged for another without conflicting with any previously drilled holes.

Biomechanics of the Locked Bone Plate

External Fixator vs Locked Internal Fixator Plate

LIFP is a construct where a screw with threaded head, akin to a pin of an external fixator (EF) is locked in the threaded hole of a bone plate, which is analogous to the frame of an EF (Fig. 4.43). The locked unit is axially and angularly stable. When this construct bears the physiological loads, the forces are transferred from one bone segment over the locked screws to the locked plate and from there again over the locked screws to the other segment (Fig. 4.44). The screw with threaded head acts as a peg

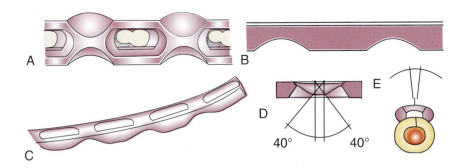

FIGURE 4.42

(A) The scalloped undersurface reduces the bone contact surface of LIFP. The plate holes are equidistant. (B) Arched profile of LIFP. (C) When the plate is shaped to fit the bone surface, it renders smooth bends. (D) The oblique undercuts on the lower side of the plate ensure that the threads of the screw do not come in contact with plate. The lag screw can be inclined up to 40° in longitudinal plane and (E) 7° in the transverse plane in both directions without impinging on the plate.[38]

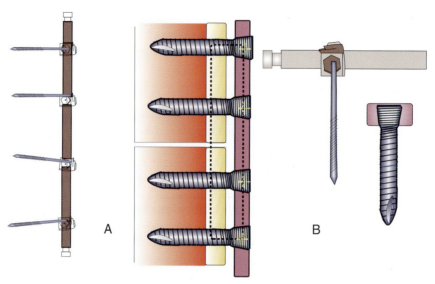

FIGURE 4.43

(**A**) Unilateral external fixator and unicortical locked plate construct are similar in function. (**B**) A locked internal fixator plate is analogous to pin-clamp-rod complex of an external fixator.

connecting the splint to the bone; unlike a conventional plate it does not compress the plate onto the bone to produce friction for achieving stability. The screw of the internal fixator is like a threaded bolt. A bolt maintains the relative position between the body of the fixator and the bone but does not press it towards the bone. In contrast to a compression screw, an internal fixator screw is exposed to bending loads and not so much to tensile forces; this is why the core diameter of locking screw is thicker than that of a conventional bone screw. The plate with locked screws forms a mono-block construct. Such a fixation is less dependent on the bone quality and on the anatomic anchoring region. Thus, a locked screw in the fixator abolishes force transmission by friction, minimizes bone contact, increases stability and eliminates the risk of loss of reduction due to toggling of the screw in the bone. Similarities and differences between EF and LIFP are presented in Table 4.2.

LIFP represents a novel, biofriendly approach to internal fixation.[40] LIFP resembles a conventional bone plate, but its biological and mechanical characteristics are different and it functions rather like a fully implanted EF, even in its secondary bone healing pattern producing abundant callus (Fig 4.44B and C). It might be considered the ultimate EF, widely spaced locked screws alluding to the EF pins and the plate functioning as the connecting bar, placed extremely close to the mechanical axis of the bone. This closeness markedly increases stability compared with a mono-lateral EF.

Furthermore, LIFP creates a substitute cortex and locks the screws in the plate; this increases stability of the fracture and equally distributes deforming loads to all the screws in contrast to those closest and farthest to the fracture site as in case of a conventional plate. This is significant when the bone is porotic or comminuted. A screw's basic function is altered to an EF pin without the disadvantage of long pin length and associated elastic deformation (compliance). It is known that EF causes least vascular damage in comparison to intramedullary nailing or conventional plate fixation.

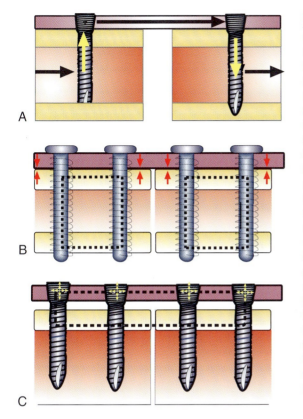

FIGURE 4.44

(A) Graphic representation of force distribution across the gap fracture borne by the locked internal fixator plate. Load transfers from bone to the plate through the locked screw head, across the fracture site, again through the locked screw head and on to the bone. This system of load transmission is unique to locked constructs. Biomechanical difference between a standard screw-plate fixation system and the locked internal fixator system. **(B)** With a conventional plate and screw system, the tightening of the screws compresses the plate onto the bone. The stability results from the friction between the undersurface of the plate and the underlying bone (red arrows). Since the screw head is free to tilt (toggle) within the plate hole, stability requires a bicortical hold of the screws (represented by the dotted rectangles). **(C)** In instance of a locked internal fixator, screw toggle does not occur as the screws are locked in the plate (golden arrows). The forces are transferred from the bone to the plate and if the locking is sufficiently stiff, there will be no force transfer to the far cortex (the plate replaces the first cortex). In biomechanical perspective, unicortical purchase of the screws is therefore sufficient to ensure stability (represented by the dotted rectangles).

Effect of Differing Forces on a Locked Screw-Plate Construct
Bending and Axial Load

Locked plate controls the axial orientation of the screw to the plate, thereby enhancing screw-plate-bone construct stability by creating an intrinsically stable single beam. In a single-beam construct there is no motion between the components of the beam, i.e. the plate and screw. Locked plate is a single-beam construct by design and acts as a fixed angle device. It enhances fracture fixation in circumstances where fracture configuration or bone quality does not provide sufficient screw purchase to achieve the plate bone compression necessary for a conventional plate-screw construct.

Locked plate changes a shear stress to a compressive force at screw-bone junction; this change improves fracture fixation because cortical bone withstands more compressive forces than shear loads (Fig. 4.45). A locked plate's fixation strength is the sum of the strength of all screw-bone junctions of the plate and is superior to that of a conventional plate; in conventional plating it is comes to single screw's axial stiffness or pull-out resistance. Moreover, angular stability evenly distributes the load over all the screws and the load is not concentrated at one screw-bone junction.

The natural angular and axial stability of locked plates adds to fixation strength. Locked plate resembles an 'internally placed external fixator' and is exceptionally rigid as it is very close to the bone and fracture site. Fixation rigidity of an EF is a function of the Schanz pin – its material, length, and

Table 4.2 External Fixator versus Locked Internal Fixator Plate[39]: Similitude and Variance

EF and LIFP are Similar in Following Aspects
Fixed angle stabilization between screws and the bar or plate
Side bar/plate is maintained at a fixed distance over the bone surface
Do not compromise periosteal blood supply
Promote secondary bone healing with callus formation
Allow modulation of construct stiffness at any stage of bone healing in external fixation and at the time of fixation in plating
Minimally invasive, biological osteosynthesis

EF and LIFP are Different in Following Aspects	
EF	LIFP
EF can be applied in various frame configurations allowing control of stiffness over a broad range.	LIFP can be applied in a limited but effective configurations.
Deflexion of Long fixator pins generate motion at the fracture site.	Screw length between plate and bone is too short to allow deflexion.
A very short pin length creates extremely rigid external fixator (atrophic non-union generators); just as very long pins construct excessively elastic external fixator (hypertrophic non-union generators).	No screw flexion; in locked construct the plate bends for flexibility. Thinner plates, made of more flexible material (titanium), and longer bridge span exhibit enhanced flexibility (bending). Thicker and shorter plates bend less.
Generates symmetric motion at far and near cortex at the fracture site.	Generates asymmetric motion; more at far cortex and less at near cortex at the fracture site.
Used in emergency treatment of fractures with severe soft tissue injuries and in multiply injured patients for emergent 'damage control' fixation.	Used as definitive treatment for periarticular fractures for anatomic joint reconstruction with angular stable screws of smaller dimension in the articular fragment. Suitable for buttressing, a minimally invasive implantation technique, and protection of fracture haematoma and local blood perfusion.
Low costs, high flexibility and the ease of application. It is ideal for emergency and combat situations.	High costs, precise technique essential for successful definitive management.
Definitive stabilization in the treatment of long bones during childhood.	Supports either secondary fracture healing by bridge plating or primary bone healing by compression.
Decent choice for definitive treatment of some distal radius fractures.	A volar locked plate offers superior early results and improved patient acceptance.
Limb lengthening and the correction of deformities in children and adolescents by Ilizarov's technique.	Useful as a support during consolidation phase of limb lengthening.

diameter and dimensions of the fixator bar; analogous to locked screw and plate. Short screw length (10–15 times shorter than that for EFs) in the locked plate construct substantially increases its rigidity. Stability across the fracture becomes a function of the mechanical properties of the plate and the amount of load applied. As a locked plate does not produce frictional force between the plate and the bone, the blood supply to the periosteum is preserved and helps rapid bone formation. Undisturbed

LOCKED INTERNAL FIXATOR PLATE

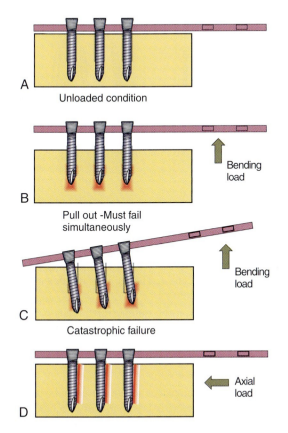

FIGURE 4.45

Effects of bending and axial loads on a locked plate design that acts like any other fixed-angle device. **(A)** Unloaded locked screw plate construct. **(B)** Bending load applied. A locked screw does not loosen and resists pull-out. Failure with pure pull-out of the screws is rare compared with 'C' and requires all screws to fail simultaneously. **(C)** Failure by a bending force causes compression of bone as well as shear between the screws and the bone. Again the strength of the construct includes the strength of the interface between all the screws and the bone as opposed to just the interface of the screw closest to the fracture gap as in conventional plating. **(D)** Axial load applied. A locked screw does not loosen; it experiences majority of the load perpendicular to its axes. When locked plate fails in bending and axial loading, large areas of bone must crush in compression. The failure of a locked plate during an axial load is the failure of the compressive strength of bone over the area of all the screws in the construct.[41]

bone perfusion decreases infection rate, bone resorption, delayed and non-union. The locked plate has superior fixation in the bone, especially in the porotic bone than a conventional plate. Screw locking does not require any axial force and plate's position is not changed when the screws are tightened. Well-tightened screws do not loosen sequentially. Stability is achieved even when the plate stays away from the bone. A plate need not closely fit the bone contour and general conformity to the bone form is sufficient in majority of fixations. To maintain osseous blood supply, the plate is placed in an extra-periosteal position, and may not have a direct contact with the bone.

Optimized Plate Anchorage with Divergent or Convergent Locked Screws

The locked screws impart angular stability to the plate similar to an angled-blade plate. The toggle seen in conventional plate is absent in locked plate construct; this prevents loss of fracture reduction. When a screw is locked in a plate, its axial pull-out resistance remains unvarying. Pull-out failure mechanism of a screw is by shearing; as the pull-out force exceeds the pull-out resistance, a screw tears out a bone 'cylinder' proportional to the size of the screw diameter. When the screws are inserted into a bone segment at divergent angles to one another, their combined pull-out force increases several times (see Fig. 3.26E–G); and more so with locked screws. The reason for this is the fixed, diverging screw axis that are secured angle-stably in the appropriately diverging screw holes of the plate (Fig. 4.46). To sum up, the locked

FIGURE 4.46

Bending the plate into a wave like form makes it possible to insert the screws divergently and convergently. This pattern of screw placement improves the pull-out resistance of the construct.

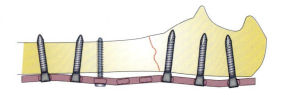

screws are angle stable, offer large resistance and do not toggle to align with the pull-out force and therefore build up a larger resistance volume. The preshaped plates for proximal humerus and radius also exemplify the property.

Unicortical Screw

Closeness of LIFP to the bone and the ability to lock the screw in the plate makes it possible to use unicortical screws without reduction in the strength of the construct or the stability of the fixation (Fig. 4.47). This locked unicortical screw functions like a conventional bicortical screw, but it requires strong anchorage for proper function within a cortex of normal thickness. Hence, it is inefficient in metaphyseal cancellous bone that has minimal cortical thickness.

Working length or the fixation strength of a screw is dependent on the number of threads of the screw that are engaged in the bone cortex; this is dependent on the thickness of the bone cortex; thicker the cortex, longer the working length. Working length depends on the total number of threads engaged; it does not matter if the screw engages one or both the cortices. Satisfactory working length is achieved when a total of 3–4 threads are fully engaged in the bone cortex.

The unicortical screws are generally used in diaphyseal bone but the places where these can be used are limited. The holding power along the long axis of a unicortical screw is less than half of a bicortical screw. The number of unicortical screws required depends on their spacing, their loading, and the quality of bone. Use of three well-spaced unicortical screws equates one bicortical application. Unicortical application is not preferred any more and in poor quality bone, biocortical engagement is recommended.

In normal bone unicortical screws demonstrate higher than normal fixation strength against three-point bending loads and axial forces. However, unicortical screws are weaker in resisting torsional loads. Cortical thickness is decisive in determining fixation strength against torsional loads because a screw's working length is proportional to bone's cortical thickness; thin cortices of porotic bone are weak in resisting torsional loads and are unsuitable for unicortical screw fixation (Fig. 4.47C and D). As demonstrated in Figure 4.47E, the advantages of bicortical fixation with regard to screw working length far outweigh the advantages conferred by healthy cortical bone.

Bicortical locked screws are superior to unicortical locked screws in all modes of loading because of the increased working length or additional amount of bone purchase; bicortical screws provide a greater interface, therefore greater stability. In situations where high torsional loads are expected, bicortical locked screws should be employed. Whether this makes the construct too rigid depends on the material of the plate, the positions of the screws and the number of screws.

Use of self-drilling and self-tapping screws facilitates percutaneous unicortical screw fixation. A self-drilling, self-tapping screw is made possible by reducing the threaded length and adding a drill and a tap section to the screw tip (Fig. 4.47F). The benefits of using these screws are as follows: surgical

LOCKED INTERNAL FIXATOR PLATE

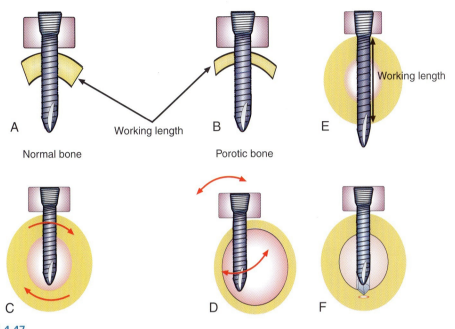

FIGURE 4.47

(**A**) The working length for a unicortical screw in healthy bone is longer (**B**) than its working length in an osteoporotic bone. (**C**) When the bone is loaded in torque the longer working length will provide a higher resistance to the torque. In normal bone unicortical screw has sufficient working length to withstand average torsional forces. (**D**) Conversely, osteoporotic bone has less resistance to torque; the working length is very short due to the thin cortex, and even under moderate torque the bone threads quickly wear out, leading to secondary displacement and instability. (**E**) In all situations, bicortical screw purchase gives maximum working length; the advantages of increased working length in a bicortical fixation far outweighs the stability offered by a single healthy cortex. (**F**) Self-drilling self-tapping locked screw. It is used only as a unicortical screw in a diaphyseal bone segment. If the cutting tip of the screw touches the far cortex, the sharp tip penetrates the far cortex and prevents the destruction of the threads in the near cortex. Self-drilling self-tapping locked screw is unavailable in many countries and its use is diminishing.

technique is simplified, screw length measurement is no longer necessary, diaphyseal and metaphyseal screws need not to be available in small increments leading to smaller inventory, and self-tapping screw tip cuts exact thread profile into the bone which improves screw-bone anchorage.

Hazards in Unicortical Insertion

Even the shortest possible self-tapping unicortical locked screw will destroy the bone threads if the screw tip touches the far cortex before the screw firmly locks in the plate hole (Fig. 4.48A); to avoid the problem, it is safer to measure the correct length of the screw after drilling.

The differences in the 'sticking-out length' of self-drilling and self-tapping screws are very important to safe guard the safety of neurovascular tissue. Self-drilling screw should not protrude beyond the bone, while self-tapping screw needs to protrude up to the first complete thread to obtain good

154 CHAPTER 4 BONE PLATES

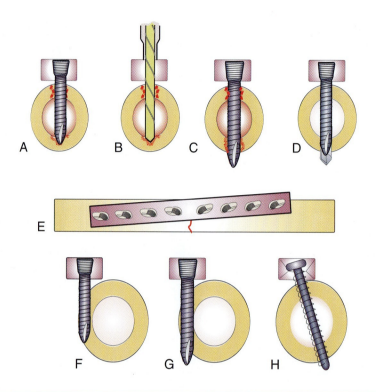

FIGURE 4.48
Length discrepancies in use of unicortical screws. **(A)** In bones with small diameter the tip of a self-tapping locked screw may make contact with the far cortex before the screw head has engaged fully in the threads of the plate hole. This destroys the bone threads in the near cortex and complete loss of fixation occurs. **(B)** To resolve the situation, far cortex is drilled through a threaded drill sleeve and **(C)** a bicortical self-tapping locked screw is inserted.[42] **(D)** The sticking-out length will vary between screw types: bicortical self-tapping screw has relatively smooth screw tip; neurovascular structures beyond the far cortex are unharmed. To provide good anchorage of the screw threads in both cortices, the self-tapping locked screw should protrude slightly beyond the far cortex. **(E)** Bicortical self-drilling self-tapping screw may be perilous; it should be used only as unicortical screw to prevent damage to the soft tissues. **(F)** Inadvertent eccentric plate position is over and again seen in MIPO. **(G)** Placing a unicortical self-tapping locked screw to secure an eccentrically positioned plate is unsafe because the screw bites only a small sector of the cortex. **(F)** Sufficient anchorage may be achieved by inserting a bicortical self-tapping screw. **(H)** A good alternative is to use a bicortical conventional cortex screw at an angle.

purchase on the far cortex (Fig. 4.48C and D). A fixed-angle unicortical locking screw may have precarious hold in the cortex (Fig. 4.48E).

Clinical conditions when unicortical fixation should be avoided are listed in Table 4.3.

Indications for Use of LIFP

Present-day locking plates are preshaped to fit the anatomic outline and permit use of both locking and conventional screws. Preshaped plates offer easy of application as there is no need to contour them, they support reduction, their aiming blocks guarantee accurate screw placement and they support less invasive approach.

The current indications for locked plate fixation are as follows:

Table 4.3 Eschew Unicortical Screw

- In porotic bone
- In thin bone cortex, e.g. in metaphyseal area
- In high torque loading on the plate
- In short main fragment
- In bones with small diameter
- In damaged bone threads in the near cortex
- Incorrect insertion of a locking screw

When in doubt, obtain bicortical purchase

1. Complex periarticular fractures, especially those with comminution of the metaphyseal region: Anatomic reduction of the articular surface with lag screw fixation remains the first priority. The metaphyseal comminution is then bridged by the plate. One may use either conventional or a locked screw to fix the diaphyseal segments.
2. Comminuted distal femoral fractures with multiplanar articular involvement: In hindrances seen in the distal femur such as previously placed lag screws or fracture lines, locked plates offer options for fixed-angle fixation while avoiding these obstacles. The coronal condylar (Hoffa) fracture at times precludes the use of conventional fixed angle devices, like the blade plate or the dynamic condylar screw.
3. Short, extra-articular metaphyseal fracture, intramedullary nails in femur and tibia fail to control short periarticular fragments and malalignment is common. Locked plate offers a superior control mechanism.
4. Tibial plateau fractures: In bicondylar type when coronal plane stability is required, the locking technique is useful. Locked plating facilitates two-column support and is valuable alternative in situations in which dual compression plating is indicated. Locked plate is a substitute to external fixation in this region as it eliminates pin site infection and improves patient comfort.
5. Fracture of distal part of the tibia
6. Periprosthetic fracture in joint replacement: Most useful in a fracture below THA and above TKA. The locked plate is superior to other devices in fixing fractures around total knee arthroplasty. Locked plates are easy to attach whereas implants like retrograde intramedullary nails, blade plate or dynamic condylar screws are hard to put around the arthroplasty because of impediments like closed femoral housing, lugs and stems of the prosthesis.
7. Fixation of corrective osteotomies: Locked plate is used in stabilizing both open and close wedge osteotomies.
8. Malunions, non-unions and failed fixation: Locked plate does not depend on friction fit between it and bone for stability and is valuable in fixation of malunions and non-unions. The locked plates in revision fixation have considerable benefit.[43] The plate provides better stability and solid fixation in normal or porotic bone compared to conventional plating, as it can function as alternate to cortical bone, offer fixed angle construct and is superior purchase.
9. Orthopaedic oncology: Stability of a locked plate is independent of the bone quality; it obtains stable fixation even in pathological bones.
10. Comminuted proximal humerus, especially in the osteopenic patient; distal part of the humerus, non-union of the humerus.
11. Distal radius, intra-articular fracture.

Use of LIFP gives the surgeon the freedom to select the most appropriate treatment method, either the compression or the locked splinting to link the fracture zone and even the freedom to combine the two in an individual patient.

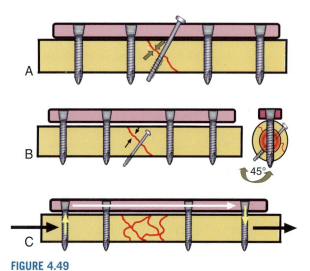

FIGURE 4.49

(A) Principle of absolute stability and compression method: interfragmentary compression with a plate dependent lag screw and a protection plate. The torque applied to tighten the lag screw leads to friction between the fractured bone ends as well as between the plate and the bone surface. The surface pressure thus created stabilizes the bone fragments in relation to the plate. The locked screws maintain the reduction. **(B)** Plate independent lag screw and fixation of the protection plate with locked screw; cross-sectional presentation of the arrangement. This technique is easier than fixing a lag screw through a plate hole. **(C)** Locked screws are axial and angular stable. LIFP is stable without any compression of the plate onto the bone. Prerequisites for using LIFP to achieve fracture fixation on principle of relative stability: long plate; adequate space between the locked screws in each main fragment to bridge the fracture zone; the bridging plate is only fixed to the main fragments proximally and distally; avoid stress concentration while leaving out three or four plate holes without screws in the fracture zone.

LIFP in Compression Mode in Accordance with the Principle of Absolute Stability[44]

LIFP with integrated holes can be used with standard plating methods, i.e. fracture fixation by compression technique to achieve absolute stability and primary bone healing. Clinical situations for such a use are:

Simple diaphysis and metaphysis fractures that require precise anatomic reduction for the superior functional outcome; simple transverse or oblique fractures with no soft-tissue injury and normal bone quality (compression plating or protection plating along with a lag screw or tension-band plate).

- Intra-articular fractures (as buttress plate)
- Delayed union or non-union
- Closed-wedge osteotomies
- Complete avascularity of the bone fragments

Lag Screw and Protection Plate

A lag screw inserted through a plate can achieve interfragmentary compression of an intra-articular fracture or of a simple fracture in the metaphysis or diaphyseal physis (Fig. 4.49A). If there is good bone quality and an open approach is possible so that accurate plate contouring can be carried out, then additional conventional cortex screws may be used to increase the friction between plate and bone. This protection plate construct helps shield the fractured bone from bending and torsional forces.

Using the LIFP with conventional cortex or cancellous bone screws requires accurate shaping of the plate in the same way as with a conventional self-compression plate. Imperfect shaping of the plate leads to a mismatch between plate and bone surface resulting in loss of reduction while tightening the screws.

When LIFP is to be fixed with conventional cortex or cancellous screws similar to a standard compression plate, it must be accurately shaped to fit the bone; inaccurate shaping may result in loss of reduction when screws are tightened. If locked screws are inserted to maintain the reduction and compression being maintained by the lag screw, no uncontrollable forces will be created because of absence of pressure of the plate on the bone surface. Thus, the risk loss of primary reduction would be abolished.

Additional stability could be achieved by using locked screws; these are preferred in porotic bone because the screws do not depend on bone health for stability. When a poorly contoured plate is used as a protection plate there is no primary loss of reduction if locked screws are deployed. A lag screw may be placed outside of a protection plate, even when the plate is being fixed with locked screws; the procedure is simpler than inserting the lag screw through the plate hole. This fixation will not disturb the main reduction (Fig. 4.49B).

LIFP in Splinting Mode in Agreement with Principle of Relative Stability
Locked screws are preferred for bridge plating; it is easier to carry out the MIPO technique with locked screws because there is no need to preshape the plate, the fragments are not pulled onto the plate, and primary reduction is maintained (Fig. 4.49C). In addition, periosteal blood supply is minimally disturbed; preserved periosteal blood supply theoretically prevents loss of periosteal perfusion, reduces infection risks and promotes fracture consolidation.

LIFP may be used to link the fracture zone using an open approach, a less or minimally invasive method to achieve fixation on principle of relative stability; the reduction could be direct, indirect, closed and approximate. The two factors that help successful fixation are use of a long plate – the longer the better and well spaced out screw positions.

LIFP in Combination of Two Methods
When the bone is fractured in two different places, the biomechanical principles of absolute stability through interfragmentary compression and relative stability by splinting can be combined in application of locked plate

- Dissimilar fracture patterns, e.g. comminution and simple in segmental fractures – simple fracture is stabilized by interfragmentary compression and comminuted segment is fixed on splinting principles.
- Intra-articular fractures with a multifragmented diaphyseal extension: The intra-articular segment is accurately reduced using interfragmentary lag screws; the rebuilt articular segment is reconnected to the diaphysis by bridging fixation.
- Intra-articular fractures with a multifragmented extension into the diaphysis: In these cases, the anatomic reduction and interfragmentary lag screw compression of the articular component is combined with a bridging fixation from the reconstructed joint block to the diaphysis.

Combinations of Different Screws
A single plate could be used to apply two plating techniques, i.e. compression using standard screws and special screws for locked fixation. In the management of fractures near a joint, locked screws are used in the joint's vicinity and conventional screws between the metaphysis and the diaphysis to apply axial compression in a simple fracture type. The splinting method can be carried out with LIFP and a conventional positioning screw or an additional reduction screw is used to pull the plate onto the bone or to reduce a displaced fragment. Additionally, the conventional screws are used to apply compression and locked screws to fix the protection plate.

A recent meta-analytical study does not make any recommendation for or against the use of locked plates for extremity fractures and concludes: 'regarding effectiveness, there were no statistically significant differences between locked plates and non-locked plates for patient-oriented outcomes, adverse events, or complications'.[45]

Contraindications

A locked plate can be used in any plating situation but it is quite unnecessary to fix a simple diaphyseal fracture by compression in a good quality bone.

Furthermore, locked plates are often unnecessary for the fixation of pelvic and acetabular fractures, partial articular fractures (buttress plate), fractures around the ankle and metastatic diaphyseal fractures treatable with intra-medullary nails. Additionally, a locked plate may be unnecessary for a calcaneal fracture fixation where a patient remains non-weight-bearing for long time after fixation.

Advantages

The theoretic advantages of improved stability (offered by locked constructs, devices that permit percutaneous insertion of plates and screws, preservation of fracture biology afforded by muscle-sparing insertion) have generally been borne out, by reportedly higher union and lower infection rates. Malalignment, non-union, implant failure and fracture, and steep learning curve still present challenges, but most recent series demonstrate lower complications with greater operative experience and better instrumentation. Future implant designs will likely improve subchondral supports, and scope of screw angulation and its lockability. Although the great majority of locked plates have been specifically anatomically designed for problematic periarticular fractures, such as those of the distal femur, proximal tibia, proximal humerus and distal radius, also available are locked small- and large-fragment straight plating sets. The indications for these plates remain undefined. It is prudent to use locked plating for problematic fractures for which unlocked plates have demonstrated an increased rate of mechanical failure (e.g. proximal humerus, distal radius, distal femur, proximal tibia). Fractures like that of humeral shaft, both-bones of forearm and lateral malleolus are often treated with conventional plates but do require locked plate fixation when the bone is severely porotic, there is a loss of a bone segment or the end segment is very short due to comminution.

Limitations

LIFP fails when it is overloaded. The locked screws slip from the threaded hole if improperly inserted – i.e. cross-threading (screw threads and plate threads are not in line with each other) occurs. They also slip when less than optimum torque is applied during screw fixation. The locked screw may break or come loose under extreme cyclic loading. A well-locked plate-screw assembly may come loose if the bone is exceptionally porotic. Use of locked plate is not an insurance against non-union and malunion.

Disadvantages

Several potential disadvantages of locked plate fixation exist. The feel for the bone quality during screw insertion and tightening, which is valuable in using conventional bone screws, is absent in a locked screw. With conventional screws, the surgeon has tactile recognition when the screw purchases the far cortex and pulls the plate against the bone. This sensation helps the surgeon know the quality of the bone and ensures that the screw is of appropriate length. There is no tactile feedback about the screw hold in the bone as the screw abruptly stops advancing as it engages the last threads in the plate hole. Screw length must be carefully determined before insertion. When there is some malalignment between the long bone axis and the plate, it is prudent to make a small incision at the plate end and the position of the plate be assessed on the lateral side of the bone by manual palpation. In such situations, despite the surgical sensation of a good tightening, a sound anchorage is not obtained with a short monocortical screw and bicortical hold should be the first choice. Locked plates can maintain fracture reduction but cannot obtain it. One possible exception is use of an anatomically preshaped locked plate in a specific technique. For example, to apply a LCP DF to stabilize a complex distal femoral fracture, the second from most distal Locking Head Screw is passed exactly parallel to the knee joint. The limb alignment is anatomical when the plate is fixed.[44]

If a non-anatomical shaped locked plate is applied in a body region with minimal subcutaneous fat, such a plate may remain prominent, cause pain and irritation forcing an early removal. Unlike a conventional screw, a locked variety does not perform a reduction of a fragment as it is being inserted and special instruments or a temporary reduction screw is essential for the manoeuvre. Higher rates of fracture malalignment occur with a locked plate than a conventional plate and more so when it is inserted by percutaneous technique. Surgeons contemplating a percutaneous approach should be experienced in conventional open techniques and should be aware of the differences. A locked screw cannot be used as a compression device. Rigidity of a locked screw plate construct could lead to delayed or non-union of a diaphyseal or metaphyseal fracture that is distracted at fixation or fracture resorption occurs during healing. The locked plate construct does not share any load with bone on either side.

If the fracture is frequently loaded, the plate may sooner or later crack or fixation may fail. This happens when a simple fracture in diaphysis is fixed with screws very close to the fracture site; the problem is short working length of the plate that could have been solved by leaving two to three plate holes without a screw (Fig. 4.50).

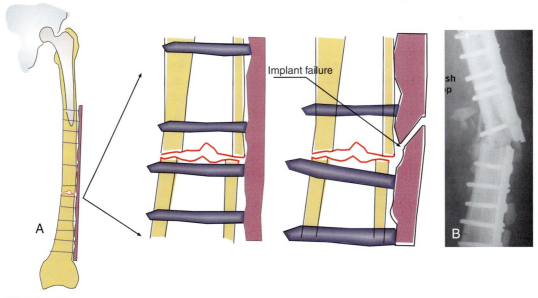

FIGURE 4.50

(**A**) An imperfectly reduced fracture within a stiff construct with a short working length can lead to catastrophic implant failure. (**B**) Radiograph representing a clinical situation of too many screws placed too close to fracture site leading to plate fatigue and failure.

If the fracture is repetitively loaded, the plate may eventually crack or fixation may be lost. This is true in cases of simple fracture patterns as also for fracture fixation in a diaphysis, and a short working length of the plate; the fault lies in locked screws placed too close to the fracture line and not leaving two to three plate holes free of screws.

The disadvantage of first-generation locked plate designs is the lack of options for the surgeon to alter the angle of the screw within the hole and achieve locking. Certain screw holes become unusable by lag screws placed for articular reduction, unique fracture geometry, anatomic variations or implanted components of a joint arthroplasty. Any attempt to contour locked plates could potentially distort the screw holes and adversely affect screw purchase. Locked plate removal may get complicated if the screw tip gets osteointegrated or the screws are cold welded to the plate due overtightening; use of torque limiting screw drivers minimize this predicament.

Far Cortex Locking

In the year 2010–2011 clinical studies of standard locked plating of distal femur fractures reported that the callus formation was deficient, inconsistent, asymmetrical, causes delayed union, late implant failure and non-union.[46, 47] This failing was attributed to high stiffness of the construct. Increasing the bridging span or use of implant made from flexible titanium alloy to decrease the stiffness of the locked plate construct did not alter the outcome. The authors observed that for a laterally applied distal femur plate, elastic bending of the plate induced more interfragmentary motion at the medial cortex than at the lateral cortex adjacent to the plate. This differential motion resulted in asymmetrical callus formation; the largest periosteal callus was seen at the medial cortex. Further animal experiments have confirmed the clinical finding that locking plates are rather stiff and do not permit the anticipated interfragmentary motion in the millimetre range; this results in poor callus formation in asymmetrical locations.

A new design of the locking screw has been developed to induce and enhance parallel interfragmentary movement at near and far cortex (Fig. 4.51). Its unthreaded shaft has varying thicknesses. The collar segment of the shaft abutting the near cortex has somewhat larger diameter to lend support during overload. This feature also confines screw shaft deflection within its elastic range and prevents screw fatigue due to excessive shaft flexion. The flexible shaft has a sufficiently small diameter to permit cantilever bending and limit peak stress in the far cortex. The threaded end of the screw maintains strong hold on the far cortex. The plate deign is same as of a standard locking plate.

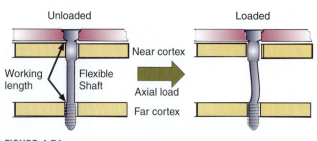

FIGURE 4.51

Far-cortex-locking concept: far cortex locking draws on a screw shaft of reduced diameter to bring about elastic flexion of the screw shaft. A far-cortex-locking screw engages into the plate and the far cortex, has no hold on near cortex which amplifies the screw's working length. The larger diameter collar segment abutting the near cortex lends support during overload.

Flexible Fixation

In the far cortex locking (FCL) construct, the screws are fixed in the plate and only in the far cortex; there is no screw hold in the near cortex. FCL construct is similar to a monolateral EF that has been applied very close to bone surface and pins holding only to the far cortex and no purchase on the near cortex (Fig. 4.52).

The screws of FCL that connect the plate and bone segments are fixed angle and at the same time flexible; the working length of these screws is comparable to that of EF pins. In contrast, the screws of a standard locked plate are rigidly fixed to near and far cortices and do not have adequate working length to offer a flexible fixation. The FCL construct provides a flexible fixation and reduces the stiffness of a locked plating construct by 80% to 88% and actively promotes callus proliferation similar to an EF.[48]

Load Distribution

Load is uniformly dispersed between FCL screws (Fig. 4.53A). Locking plates do not transmit load by plate-to-bone compression but pass it on through fixed angle screws. This mode of load transfer induces stress concentration at the screw bone interface, particularly at the outermost locking screw. In porotic bone this stress concentration increases the fracture risk at the end of the locking plates; in conventional compression plates such a risk is minimal. All FCL screws undergo identical degree of flexion, and strain is spread over the complete working length of FCL screw shafts in the plate assembly. In a standard locking screw, strain is concentrated close to the near cortex and segment between near and far cortex carries no load (Fig. 4.53B). Each FCL screw-bone interface in the far cortex equally shares the load. As the load increases, it is also shared at the near cortex. When FCL screws are used in a construct there is no stress riser at the outermost screw; such a stress riser always exists in a standard locked plate construct.

Progressive Stiffness

FCL constructs initially show low stiffness as all the load is directly transferred from the plate to the far cortex through flexible screw shafts. When load rises, because of elastic flexion, the FCL screw musters additional support at the near cortex and the construct stiffness increases six folds.

This biphasic stiffness profile is analogous to the non-linear behaviour of Ilizarov fixators that become more and more stiff as the loads increase. In practice, the low early stiffness of an FCL plate allows interfragmentary

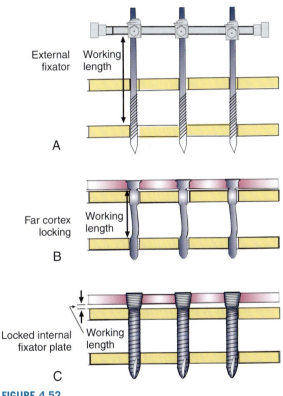

FIGURE 4.52

Working length of fixation constructs. (**A**) Equivalent to the length of Schanz pins of an external fixator. (**B**) Flexible shafts of FCL screws provide a sufficient working length for flexible, fixed-angle connection of a locking plate to a diaphysis. FCL screws reduce the initial axial stiffness of LIFP by 88%. (**C**) Note the short working length of the locked screws of LIFP, the reason for its high stiffness.

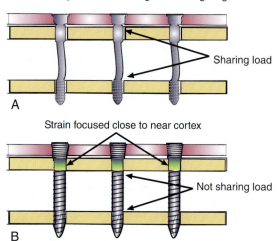

FIGURE 4.53

(A) Each far cortical locking (FCL) screw exhibits equal amounts of flexion, whereby strain is distributed over the entire working length of the FCL screw shaft. (B) In contrast, standard locked plating screws exhibited focused strain adjacent to the near cortex, whereby the screw segment between the near and far cortex remained functionally latent.

motion in period immediately after the surgery when weight bearing is minimal and healing is in early phase. The a FCL screw could be so designed to permit interfragmentary motion within 0.2- to 1-mm range to promote best possible secondary bone healing. In an eventuality of an elevated loading in initial healing phase, the near cortex support protects the fracture site from excessive motion.

Parallel Interfragmentary Motion

Axially loaded conventional bridge plating construct undergoes plate flexion (i.e. elastic plate bending). This flexion facilitates interfragmentary motion because the plate acts as a hinge and allows interfragmentary motion in gradually increasing quantity towards the far cortex opposite the plate (Fig. 4.54A). The moment pattern leads to asymmetrical gap closure, whereby interfragmentary motion at the near cortex is suppressed and more so in locked plating construct where it effectively prevents motion at the plate bone interface. It has also been shown in an animal model that asymmetrical gap closure with locking plates caused asymmetrical callus formation with more callus formation at the far cortex than the near cortex. In an FCL construct the flexible shafts of FCL screws act as cantilever beams and undergo S-shaped flexion to induce nearly parallel interfragmentary motion at both the cortices (Fig. 4.54B).

Clinically, the more or less parallel interfragmentary motion provided by FCL construct contributes to symmetrical callus formation across the entire facture site.

FCL construct is comparable in strength to a standard locked construct. In animal models it has been confirmed that FCL construct actively promotes fracture healing by providing flexible fixation and parallel interfragmentary motion. Results of prospective comparative clinical studies are awaited to assess the benefits of the FCL fixation over standard locked plating.

The laboratory findings of FCL have been converted to clinical practice; first generation of FCL screws are available for clinical use (Fig. 4.55 & 4.56). Additional clinical research, however, is essential to verify that the biomechanical benefits of FCL documented in the laboratory setting are borne out clinically in the form of predictable callus formation.

PLATE REMOVAL

A plate may be removed as soon as healing is complete; this particularly applies to patients with normal bones. Once the fracture is fully healed, the plate has no further function. When the screws remain

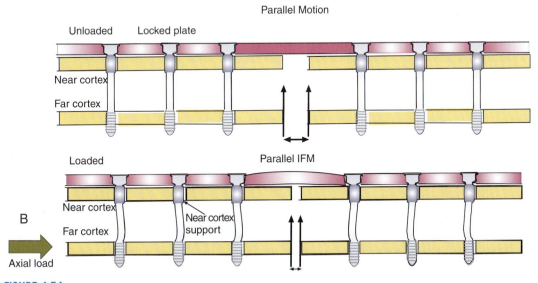

FIGURE 4.54
(**A**) Standard locked construct exhibits asymmetrical gap closure, whereby interfragmentary motion (IFM) at the near cortex is minimal, 5 times less motion at the near cortex than at the far cortex. IFM at near cortex may be too small to promote callus formation. (**B**) Far cortex locking construct induces symmetrical (parallel) IFM by cantilever bending of FCL screws. Interfragmentary motion in response to partial weight bearing is within the 0.2- to 1-mm range known to stimulate callus formation.

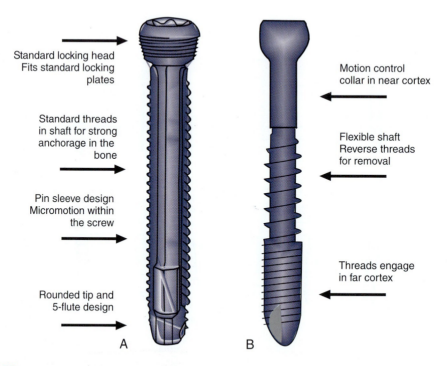

FIGURE 4.55

(A) Dynamic Locking Screw of AO Foundation.[49] (B) Zimmer's MotionLoc Screw.[50] MotionLoc screws are only intended for use in the diaphyseal side of a fracture where screw purchase in the far cortex opposite the plate can be obtained. These should not be used in the metaphysis or epiphysis of the bone. To maximize the effectiveness of the MotionLoc screws, the plate should not be compressed to the bone but be elevated off the bone surface by inserting two suitable spacers before plate application. However, the gap between the plate and the bone should not be greater than 3 mm as this may place undue stress on the screw and cause failure. Standard locking screws should not be used in same fracture segment where MotionLoc screws are installed as this may lead to a stress riser and potential failure to increase interfragmentary movement. Dynamic Locking Screws may be used in the metaphysis as well as in the diaphysis.

tight the plate supports a part of the load and the bone cortex tends to atrophy from disuse. It turns osteopenic and becomes weaker than the normal bone. The changes occur primarily directly beneath the plate. This is the so-called 'stress protection' phenomenon. Re-fracture is therefore most likely in the bone immediately adjacent to the edge of a plate (Fig. 4.57A–C); this is the result of stress concentration and the osteopenic changes. Stress protection is manifested by an increase in the diameter of the medullary cavity.

Another reason for plate removal is the possibility of corrosion, either directly or because of fretting between the plate and the underside of screw heads; such an effect is more likely when the implants are made of stainless steel. If a locked plate is not shaped to fit the local structures, it may become prominent in an area that has least amount of subcutaneous fat and can cause pain and discomfort and require its removal. Removing a plate before complete fracture consolidation, increases the rate of re-fracture and this can be avoided by preventing unnecessary disruption of vascular supply to the bone and delaying removal till its re-establishment; waiting for consolidation of fracture and remodelling; and by limiting intensity of physical activity for 16 weeks after plate removal, when the screw holes cease to behave as stress risers. In the upper limb, a metallic implant can be left in place. Removal should be considered in the presence of inflammatory reactions or if the implants bother the patient mechanically (Fig. 4.57D). Plate removal from the humerus may jeopardize the radial nerve and should only be undertaken if significant clinical symptoms or complications are present. A major concern in removal of forearm plates is possibility of injury to superficial radial or to interosseous nerves; a 12% incidence has been reported; their frequency is inversely proportional to surgeon's experience. Forearm plate removal carries the highest overall complication rate at 40%. Another study found re-fracture rates of up to 20% depending on the type of plate that was initially used, with removal of narrow large fragment plate having the worst prognosis.[51] In the lower limb a plate should be removed; however, isolated screws may be left permanently. In elderly patients, asymptomatic implants in the upper and lower limbs are usually left in place.

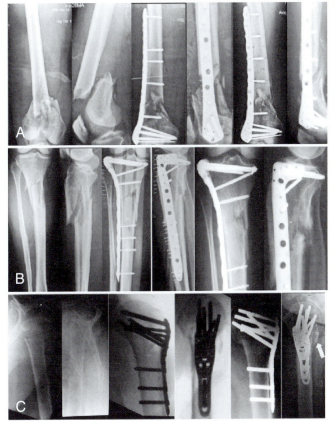

FIGURE 4.56

MotionLoc[50] screws in clinical use; these are deployed only in the shaft of the bone—(**A**) in distal femur, (**B**) in proximal tibia. Clinical example of use of Dynamic Locking Screws[49] (**C**), these are used in shaft and metaphyseal regions.

It is difficult to tell if a fracture has healed when held under rigid compression. A plate may be removed after an arbitrary period based on clinical judgment and experience. The guidelines cited in Table 4.4 for removal of plates are widely accepted.

Bone re-fracture following removal of a plate is a recognized possibility, unless steps are taken to limit weight bearing for a reasonable time. Plate-induced osteopenia can predispose the bone to re-fracture after plate removal as remodelling of the cortices during healing leads to a bone of lower strength. Other discontinuities are also present because of removal of screws. Discontinuous structures under load give rise to concentrations of stress (see page 15). The presence of drill holes weakens the bone; the weakening effect of the holes is much greater than would be expected. The resistance to

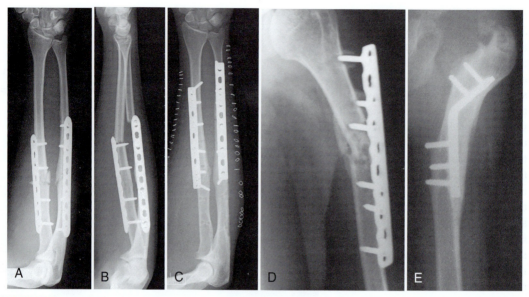

FIGURE 4.57

(A) Both fractures of the forearm bones were fixed with locking plates. (B) Thirty-two months later during a soccer match a fall on outstretched arm caused refracture of both bones through 'stress-risers', the distal screw holes in both the bones. (C) New fractures were fixed with conventional plates. (D) Discomfort and prominence of the plate under the deltoid prompted its removal. (E) In children exuberant callus formation is common; plate removal at times is a formidable task.

Table 4.4 Timing of Plate Removal. Recommendations for Removal of Plates in the Lower Limb

Bone/Fracture	Time After Implantation in Months
Malleolar fractures	8—12
The tibial pilon	12—18
The tibial shaft	12—18
The tibial head	12—18
The femoral condyles	12—24
The femoral shaft:	
Single plate	24–36
Double plate	From month 18, in two steps (interval 6 months)
Pertrochanteric and femoral neck fractures	12–18
Upper extremity	Optional
Shaft of radius/ulna	24–28
Distal radius	8–12
Metacarpals	4–6

torsional loading is reduced by 50%. The capacity of bone to absorb energy to prevent fracture is reduced to 25% of normal. The resistance to bending loads is similarly reduced. Following plate removal, the bone should be protected from excessive stress until the post-healing cortical osteopenia gradually disappears as the bone takes the total load of the limb and remodelling of the bone occurs to normal dimensions. Once the screw holes are filled by radiolucent bone, they stop being a weak spot. Although in experimental animals the screw holes fill up in about 8 weeks, it is customary to delay strenuous activity after plate removal in humans for a period up to 16 weeks.

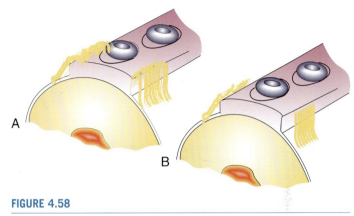

FIGURE 4.58

(**A**) Bone grows over the edges of plate. (**B**). Remove only minimum required amount because extensive removal weakens the bone.

There is more need for protection of the patient at the time of plate removal than after plating because (a) the re-fracture strength of the bone is less than the initial plated bone strength and (b) the injury is no longer acute and therefore the functional level must be tempered by planned treatment, rather than the patient's symptoms. It takes a long time before the bone recovers from the weakening effects of plate removal. Advanced age of the patient and weight bearing bones are two factors that delay recovery. Since muscle actions associated with physiotherapy or functional activities load the bones enhancing blood supply, the recovery phase may extend from 3–4 months. This recovery can be sufficient for an unprotected return to the activities of daily living.

Bone growth over the plates and into the holes and screws cause difficulty in implant removal (Fig. 4.58). Titanium implants in particular are associated with a marked bone in-growth. Plate removal of a doubly plated fracture should be staged over a time to reduce the risk of re-fracture. The removal should be done at two operations, 4–6 months apart, with cancellous bone grafting recommended at each operation.

Removal of LIFP

Compared with conventional plates, removal of angle stable locked plates may be more difficult as the callus may grow into the plate holes. Implant removal may require longer skin incision than the initial surgery. The locking screws made of titanium are hard to remove because cold welding may take place between the screw and plate (Fig. 4.59A–D).

Fan Blade Effect

Removal of last locking screw or tightening of first inserted locking screw may rotate the plate like a blade of an electric fan (Fig. 4.59E and F). To avoid damage to the surrounding soft tissue the opposite end of the plate must be steadied with a Kirschner wire, a screw or a drill bit. Another strategy is first to loosen all the screws and then remove them one by one.

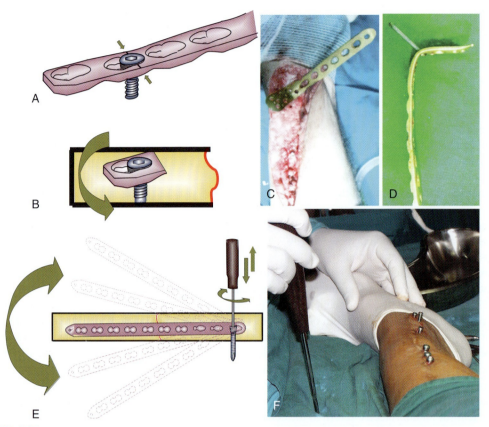

FIGURE 4.59

(**A**) Each side of a locking plate is cut to remove a cold-welded screw. (**B**) A plate is transversely cut around the cold-welded screw; soft tissues are protected with saline-soaked gauze and constant irrigation while suction removes the metal debris. The plate segment is held in pliers and turned round to remove the screw. (**C**) All the screws were removed from the plate except one that had jammed (cold welded). The plate was bent to be used as a handle and the entire plate was rotated to unscrew the jammed screw from the bone. (**D**) The jammed screw and the bent plate (**E**) The plate may swing like an electric fan's blades while removing the last or inserting the first locked screw. Loosening and leaving a screw halfway in the hole in the distal fragment stalls this effect.[53] (**F**) another tactic is first to loosen all the screws then remove one by one.

REGIONAL CONSIDERATIONS

Preshaped Plates

Since the era of modern plating began, precontouring (prebending) of a plate, i.e. preoperative or intra-operative bending of a plate to the shape of the bone has been part of surgical acumen. Preshaped plates,[52] ones that are designed and shaped during manufacture to fit a specific anatomical site so that intra-operative contouring of the plate is usually not needed, are natural evolution from the basic bone plates, viz. Sherman, Lane, Lambote and AO.

Currently the MIPO technique is in vogue. It facilitates slipping an implant under the skin through a small incision away from the fracture site and then along a bone surface across the main injury area to fix the fragments. The tactic is very useful when the skin is badly contused; an LIFP or a conventional plate could easily be used without risking a skin breakdown. A preshaped plate is a welcome design for this new technique.

Characteristics of a preshaped plate are that the geometry matches the anatomy of the patient with a little or no bending. Depending upon the need, screw holes are strategically deployed to obtain maximum purchase. All the biomechanical needs of the region are addressed at the designing stage. A preshaped plate not only reduces operation room time spent in contouring a plate but also minimizes soft-tissue irritation and soft tissue dissection. Unlike straight plates, a preshaped plate acts as guide or template for restoring the patient's original anatomy when reconstructing a highly comminuted fracture, a malunion or a non-union. Preshaped plates for epi-metaphyseal fracture are thinner than others. Therefore, have less interference with soft tissues. Thinner plates allow the use of screws of smaller size, in divergent or convergent pattern with guiding blocks for accuracy; these are most useful near a joint. Nearly all of preshaped plates are locking internal fixator plates. Preshaped plates are gaining popularity and are available for almost all body regions.

The Femur

Subtrochanteric Fracture

Plating has a place in the treatment of subtrochanteric femur fractures. The indications for plating of some subtrochanteric fractures are as follows:

1. Fractures with trochanteric extension. Plate fixation prevents varus malalignment seen with the extended fracture patterns treated by intramedullary nailing.
2. Reverse obliquity fracture. A lateral plate when connected to the distal fragment reduces the reverse obliquity to its anatomic location and prevents varus malalignment; it is difficult to control varus by intramedullary nailing.
3. Subtrochanteric fractures associated with indwelling intramedullary hardware, screws from previous surgery or total joint components blocking the femoral canal are indications for plating.

A 95° condylar plate or its condylar compression screw (CCS) variant are fine implants to manage these difficult fractures. Similarly, use of anatomically preshaped locking internal fixator plate produces excellent alignment in the sagittal plane (Fig. 4.60); plate does not address the coronal plane alignment, i.e. rotation and shortening; attention to details is necessary to achieve correct alignment. 'Biologic plating', i.e. indirect reduction and MIPO, is technique of choice to achieve relatively stable fixation; this kind of fixation does not reduce all of the fragments but does obtain early union; full weight bearing is delayed for the first 6–8 weeks.

Femoral Shaft

Plating is an excellent method of treating fractures of the femoral shaft in patients under 60 years of age. Fractures of the shaft of the femur at all levels may be treated by plating but it is specially indicated for those situated at and distal to the junction of the middle and lower third of the shaft.

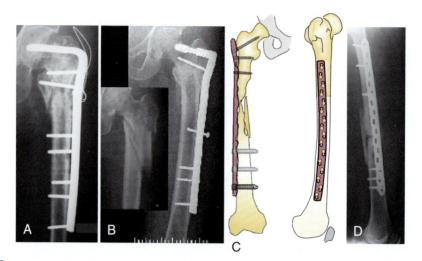

FIGURE 4.60

Plate fixation of subtrochanteric fracture. **(A)** 95° condylar plate. **(B)** Condylar compression screw with long plate. **(C)** Sketch of a preshaped LIFP. **(D)** Sketch and radiograph of preshaped and side specific plate for diaphyseal fracture. All the constructs create relative stability at the fracture site.

There are indications for plating shaft of femur. Minimal invasive tactics and LIFP have changed the perspective of plate fixation of fracture of shaft of femur. Open reduction and internal fixation with plate has been transformed to closed extramedullary plating technique, which is comparable to a closed intramedullary nailing. Intramedullary nailing is indeed the treatment of choice but there are many occasions when plating is indicated.[53] Some instances are as follows:

- Multiple injured patient with chest injury
- Ipsilateral shaft and femoral neck fracture
- Fracture shaft of femur in adolescence
- Associated neurovascular injury
- Delayed case that requires more dissection to align the canal
- Use of fracture table is unsuitable, e.g. associated pelvic and acetabular fractures, unstable spine, ipsilateral tibia fracture
- Very narrow or deformed medullary canal
- Some non-unions
- Associate abdominal injury; plating to follow emergent laparotomy
- Periprosthetic fracture
- Lack of equipment for intramedullary nailing
- Non-availability of image intensifier
- As an alternative to external fixation for damage control

A plate is applied on the tension (lateral) side of the femur. A broad heavy-duty plate, either a conventional type or a locking variety, is used and at least seven cortices proximal and distal to the limits of fracture are engaged. Preshaped plates with anterior bowing to match that of the shaft are best suited for plating; accurate positioning of a long straight plate is not easy. Preshaped femoral plate has a curvature that adapts to the anterior bow of the femoral shaft and hence it is side specific (Fig. 4.60D).

Distal Femur

A CCS or a 95° angled blade plate (ABP) has been the device of choice as it maintains reduction of the segments that are usually intra-articular (see Fig. 4.9). The implant firmly fixes the metaphysis to the shaft and helps early mobilization.

The two prevalent methods of inserting the condylar screw/blade plate at two-third and one-third junction of the lateral condyle produce a degree of external rotation because the plate rotates over the outer surface of femoral shaft as the placement screws are tightened. This rotation is minimized if the plate is inserted at three-fourth–one-fourth junction (Fig. 4.61).[54]

Additional advantages of method 3/4–1/4 are that its use does not require a patellofemoral Kirschner wire. Insertion of condylar screw perpendicular to the bone is sufficient for accurate placement. There is no risk of penetration of the condylar screw within the intercondylar fossa. Whenever a longer plate is required, it automatically aligns with the femoral shaft whereas in the previous methods it would lead to some anterior prominence of the plate due the curvature of the lower end of femur (Fig. 4.62).

In clinical practice, the ABP and CCS have the same indications in the treatment of fractures of distal femur and the results obtained are equivalent even in the porotic bone (Fig. 4.63 A and B). Whether to use a blade plate or a screw plate is often debated. The fact that a technique is difficult to master is not a good argument if results are better when the technique is properly mastered. Recent biomechanical assessment concludes that the width and U-profile of the ABP does not offer any better rotational stability of the condylar block than CCS.[55] Contrary to the belief CCS provides superior purchase and rotational stability than ABP, though the difference in measurements

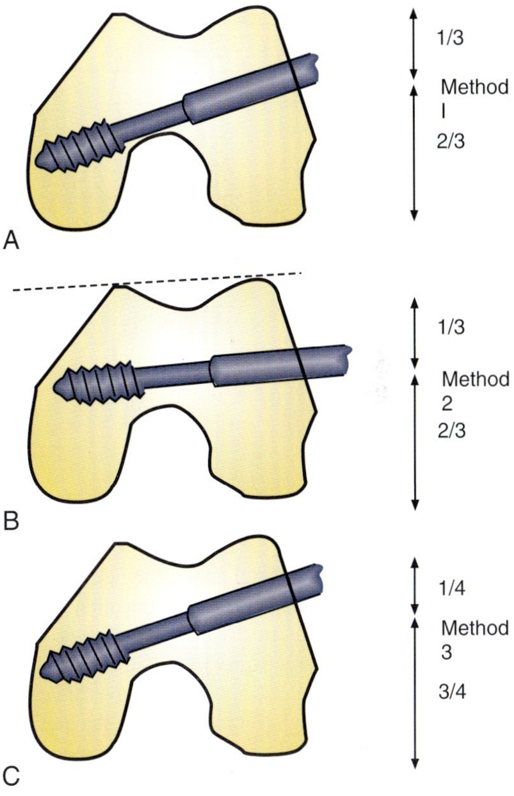

FIGURE 4.61

Three methods of condylar screw insertion. In the first two, the screw is inserted by 1/3–2/3 protocol. (**A**) Method 1: screw is inserted at right angle to the lateral surface of the condyle. The condyle may externally rotate through a range of 7.3–15.7°. The screw can damage the origin of anterior cruciate ligament as it traverses the intercondylar notch. (**B**) Method 2: screw is passed parallel to the line passing touching the uppermost points of the condyles. The condyles may internally rotate but to a lesser degree. A K-wire is usually placed in the joint to visualize the level of condyles. (**C**) Method 3: Screw is inserted by 1/4–3/4 protocol. Screw is passed at right angles to lateral surface of the condyle. External rotation is minimal. This is the recommended method now.[54]

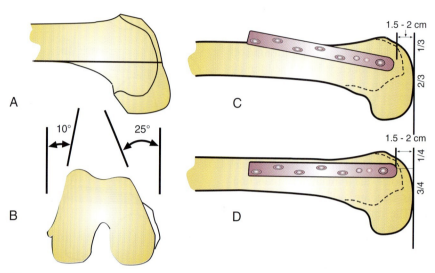

FIGURE 4.62

(**A**) Lateral projection of distal femur. Line drawn along the posterior cortex divides the condyles in two halves; the anterior half of the condyle is a continuation of the femoral shaft, while the posterior half appears attached to the posterior cortex. (**B**) The distal femur is trapezoidal. It is narrow anteriorly and broader posteriorly; the length of screw should be chosen with this fact in mind. (**C**) If a long plate is required for fixation of a supracondylar fracture, e.g. fractures not seen on radiographs are encountered, the curvature of femur might cause the plate to overhang in the mid-thigh if it is applied by the prevailing methods (protocol 1/3–2/3, methods 1 and 2). (**D**) When the plate is applied near the anterior aspect (protocol 1/4–3/4, method 3), a longer plate is practically aligned with long axis of the shaft.[55] A condylar plate must be placed into the anterior half of the condyles to allow the curved proximal segment of the plate to lie on the femoral shaft.[54]

is statistically insignificant. This is probably due to good purchase of the large sliding screw in the condyles and the compression effect. To place a CCS, correct positioning is mandatory in frontal and transverse plane but there is some freedom in sagittal plane. Use of a drill bit in place of a chisel is less likely to disturb the reduction. If required, only the broken plate of CCS may be replaced to regain stability. A Lag screw through the distal most round hole of is mandatory for stability in both the implants; its omission or removal inflicts instability. However, for a fracture of femoral condyle with a petite distal fragment, which may even be shorter than 4 cm, the use of ABP is recommended. ABP's U-shaped blade gives better rotational stability than CCS.

In conclusion, from technical and mechanical view point, the CCS is the preferred implant to fix the distal condylar segment even in porotic bone, provided the distal block is not shorter than 4 cm.

The Condylar Plate

Condylar locking internal fixator plate for fixation of distal femur fractures is the contemporary implant and has largely replaced intramedullary nails, blade plates and condylar screws. The plate offers angular stable screw placement for short, comminuted or osteoporotic distal femoral articular fractures, which is an improvement over earlier implants (Fig. 4.63C).

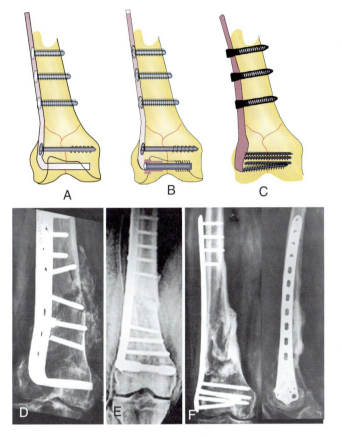

FIGURE 4.63
(A) Properties of 95° angled blade plate (95-ABP) and condylar cancellous screw (CCS) are identical even in the osteoprotic bone. The width and 'U' profile of the 95-ABP does not provide superior rotational control. (B) Contrary to the belief, CCS provides superior rotational stability though statistically insignificant. It has good purchase due to size of its threads and produces a compression effect, though statistically insignificant. In both the implants a lag screw through the plate is mandatory for stability: absence of lag screw inflicts instability. (C) The condylar plate with locking screw capability and integrated holes is biomechanically superior to a conventional condylar buttress plate, 95° angled blade plate, a condylar cancellous screw and a retrograde nail. Preshaped to fit the local anatomy, longer plates are preferred to the short ones. Radiographs showing fixation of distal third of femur using (D) 95° condylar plate (E) 95° condylar compression screw. (F) Locking condylar plate; lateral view shows how a preshaped plate snugly fits the femoral curvature.

The plate is designed for porotic, comminuted fractures, intra-articular and periarticular fractures of distal femur. A fixed or variable angle locked screw option allows for stable fixation of periprosthetic fractures and are adaptable to all total knee designs, including ones with a closed box or a stem.

It may be straight or curved with integrated plate holes. Curved plates are preshaped to reflect the anterior convexity (radius of curvature 1100 mm) of the femur and come in right and left versions. The design of the plate's undersurface ensures reduced contact with the bone surface and inflicts minimal periosteal injury. Locking screws in the head of the plate form a stable angular screw-plate construct. Integrated holes in the shaft area permit use of either standard or locked screw. The plate may be inserted either through a conventional open technique or a minimally invasive incision with percutaneous screw placement.

Biomechanical studies have compared function of locking condylar buttress plate to an unlocked condylar buttress plate, 95° ABP, a retrograde nail and a dynamic condylar screw.[54] The locking femoral buttress plate was biomechanically superior in its ability to resist applied loads and had less irreversible deformation.[56] These biomechanical studies demonstrate that a locking plate provides enhanced stability.[57] All the three devices are in popular use. Figure 4.63D–F shows their clinical application.

The Tibia

Plates are generally passed percutaneously either from proximal or distal end and blocking K-wire technique[58] facilitates freehand, accurate and percutaneous insertion of a plate in fixation (Fig. 4.64). The technique eliminates the need of a specialized jig. Often used in the distal tibia, a fracture is reduced with the assistance of an EF or a femoral distractor. A 2-cm long vertical incision is made distal to the medial malleolus and a full-thickness, subperiosteal flap is created using a tunneller or a periosteal elevator.

Under fluoroscopic guidance, terminally threaded, 1.6 mm K-wires are placed percutaneously in the bone at right angles to the long and short axes of the plate, both anteriorly and posteriorly, in relation to plate's desired final position; Viewing under image intensifier, 1.6 mm K-wires with threaded end are inserted percutaneously at the bone edge in relation to plate's desired final position angles; care is taken to avoid injury to saphenous vein and nerve. The previously inserted 'blocking' K-wires guide

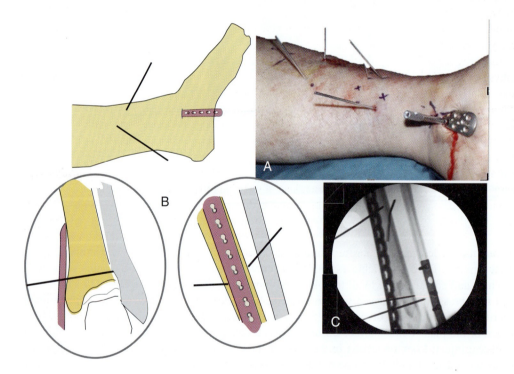

FIGURE 4.64

The blocking K-wires ensure anatomic accuracy of plate placement, a limiting feature of percutaneous plating technique particularly in the absence of a plate-specific jig. The technique is part of the surgical protocol utilizing temporary external fixation to maintain reduction and is directed at the preservation of the periarticular soft tissues of the tibia. Use of K-wires is a familiar procedure to fracture surgeons. **(A)** Sketch and clinical photograph of placement of blocking K-wires. **(B)** Sketches showing two views of K-wires guiding the plate. **(C)** Image intensifier snap-shot during surgery.

the plate to precise position and prevent its deflection by soft tissues. Fluoroscopy time and radiation exposure is reduced; however, plate placement and final fracture reduction is confirmed by fluoroscopy. The blocking K-wire technique is also applicable to treatment of tibial plateau fractures.

Plating is absolutely indicated for the tibial shaft fractures associated with a displaced intra-articular fracture of the knee and the ankle.

Proximal Tibia

The tibial plateau fracture requires accurate open reduction and fixation. Buttress plating is almost always necessary to support epiphyseal–metaphyseal fragments. Indirect reduction techniques are used to plate these fractures.

MIPO has been advocated for low-energy as well as high-energy fractures. Simple split and split-depression fractures confined to the lateral plateau are dealt through a single-incision anterolateral approach; a straight incision is made from the anterolateral joint line distally to 6–8 cm. A midline incision also allows good access to the medial and lateral condyles. Fractures of medial condyle with posterior displacement are approached by dual or posterior–medial incisions. Use of percutaneous reduction techniques, such as the application of femoral distractors, Kirschner-wire joysticks, and percutaneously applied reduction forceps minimize soft-tissue injury as the major condylar fragments are manipulated.

Laterally based locking plates provide adequate stability in the presence of metaphyseal or metadiaphyseal comminution. Additional interfragmentary screws may be necessary to prevent secondary loss of reduction because locked plates do not apply compression. When the condylar fragments are not comminuted and are well reduced, a laterally based locking plate alone can control the medial condyle. Anatomical cortical contact between the fracture fragments is essential for effective fixation only from the lateral side; when such a contact is in doubt an additional medial approach is made to apply a small locking plate or an antiglide plate. Use of only laterally based locking plate may not control subsidence and malalignment of the intercondylar fracture, more so when applied to a fracture pattern that consists of comminution, with buckling of the cortex on one side and gapping of the fracture or a tension failure on the opposite side; the fracture pattern is prognostic of late malalignment.[59]

The lateral tibial condyle is located slightly higher than the medial joint surface. The plate on the lateral side should be placed at a lower level to avoid damage to medial joint surface by screw penetration (Fig. 4.65).

Plating is employed to fix fractures of the tibial diaphysis. Narrow plates are used; heavy-duty broad plates are never used. Plates are usually applied on the subcutaneous surface of the tibia, mainly for the operator's convenience. Plates may also be applied on the lateral surface. It is essential to engage six cortices on either side of the fracture.

To compress a tibial diaphyseal fracture, eccentric insertion of a screw on each side of the fracture is recommended. Placement of a single screw in each fragment may act as a fulcrum around which the

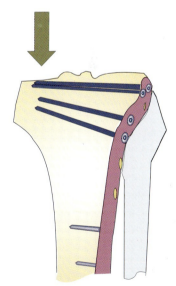

FIGURE 4.65

Medial joint surface is at risk of being penetrated by locking screws inserted just below the lateral joint surface; lateral plate should be placed at lower level to avoid the discomfiture.

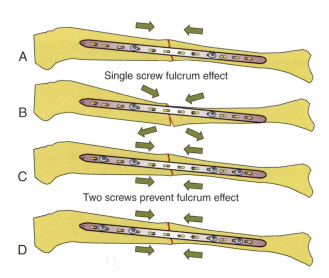

FIGURE 4.66

(A) Single screw in each fragment is a typical practice. (B) When tightened a fulcrum effect may be produced. (C) To avoid the fulcrum effect, prior to compression, two screws are inserted in eccentric position in each fragment. (D) Two screwdrivers, one on each side of the fragment are used at the same time to compress the fracture from both sides. This technique is consistent with biological plating as it limits the extent of surgical exposure and avoids use of plate holding forceps: both factors help in maintaining bone vitality.[60]

fragments can rotate if the plate is placed in a too anterior or too posterior position or there is comminution of either cortex (Fig. 4.66A and B). A simple method circumvents fulcrum effect; instead of one, two eccentric screws are inserted in each fragment, prior to compression. Two screwdrivers are used at the same time to compress the fracture from both sides (Fig. 4.66C and D). This technique is consistent with biological plating as it limits the extent of surgical exposure and avoids use of plate holding forceps: both factors help in maintaining bone vitality.

Management of tibial shaft fractures by minimally invasive surgery and a relatively stable fixation provides excellent results. When plating is indicated, bridge plating method is often used. Bridge plating draws on the locking plate as an internal, extramedullary splint, fixed to proximal and distal intact fragments. The intermediate fracture zone is left untouched, bypassed by the plate. Anatomical reduction of comminuted fragments is not necessary. Direct exposure of these fragments damages their soft-tissue attachments that provide blood supply as well as aid in their realignment as length is restored. As and when soft-tissue attachments are preserved, healing is predictable. Correction of length, rotation and axial alignment of the main shaft fragments can usually be achieved indirectly, using traction and soft-tissue tension. Relative stability at fracture site, provided by the bridging plate, supports indirect healing (callus formation).[61]

In general, when there is medial comminution and severe soft tissue injury, it is prudent to use a locking plate. The plate is introduced subcutaneously from proximal or distal incisions, leaving the skin intact over the fracture area. Stab incisions are made with caution to avoid damage to great saphenous vein and saphenous nerve.

Tibial Locked Internal Fixator Plate

LIFP metaphyseal plate for lower end of the tibia (LCP tibial plate[27]; Fig. 4.67) is precontoured to meet the shape and thickness requirement of the area and mode of application. Its bullet tip enables easier application of a minimally invasive surgical technique. The thinned plate profile, especially designed for the distal end, provides easy contouring of the plate and takes the peculiarities of the metaphyseal

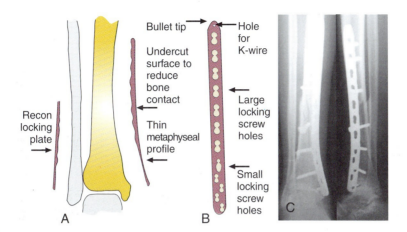

FIGURE 4.67

(A) Locked internal fixator metaphyseal plates for lower end of the tibia and fibula. (B) Preshaped plate has a bullet tip at one end for easy insertion and its distal thinned plate profile facilitates contouring. Assortment of holes has variegated functions.[27] (C) Radiogram showing fixation of fracture of distal third of tibia with a preshpaed plate.

area into account. The dense net of integrated holes in the thinned plate area of the distal end covering the malleolar region allows a closer insertion of the screws and therefore, provides a higher purchase with a better stability. The integrated holes provide a choice of dynamic compression and angular stability in one implant. The angulation (11°) of the two outermost hole units towards the centre of thinned plate area allow a closer juxta-articular plate placement. A single smaller hole is intended for temporary fixation with a K-wire. The undercuts on the surface abutting bone face maintain good vascularization of the periosteum. Plates with similar design are available for fractures in the metaphyseal areas that reach into proximal tibia, the proximal and distal shat of the humerus, fibula and proximal and distal radius as well as ulna.

The Calcaneus

LIFP for calcaneus has a low profile design to facilitate its placement on the lateral side of the heel where the soft tissue cover is tenuous (Fig. 4.68). The plates and screws are made of titanium and are self-tapping. The locking mechanism in uniaxially locked screws has a non-conically shaped complete thread at the screw holes; a plate with polyaxially locking screws is also available.

The Humerus

The average cortical thickness of the humerus shaft is a useful guide to decide adequacy of the bone strength for purchase of conventional screws and plate in fracture fixation. Average cortical thickness of 4 mm or more is essential for secure plate-screw fixation; lesser values allude to its possible failure (Fig. 4.69). To calculate the average cortical thickness, two parallel lines are drawn. The first line is drawn where the two cortices of proximal humerus become parallel; the second line is drawn 20 mm distally. The thickness of cortical bone is measured at four cortices and average value is arrived at.

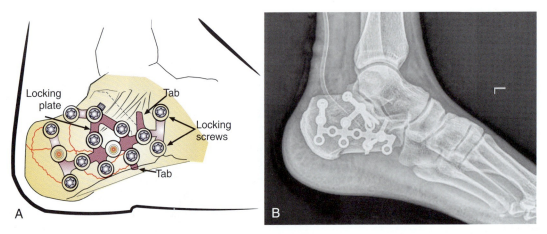

FIGURE 4.68

(A) Line sketch of a calcaneus locking plate.[62] After anatomical reduction, the interlocking plate is modeled and applied to the calcaneal wall. The tab over the calcaneal neck is precisely bowed with special forceps to keep the anterior process fragment in the anatomical position. The second tab is also bowed towards the bone, to keep a plantar triangular fragment in position. Six to seven screws are usually placed into the calcaneal bone: Two to three from the subthalamic area into the sustentaculum. The very first is a 3.5-mm conventional screw which is inserted as a compression screw to eliminate any gap in the subtalar joint. The second screw fixes the lateral part of the posterior facet. Two locking screws are then inserted into the anterior process fragment close to the calcaneocuboidal joint. Finally, two screws are inserted into the tuberosity fragment far dorsally.[63] (B) Radiogram showing fixation of calcaneus fracture.

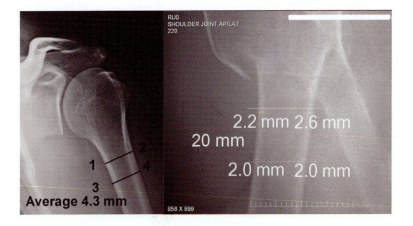

FIGURE 4.69

Cortical thickness of ≥4 mm is considered essential for adequate screw purchase of conventional screw-plate system. Locking internal fixation plate is an option to fix a fracture with cortical thickness of ≤ 4 mm.[64]

The Proximal Humerus

Fracture fixation using locked plate has become an established treatment for displaced fractures of proximal Humerus as it has shown better outcome and biomechanical superiority even in porotic bone. The fixed-angle screws act as oblique struts to support the humeral head fragment and resist varus displacement. Precontoured and anatomically shaped plate has multiple holes in the section abutting the head (Fig. 4.70). These locking screw holes are divergently directed in a fixed trajectory to improve the fixation. The screws are directed at various angles in the head, ascending and crossing to achieve purchase in the areas of highest bone density in the posterior, medial and cranial zones of the humeral head to minimize pull-out; biomechanical advantages of crossing head are well recognized (see page 96). Inferomedial screws are very important, as mechanical failures are likely when these are not properly positioned. Plates also have several holes of 2 mm diameter at the proximal end through which sutures are passed to repair and stabilize the rotator cuff. The blunt-ended screws are advantageous compared with the pointed screws in the prevention of glenoid erosions in case of screw perforations. Newer designs allow positioning according to surgeon preference within a 40° arc in the humeral head. A prospective randomized clinical observational study has concluded that there is no advantage of polyaxiality over the well-chosen fixed trajectories; most of the surgeons select the same path for the polyaxial screws as previously present in the fixed-angle plate. Moreover, it is likely that the screws may be placed in another directions into a hollow, osteopenic zone and do not help in maintaining the reduction; proper reduction and fixation of fracture is what matters when adequate number of long-enough screws are used.

Shaft of Humerus

The advantage of early mobilization supports surgical stabilization of humeral shaft fractures in principle. The literature supports plate osteosynthesis as both the safest and biomechanically superior method of fixation for the acute diaphyseal fracture.[67] When indicated, a broad heavy-duty plate is used for a normal bone; for most adults the thickness should be >3.5 mm (a large-fragment plate); a narrow plate is used only when the humerus is very thin (Fig. 4.71). In porotic bone locked screws offer better purchase and an LIFP is used. The plate is usually placed on the dorsal surface of the humerus but can also be placed on the volar side; dorsal incisions are cosmetically more acceptable. Screws should engage a minimum of six cortices per main fragment.[68]

Distal Humerus

Kirschner-wire fixation alone does not provide required stability to treat bicolumnar distal humeral fractures. In addition, postoperative elbow immobilization of 3–4 weeks leads to unacceptable stiffness. Application of two plates provides adequate stability to obtain bony healing and early mobilization; there is disagreement on their preferred location.

Orthogonal Plating

Orthogonal or 90–90 plating or perpendicular plating means placing one plate on the medial column of the distal humerus and the other plate along the posterolateral aspect of the lateral column of humerus (Fig. 4.71D). Use of two plates, one on each column produced enough stability to commence

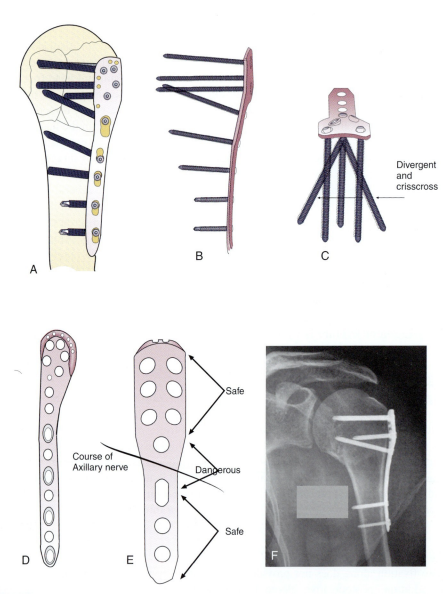

FIGURE 4.70

(**A**) The Proximal Humerus Locking Plate[65] (PHLP) is contoured to the anatomy of the lateral aspect of the proximal part of the humerus and works as an internal fixator by angular stability. The screw arrangement of the locking screws in the humeral head is three-dimensional. Additional smaller holes are used for fixation of sutures or wires, allowing reattachment of the greater or lesser tuberosities in comminuted fractures to neutralize the tension forces of the rotator cuff muscles. (**B**) Profile of PHLP showing angulation of the locking screw. (**C**) End-on view of the same plate showing crossing of the locking screws. (**D**) Periarticular proximal lateral humeral locking plate®.[50] (**E**) SuturePlate®[66] and schema showing danger zone for insertion of locked screws in minimally invasive surgery; Axillary nerve is at risk in this region. Radiograph of proximal humerus showing fracture fixation with a locked preshaped plate.

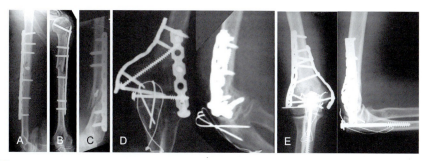

FIGURE 4.71

Radiographs showing plating of humeral shaft. **(A)** Posterior placement. **(B)** Anterolateral placement. **(C)** LIFP near the epiphysis Anteroposterior and lateral views of elbows treated with **(D)** Orthogonal (90°–90°) plating. **(E)** Parallel plating of distal humeral fracture.

immediate movements of the joint and achieve bony healing.[69] Fixation of the bone fragments relies on the stability of the hardware construct rather than on screw purchase in the bone.

Parallel Plating

Fixation failure at supracondylar level because of suboptimal anchorage of the articular fragments to the shaft caused by the limited number and inadequate length of screws that can be placed in the distal fragments led to development of parallel plating.[70] The technique links both columns of the distal humerus, to provide the necessary structural stability for fracture healing.

The interdigitation of the distal screws is like a keystone of an arch, being the structural link necessary for adequate fixation. Thus, fixation of the bone fragments relies on the stability of the hardware construct rather than on screw purchase in the bone (Fig. 4.71E). The biomechanical analysis of these constructs showed that in good quality bone the choice of implant or type of construct did not matter. When bone-mineral density was low (<420 mg/cm^3) both constructs in locking plates provided superior resistance against screw loosening compared with the non-locking conventional reconstruction plates. The orthogonal system compared to the parallel placement was significantly more stable in compression and external rotation and showed higher resistance to axial plastic deformation; locked plates are recommended for comminuted and osteoporotic bones.

The Radius and Ulna

Fractures of Radial Head

Two- to four-fragment fracture of radial head may be reconstructed using thin locked plate; 2.0-mm locking plate fixation offers adequate stability and are non-irritant to soft tissue in their superficial location.[71] Crossed screws and triangulation principles are utilized in these plates (Fig. 4.72); locked screws enhance the triangulation effect (see Fig. 3.26).

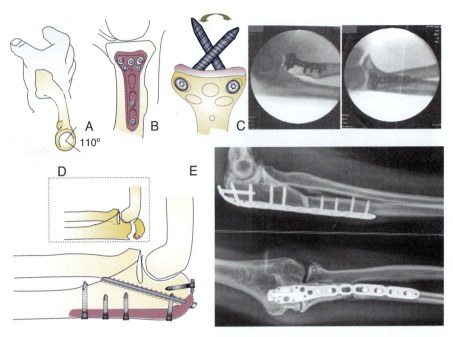

FIGURE 4.72

(**A**) The radial head plate fits within the 'safe zone' of the radial head, which is the area between 1 O'clock and 4 O'clock on the clock face. (**B**) The plate has multiple screw holes in two rows to capture and hold the radial head fragments. The three holes in the longitudinal section of T offer strong distal purchase; radiographs showing application of the plate (**C**) The locked screws holes are designed in crossing pattern to improve their holding power; radiographs showing application of plate to fix a fracture of radial head and neck. (**D**) Hook plate fixation of fracture of olecranon process of the ulna. Inset, the fracture pattern. (**E**) Preshaped plate for olecranon. Plates are side specific to match the ulnar bow.

The Proximal Ulna

The presence of articular surface in the proximal olecranon process dictates only unicortical screw purchase and a locked screw becomes mandatory. Indications for locked plating of proximal ulna include simple and complex extra- and intra-articular olecranon fractures. Pseudoarthrosis of the proximal ulna and repair of the olecranon after osteotomies in distal humerus surgery may also be fixed with locked plating. Plates are usually placed on the dorsal face of the ulna to create a tension-band effect and to achieve high biomechanical stability. Posterior plating is considered to be biomechanically superior to dual plating applied from the medial and lateral aspects.[72] The proximal ulna has a 4° valgus angulation; the plate must be preshaped to accommodate this bend. Preshaped plates for proximal ulna offer an anatomical fit (Fig. 4.72D and E). Several notches in the plate shaft allow the plate to be contoured to the individual anatomy of the bone. Use of axial intramedullary screws in comminuted proximal ulnar fractures is an added advantage; however, the tab for axial screw can be cut off if not required.

Fractures of Diaphysis of the Radius and the Ulna

In plating of diaphyseal fractures of radius and ulna it is essential to maintain length, axial and rotational alignment of both the bones and restore configuration of each bone; encroachment of interosseous space either by a plate or by callous should be avoided; only this will re-establish full pronation and supination (Fig. 4.73). In the middle and upper third of the radius the plate is applied on the dorsal surface of the bone, as this is the tension side. A plate placed on the anterior aspect encroaches on the interosseous space during pronation and limits this important motion. In the upper third it may abut against the coronoid process of the ulna and block the pronation permanently. In the distal third of the radius a plate fits snugly on flat volar surface and has excellent soft tissue coverage. In fixation of ulnar shaft fractures the plate location depends on the fit of the plate to the bone and is often placed on the subcutaneous dorsal surface and rarely on the anterior aspect.

A longer plate is preferred over a shorter one. A transverse fracture may be fixed with a four-hole plate but it is safer to engage a minimum of five cortices on each side of the fracture. In an oblique or comminuted fracture a longer plate with 7–9 holes is preferred. Screws should not be placed closer than 1 cm from the fracture. Locked plates have advantage that plate contouring is not required to maintain the radial bow.

Bone grafts may be added when more than one third of the circumference of the cortex is comminuted. The graft should be placed on the tension side of the bone. After removal of a bone plate there is considerable decrease in the strength of the forearm bones with an increased risk of re-fracture in the event of overloading.

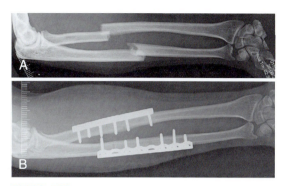

FIGURE 4.73

(**A**) Fracture of upper third of radius and middle third of ulna. (**B**) Open reduction and internal fixation with conventional plates and screws.

Distal Radius

Healthy and active elderly patients are growing in number; they are less likely to accept a malunion as it is associated with pain, stiffness, weak grip strength and carpal instability in a significant percentage of patients; only restoration of normal anatomy after fracture of distal radius can provide optimal function. Common reasons of instability of this fracture are shown in Table 4.5; plating ensures more consistent correction of displacement and maintenance of reduction.

Volar locking plates are preferred over the dorsal ones; two types of volar locking plates are available: Fixed and variable angle. A contoured volar plate for both volar and dorsal displaced fractures of distal radius uses fixed angle technology to get optimum support for the often-problematic distal radius fractures (Fig. 4.74). The vertical arm of the T-plate has holes to accept conventional cortical screws for fixation to the shaft. The transverse arm anatomically fits the volar surface of distal radius, supports marginal fragments and all aspects of the subchondral plate. It has holes in two rows for locked pegs and screws: proximal row is

Table 4.5 Five Predictors of Instability[73]

- Patient over 60 years of age
- Intra-articular fracture
- Dorsal comminution
- Dorsal angulation of more than 20°
- Associated ulnar fracture

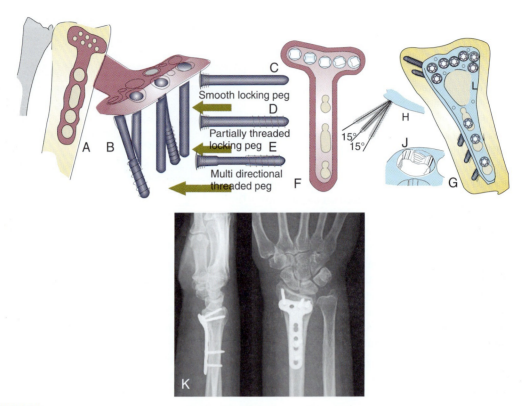

FIGURE 4.74

Locked screw technology makes it possible to use pegs to support fragile dorsal cortex of distal radius. **(A)** Precontoured plate, e.g. DVR®[74] is useful for grossly comminuted distal radius fractures. **(B)** Close up view of the plate shows three types of pegs. Locking pegs facilitate the creation of a scaffold that supports the reduction of the fracture and provide a strong peg to plate interface. **(C)** Blunt tip is forgiving and prevents extensor tendon damage in case of dorsal protrusion. **(D)** Partially threaded pegs help capture dorsal comminuted fragments. **(E)** Multidirectional pegs, with a cone of 20° angulation and threaded locking pegs allow maximum intra-operative flexibility. **(F)** Variable angle LCP® volar extra-articular distal radius plate[27]; variable angle locked screw may be inserted in the cloverleaf shaped holes in the head of the plate. Combi holes in the longitudinal limb allow use of locked screws and offer angular stability in the threaded section, or compression with conventional screws in non-threaded section. **(G)** Variable angle LCP® two column volar distal radius plate[27] two columns allow independent fine countering of a radial and intermediate columns; plate is available in right and left version. **(H)** Screws can be angled anywhere within 30° cone around the central axis of the plate hole. **(J)** Four columns of threads in the variable angle locked hole provide four points of threaded locking between the plate and screw, forming a fixed angle construct at a desired screw angle. The plates are indicated for fixation of complex intra- and extra-articular fractures and osteotomies of the distal radius in adults, skeletally mature adolescents. They are also indicated for fractures in adolescent distal radius such as intra-articular fractures exiting the epiphysis; intra-articular fractures exiting the metaphysis; physeal crush injuries and any injuries which cause growth arrest to the distal radius. **(K)** Radiograph showing a fixed trajectory plate for distal radial fracture; note the deep placement of screw in the styloid.

normally used. All the peg holes on the proximal peg row are always filled because these provide the stability crucial to prevent dorsal re-displacement of the fractures. The proximal row pegs follow anatomical contour and support dorsal aspect of subchondral plate. A peg in the first hole on the ulnar side stabilizes the lunate fossa. Smooth pegs offer the strongest support to subchondral bone and are routinely used but a threaded peg is required to capture dorsal comminuted fragments The distal row of peg holes provides additional support to the central and volar aspect of the subchondral plate and are used when there is extensive comminution or severe osteoporosis. Both, the transverse and vertical limbs have small holes to insert Kirschner wires for temporary fixation and plate alignment. The implant is of value in 'complex articular fracture of the distal radius', i.e. subgroup C3.2 according to the Comprehensive Classification of fractures. Right- and left-sided implants are available in five sizes.

Variable angle locked plates allow an independent trajectory to be selected for each screw or peg (Fig. 4.74F–J). They display all the advantages of fixed-angled locked plates but have the benefit of matching the distal fixation to the variable geometry and surface contour of the distal radius. Polyaxial plates do tend to be thicker and more prominent than the standard locked plate design and differ radically from manufacturer to manufacturer.

Fragment-Specific Implants

Fragment-specific implant is designed to independently stabilize each major fracture fragment (Fig. 4.75). Use of a combination of small implants designed to conform the complex three-dimensional geometry of the distal radius enhances subchondral support and rigidity; implant placement in orthogonal planes also enhances construct rigidity. L-shaped plate is applied on dorsal surface to support lunate fossa fracture.

Fluoroscopic Evaluation of Locked Screw Placement

Image intensification fluoroscopy is an essential adjunct to facilitate application of volar fixation devices in the radius, and all procedures are carried out with fluoroscopic assistance. Standard anteroposterior and lateral views of the distal radius do not provide an accurate view of the articular surface; tangential views are required to assess screw placement into subchondral bone and avoid penetration of articular cartilage.[75]

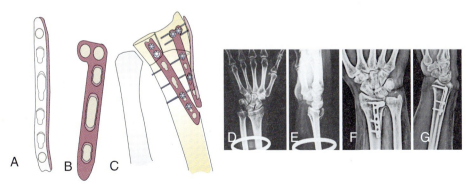

FIGURE 4.75

(**A**) Dedicated radial column plate is preshaped; however additional contouring may be necessary.[27] (**B**) L plate for dorsal application, often used to fix lunate fossa fragment. (**C**) Reconstruction of distal radius using an array of fragment specific plates. (**D and E**) Lunate fossa fracture and dorsal cortex comminution. (**F and G**) Application of L plate on dorsal surface to maintain reduction.

186 CHAPTER 4 BONE PLATES

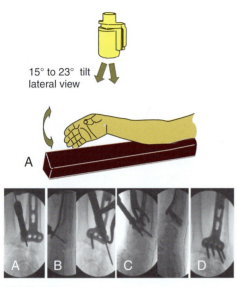

FIGURE 4.76

(**A**) Tilted lateral view provides a clear joint line visualization. Live continuous fluoroscopy is practical way to visualize as it provides an infinite number of tilt lateral views. Fluoroscopic evaluation of screw placement in the lower end of radius in anteroposterior and lateral views. (**B**) Possible position of the Ulnar screw is estimated first. (**C**) Assessment of styloid screw. (**D**) after insertion of all the screws in distal radius.

The distal radial articular surface has an average radial inclination of 22° and an average volar tilt of 14°. A tangential anteroposterior radiograph is obtained by placing the wrist in full pronation and elevating it 10–15° from a horizontal position. A tangential lateral view is obtained by elevating the forearm 22° (Fig. 4.76). These views allow optimal visualization of the articular surface, which ensures correct placement of distal screws or pegs into subchondral bone. Multiple tangential views are required for evaluation of intra-articular screw placement during locked volar plating of the distal radius. Lower angle tilt (15–23°) lateral views are more specific for the ulnar screws, and higher angle views (23–35°) are more specific for the radial screws.[76] Whenever possible the ulnar screws are placed first, using lower angle tilt lateral views to evaluate for intra-articular placement (Fig. 4.76B). The styloid screw may be placed last and can then be evaluated on the PA and tangential PA views. Live continuous fluoroscopy is practical way to visualize, as it provides an infinite number of tilt lateral views.

It is also important to avoid prominent screws that may penetrate dorsally into tendon compartments. In this regard, fluoroscopy is not 100% reliable.[77] It is less sensitive in determining screw position, especially in the ulnar aspect of the dorsal radius, the intermediate column. Printed image intensifier images have limited sensitivity for the diagnosis of dorsal cortical penetration of a volarly inserted screw, particularly among less experienced observers and for the evaluation of the most ulnar screw positions. In addition, a learning curve exists in applying these devices and interpreting fluoroscopic images. Surgeons with less experience are less likely to detect and exchange a dorsally prominent screw. A low threshold for screw exchange is recommended when the possibility of screw prominence exists. Because locked plate devices rely on the plate-screw interface rather than the bone-screw interface for fixation, a technique in which locked screws are not drilled through the dorsal cortex of the radius is recommended. Use of locked screws as opposed to smooth locked pegs for AO C3 intra-articular distal radius fractures, particularly subchondral and in the ulnar side of the lunate fragment, optimizes construct stability.[78] This may shorten the post-surgery treatment period and may reduce the overall treatment costs.

Distraction Plating for Distal Radius Fracture

Distraction plating is an effective treatment for distal radius fractures that are severely comminuted, osteoporotic, and of AO C-2 or C-3 type (Fig. 4.77). A 3.5-mm or 2.4-mm locked plate is placed dorsally from the radial diaphysis to the metacarpal across the radiocarpal joint. It is secured by at least three bicortical locked screws at either end of the plate after reducing the fracture by traction taking care to avoid over distraction at the radiocarpal joint; separation of more than 5 mm causes loss of digital motion; the digits are assessed to confirm full passive flexion to avoid extrinsic extensor tightness. Supplemental fixation with Kirschner wires is used to secure and support the articular fragments. Hand function is encouraged after a week in a short comforting support. Plate is removed after fracture consolidation, at around 4 months and wrist motion is then initiated.[79] Distraction plating is a treatment option and not a panacea for the fixation of distal radius fractures. It appears to provide acceptable results based on the ability to restore functional range of motion and achieve acceptable radiographic outcomes.

The Hand

There is a growing trend amongst hand surgeons to use locking plate for internal fixation of difficult acute fractures and complex delayed and non-unions. locking plates are used for periarticular metacarpal and phalangeal fractures, especially those with metaphyseal comminution, complex multifragmentary diaphyseal fractures with bone loss (i.e. open, combined injuries of the hand), osteopenic and other pathologic fractures, fixation for arthrodeses of the small joints of the hand, non-unions and corrective osteotomies in the hand (Fig. 4.78 and 4.79).

The Clavicle

The traditional complacency regarding diaphyseal clavicle fractures has given way to the realization that displaced comminuted fractures are at risk for non-union and symptomatic malunion.[82] Plating is indicated for acute clavicular fracture in following situations: displaced fractures, bilateral happening, associated with multiple rib fractures, scapula fractures, other lower and upper limb fractures; also in painful non-unions.

The use of LIFP in clavicle fracture fixation has lower complication rates and higher rates of return to work and exercise as compared to use of conventional plates. A few designs of clavicle plate are illustrated (Fig. 4.80). Site-specific preshaped locking plates are advantageous, well-situated and less prominent after healing, leading to lower rates of hardware removal after union. Figure 4.80D and E show placement of a preshaped plate that fits the superior surface of the clavicle; accompanying radiograph shows reduction of displaced clavicle.

The Rib

Non-operative treatment for multiple or flail chest is painful and has many complications like post-traumatic pneumonia, empyema, respiratory insufficiency and long-term pain from fracture malunion and non-union. However, patients who had been treated by plate fixation in acute stage benefited; early experience of application of locking plates and locking intramedullary implants applied by the MIPO technique has shown low morbidity and virtually no mortality. Indications for plate fixation are extensive flail chest, respiratory failure,

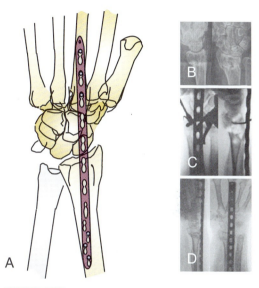

FIGURE 4.77

Distraction plating for a C type fracture of osteoporotic distal radius in elderly patients using a 12-hole, small-fragment locking compression plate placed on the dorsal surface. 3 bicortical screws are placed in the radial diaphysis and 3 bicortical screws are placed into the third metacarpal. Radiographs showing (**B**) comminuted fracture of distal radius. (**C**) Distraction plate in position and articular surface is being reconstructed. (**D**) Healed fracture.

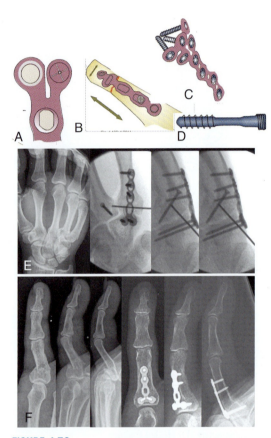

FIGURE 4.78

(A) In Synthes[27] system, the locking screw angle is monoaxial. (B) Plate has polyaxial (i.e. variable angle) locking interfaces. The oblong gliding holes are placed length and breadth wise; the combination permits correction in two planes. (C) Screw holes are offset to reduce screw collision during polyaxial locking within a 20° cone and to avoid fracture propagation with drilling.[80] (D) Cobalt-chrome multidirectional locking screw creates a new path in the plate; narrow shaft matches bending stiffness with 2.5-mm locking crews.[81] (E) A fracture of base of 5th metacarpal is stabilized using locked plate in bridging mode. (F) Fracture of proximal phalanx fixed with a locking plate.

inability to wean from ventilator and thoracotomy for other reasons. Low-profile plates of 1.5 mm thickness are made of titanium alloy for flexibility and strength (Fig. 4.81). The plates are preshaped to fit average rib profile and are color coded to reduce the operative time. Locking and conventional screws are available; conventional screws are used for temporary fixation and are replaced by locking screws at the end of fixation. Locking fixation seems to be advantageous in rib stabilization, as no cases of nonunion, hardware dissociation or hardware migration were observed in a reported series.[84] Figure 4.81D shows clinical photograph of rib plate application.

Paediatric Applications

After introduction of MIPO plates are increasingly being used for paediatric patients in trauma, limb lengthening, non-unions, poor quality of bone, fixation of allograft after segmental resection and epiphysiodesis. Plating, especially use of LIFP is gaining popularity in fixation of femoral diaphyseal fractures, as it keeps away from epiphyseal area. Plating is an alternative to external fixation because it offers greater biomechanical stability, circumvents pin tract infections and there is no re-fracture after removal. Bridge plating technique is a valuable in paediatric patient group. Conventional as well as LIFP may be used for bridge plating; LIFP has advantages of unicortical screw fixation, elimination of the need to measure screw lengths, and curtails surgical time. Plating is valuable for fixation of fractures of metadiaphyseal region; specifically, preshaped LIFP provides superior fracture stability in short fragments, provides improved control of alignment and avoids the susceptible physeal zone. Locked plating is also valuable for periarticular fractures with short segments, such as in the subtrochanteric and supracondylar regions of the femur, where the screws must be so placed as to avoid the physis (Fig. 4.82).

Limb Lengthening and Bone Transport

Submuscular plating has been used for support after distraction osteogenesis (Fig. 4.83), for distraction over a plate, and for distraction over an old implanted plate for post-traumatic limb length discrepancy. Submuscular

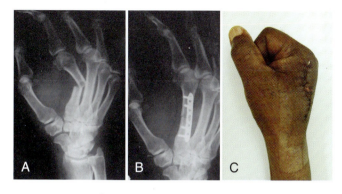

FIGURE 4.79

(A) Radiograph of hand. A transverse fracture of 2nd metacarpal. (B) Fixation with a locking plate. (C) Function on 3rd post-operation day.

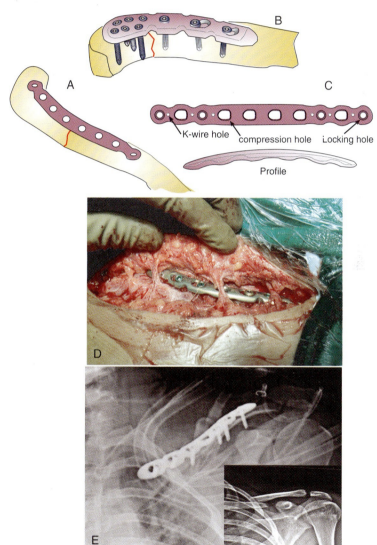

FIGURE 4.80

Three designs of LIFP for clavicle fracture fixation. (A) Plate for medial three fifths of the clavicle shaft.[83] (B) Plate for lateral two fifths of the bone.[35] Both the plates are specific for left and right side. Notches in the plate allow additional plate contouring. Tapered tip helps submuscular plate insertion. (C) Plate design for anterior placement on the clavicle.[83] (D) Preshaped locking plate on superior surface of the clavicle. Note the preserved supraclavicular nerves. (E) Radiograph showing well reduced fracture; inset injury radiograph.

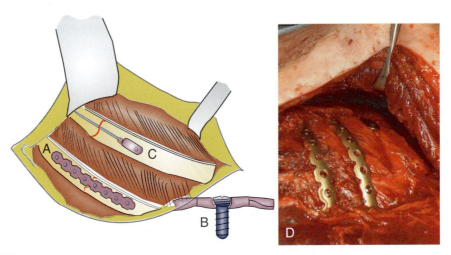

FIGURE 4.81

Rib fracture fixation. (**A**) A locked plate is applied over the rib periosteum; the periosteum of the rib is preserved. A special drill bit with a stop designed to prevent over drilling is used. A screwdriver with self-retaining blade helps in quick fixation. A universal 8-hole plate is often applied. Preshaped rib-specific plates are available for 3–9 ribs; these are color coded for right and left sides. Use of these plates minimizes intra-operative bending. (**B**) Enlarged view of low-profile 1.5-mm thick plate with self-tapping blunt tipped locking screw. (**C**) An intramedullary splint that needs only one screw to be fixed is available in three widths; its application procedure is minimally invasive.[85] (**D**) Intra-operative photograph of a patient showing the rib plates to stabilize multiple fractures.

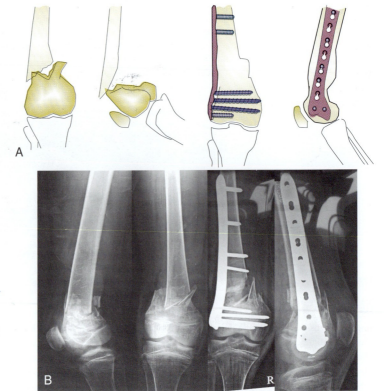

FIGURE 4.82

(**A**) Tracings of radiographs showing supracondylar fracture of femur before and after fixation with a distal femoral locking plate. (**B**) Radiographs of another patient with a distal femoral locking plate in place.

plating over the distraction callus is a new option that permits early removal of the fixator with fewer complications.[87] It shortens EF time to half, precludes bone grating and is easily acceptable by the patient.

Epiphysiodesis[88]

Conventional plates shaped like the figure '8' are used as lateral tension band plates for gradual correction of angular deformities using the guided growth principle (Fig. 4.84); locking plates do not offer any definite advantage.

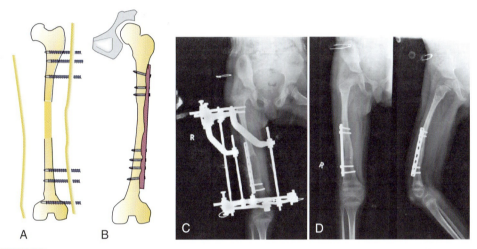

FIGURE 4.83

(**A**) Tracing of radiograph of femoral lengthening conducted with a monolateral external fixator; (**B**) after the target length was achieved, submuscular plating under the fluoroscopic guide was carried to maintain the distracted segment and remove the fixator. (**C**) Radiographs femoral lengthening conducted with a circular fixator (**D**) Anteroposterior and lateral views of femur showing lateral plating to protect the regenerated bone. The plate may also be placed submuscular on medial side when the external fixator is present on the lateral side, and is biomechanically optimal in the presence of femoral defect.[86]

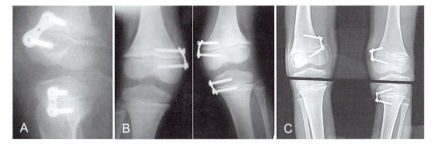

Figure 4.84

(**A**) Conventional plates, known as '8-plates' as they resemble the number. (**B**) '8' plates and screws are applied across the physis to retard growth of half of the epiphysis to achieve correction of angular deformity. (**C**) As the child grows the angular deformity corrects and parallel screws become divergent indicating growth of the physis on the opposite side.

REFERENCES

1. Perren SM. Evolution of the internal fixation of long bone fractures: the scientific basis of biological internal fixation. Choosing a new balance between stability and biology. J Bone Joint Surg Br 2002;84:1093–110.
2. Müller ME, Allgower M, Schneider R, Willenegger H. Manual of internal fixation. 3rd ed. Berlin: Springer-Verlag; 1991.
3. Black J, Dumbleton JH. Clinical biomechanics. New York: Churchill Livingstone; 1981.
4. Perren SM, Allgower M, Burch HB, et al. The concept of biological plating using the limited contact-dynamic compression plate (LC-DCP). Injury 1991;22(Suppl. 1):1–41.
5. Tencer AF, Johnson KD. Biomechanics in orthopaedic trauma: bone fracture and fixation. London: Martin Dunitz; 1994.
6. TriMed, Inc. 27533 Avenue Hopkins, Valencia, CA 91355 USA.
7. Mast J, Jacob R, Ganz R. Planning and reduction technique in fracture surgery. Berlin: Springer-Verlag; 1989.
8. Mears DC. Materials and orthopaedic surgery. Baltimore: Williams & Wilkins; 1979.
9. Gozna ER, Harrington IJ, Evans DC. Biomechanics of musculoskeletal injury. Baltimore: Williams & Wilkins; 1982.
10. Brunner CF, Weber BG. Special techniques in internal fixation. Berlin: Springer-Verlag; 1981.
11. Harder Y, Martinet O, Barraud G-E, Cordey J, Regazzoni P. The mechanics of internal fixation of fractures of the distal femur: a comparison of the condylar screw (DCS) with the condylar plate (CP). Injury 1999;30:S-A31–9.
12. Perren SM. The concept of biological plating using the limited contact–dynamic compression plate (LC-DCP). Injury 1991;22:1–41.
13. Radin EL, Rose RM, Blaha JD, Litsky AS. Practical biomechanics for the orthopaedic surgeon. 2nd ed. New York: Churchill Livingstone; 1992.
14. Hipp JA, Cheal EJ, Hayes WC. Biomechanics of fractures. In: Browner B, editor. Biomechanics of fractures in skeletal trauma — fracture, dislocation and ligamentous injury. Philadelphia: WB Saunders; 1992. p. 95–125.
15. Schwawecker F. The practice of osteosynthesis. Chicago: Yearbook; 1974.
16. Stoffel K, Klaue K, Perren SM. Functional load of plates in fracture fixation in vivo and its correlate in bone healing. Injury 2000;31:S-B37–50.
17. Kubiak EN, Fulkerson E, Strauss E, Egol KA. The evolution of locked plates. J Bone Joint Surg 2006;88-A(Suppl. 4):189–200.
18. Egol KA, Kubiak EN, Fulkerson E, Kummer FJ, Koval KJ. Biomechanics of locked plates and screws. J. Orthop Trauma 2004;18:488–93.
19. Sequin F, Texhammar R. AO/AS IF instrumentation. Berlin: Springer-Verlag; 1981.
20. Rozbruch, SR, Müller U, Gautier E, Ganz R. The evolution of femoral shaft plating technique. Clin Orthop 1998;354:195–208.
21. Gautier E, Sommer C. Guidelines for the clinical application of the LCP. Injury 2003;34(Suppl. 2):B63–76.
22. Stoffel K, Dieter U, Stachowiak G, Gachter A, Kuster M. Biomechanical testing of the LCP – how can stability in locked internal fixators be controlled? Injury 2003; 34:S-B11–19.
23. Sommer C, Babst R, Müller M, Hanson B. Locking compression plate loosening and plate breakage: a report of four cases. J Orthop Trauma 2004;18:571–7.
24. Miller DL, Goswami T. A review of locking compression plate biomechanics and their advantages as internal fixators in fracture healing. Clin Biomech 2007;22:1049–62.
25. Frigg R, Frenk A, Wagner M. Biomechanics of plate osteosynthesis. Tech Orthop 2007;22(4):203–08.
26. Sonderegger J, Grob KR, Kuster MS. Dynamic plate osteosynthesis for fracture stabilization: how to do it. Orthop Rev 2010;2:e4.
27. Synthes, West Chester, PA.

28. Cronier P, Pietu G, Dujardin C, Bigorre N, Ducellier F, Gerard R. The concept of locking plates. Orthop Traumatol Surg Res 2010;96S:S17–36.
29. Tornier, SAS Montbonnot Saint Martin France
30. Numelock II, Stryker, Selzac, Switzerland
31. NewClip® Newclip Technics, Haute-Goulaine, France
32. POLYAX, DePuy, Warsaw, IN
33. Biotech international, Salon de Provence, France
34. NCB® Zimmer Winterthur Switzerland
35. Kinetikos Medical Incorporated, Carlsbad, CA 92009
36. Litos, Hamburg
37. Haidukewych G, Sems SA, Huebner DD, Horwitz, Levy B. Results of polyaxial locked-plate fixation of periarticular fractures of the knee. J Bone Joint Surg Am 2007;89:614–20.
38. Ruedi TP, Buckley RE, Moran CG. AO principles of fracture management, Vol 1. Davos Platz: AO Publishing; 2007. p. 229.
39. Schmal H, Strohm PC, Jaeger M, Sudkamp NP. Flexible fixation and fracture healing: do locked plating 'internal fixators' resemble external fixators? J Orthop Trauma 2011;25:S15–20.
40. Frigg R. Locking compression plate (LCP). An osteosynthesis plate based on the Dynamic Compression Plate and the Point Contact Fixator (PC-Fix). Injury 2001;32:S-B63–6.
41. Dickson KF, Munz JW. Locked plating: biomechanics and biology. Tech Orthop 2007;22(4):E1–6.
42. Sommer C, Gautier E, Muller M, Helfet DL, Wagner M. First clinical results of the locking compression plate (LCP). Injury 2003;34(Suppl. 2):B43–54.
43. Charlson MD, Weber TG. Role of locked plating in revision fixation. Tech Orthop 2003;17(4):515–21.
44. Wagner M, Frenk A, Frigg R. Locked plating: biomechanics and biology and locked plating: clinical indications. Tech Orthop 2007;22(4):209–18.
45. Anglen J, Kyle RF, Marsh JL, Virkus WW, Watters III WC, Keith MW, Turkelson CM, Wies JL, Boyer KM. Locking plates for extremity fractures. J Am Acad Orthop Surg 2009;17:465–72.
46. Lujan TJ, Henderson CE, Madey SM, Fitzpatrick DC, Marsh JL, Bottlang M. Locked plating of distal femur fractures leads to inconsistent and asymmetric callus formation. J Orthop Trauma 2010;24:156–62.
47. Henderson CE, Lujan TJ, Kuhl LL, Bottlang M, Fitzpatrick DC, Marsh JL. Healing complications are common after locked plating for distal femur fractures. Clin Orthop Relat Res 2011;469:1757–65.
48. Bottlang M, Feist F. Biomechanics of far cortical locking. J Orthop Trauma 2011;25:S21–8.
49. Stockle U, Acklin Y, Sommer Ch, Nork S. Dynamic locking screw brochure. Davos: AO Foundation; 2011.
50. Zimmer, Warsaw, Indiana, USA
51. Jamil W, Allami M, Choudhury MZ, Mann C, Bagga T, Roberts A. Do orthopaedic surgeons need a policy on the removal of metalwork? A descriptive national survey of practicing surgeons in the United Kingdom. Injury 2008;39:362–7
52. Ruedi TP, Buckley RE, Moran CG. AO principles of fracture management 2E. Davos Platz: AO Publishing; 2007. p. A11.
53. Bavonratanavech S. Plating for shaft femur fractures – a new surgical technique. Guest lecture at Traumacon. 2012, August 16–19. Mumbai, India.
54. Maier A, Cordey J. Regazzoni P. Prevention of malunions in the rotation of complex fractures of the distal femur treated using the Dynamic Condylar Screw (DCS): an anatomical graphic analysis using computed tomography on cadaveric specimens. Injury 2000;31:S-B63–9.
55. Harder Y, Martinet O, Barraud G-E, Cordey J, Regazzoni P. The mechanics of internal fixation of fractures of the distal femur: a comparison of the condylar screw (DCS) with the condylar plate (CP). Injury 1999;30:S-A31–9.

56. Marti A, Fankhauser C, Frenk A, Cordey J, Gasser B. Biomechanical evaluation of the less invasive stabilization for the internal fixation of distal femur fractures. J Orthop Trauma 2001;15:482–7.
57. Zlowodzki M, Williamson RS, Zardiackas LD, Kregor PJ. Biomechanical evaluation of the less invasive stabilization system, angled blade plate, and retrograde intramedullary nail for the fixation of distal femur fractures: an osteoporotic cadaveric model in Orthopaedic Trauma Association 18th Annual meeting final program. Rosemont, IL: Orthopaedic Trauma Association; 2002. p. 178–9.
58. JC, Bowen TR. Blocking wires facilitate freehand percutaneous plating of periarticular tibia fractures. J Orthop Trauma 2006;20:414–18.
59. Phisitkul P, Mckinley TO, Nepola JV, Marsh JL. Complications of locking plate fixation in complex proximal tibia injuries. J Orthop Trauma 2007;21:83–91.
60. Naina F. Anterior or posterior angulation in compression of a diaphyseal fracture. SICOT news letter 1996.
61. AO surgical reference Tibia shaft 42-C1 CRIF. [Accessed 2012 1 September 1]. Available at https://www2.aofoundation.org/wps/portal/surgery?showPage5diagnosis&bone5Tibia&segment5Shaft
62. Clinical House (Synthes®) Inc., Bochum, Germany.
63. Zwipp H, Rammelt S, Barthel S. Calcaneal fractures—open reduction and internal fixation (ORIF). Injury 2004;35:S-B46–54.
64. Tingart, MJ, Apreleva, M, von Stechow, D, Zurakowski, D, and Warner, JJ. The cortical thickness of the proximal humeral diaphysis predicts bone mineral density of the proximal humerus. J Bone Joint Surg [Br] 2003;85B:611–17.
65. Synthes, Switzerland)
66. Suture Plate™ Arthrex, Naples, USA
67. Niall DM, O'Mahony J, McElwain JP. Plating of humeral shaft fractures—has the pendulum swung back? Injury 2004;35:580–6.
68. Ziran BH, Kinney RC, Smith WR, Peacher G. Sub-muscular plating of the humerus: An emerging technique. Injury 2010;41:1047–52.
69. Jupiter JB, Neff U, Holzach P, Allgöwer M. Intercondylar fracture of the humerus. J Bone Joint Surg Am 1985;67:226–39.
70. Sanchez-Sotelo J, Torchia ME, O'Driscoll SW. Complex distal humeral fractures: internal fixation with a principle-based parallel-plate technique. J Bone Joint Surg Am 2007;89:961–9.
71. Burkhart KJ, MD, Muelle LP, Krezdorn D, Appelmann P, Prommersberger KJ, Sternstein W, Rommens PM. Stability of radial head and neck fractures: a biomechanical study of six fixation constructs with consideration of three locking plates. J Hand Surg 2007;32A:1569–75.
72. Erturer RE, Sever C, Sonmez MM, Ozcelik IB, Akman S, Ozturk I. Results of open reduction and plate osteosynthesis in comminuted fracture of the olecranon. J Shoulder Elbow Surg 2011;20:449–54.
73. Lafontaine M, Hardy D, Delince P. Stability assessment of distal radius fractures. Injury 1989;20:208–10.
74. DePuy International, Leeds, England
75. Nana AD, Joshi A, Lichtman DM. Plating of the Distal Radius. J Am Acad Orthop Surg 2005;13:159–71.
76. Soong M, Got C, Katarincic J, Akelman E. Fluoroscopic evaluation of intra-articular screw placement during locked volar plating of the distal radius: a cadaveric study. J Hand Surg 2008;33A:1720–3.
77. Thomas AD, Greenberg J. Use of fluoroscopy in determining screw overshoot in the dorsal distal radius: a cadaveric study. J Hand Surg 2009;34A:258–61.
78. Martineau PA, Waitayawinyu T, Malone KJ, Hanel DP, Trumble TE. Volar plating of AOC3 distal radius fractures: biomechanical evaluation of locking screw and locking smooth peg configurations. J Hand Surg 2008;33A:827–34.
79. Richard MJ, Katolik LI, Hanel DP, Wartinbee DA, Ruch DS. Distraction plating for the treatment of highly comminuted distal radius fractures in elderly patients. J Hand Surg 2012; 37A:948–56.
80. The Medartis, Basel, Switzerland.
81. DePuy, Warsaw, IN, USA.

82. Bravo CJ, Wright CA. Displaced, comminuted diaphyseal clavicle fracture. J Hand Surg 2009; 34(10):1883–5. doi: 10.1016/j.jhsa.2009.10.012.
83. Acumed 5885 NW Cornelius Pass Road Hillsboro, OR.
84. Althausen PL, Shannon S, Watts C, Thomas K, Bain MA, Coll D, O'mara TJ, Bray TJ. Early surgical stabilization of flail chest with locked plate fixation. J Orthop Trauma 2011;25:641–8.
85. Synthes® CMF, West Chester, PA, USA.
86. Nayagam S, Davis B, Thevendran G, Roche AJ. Medial submuscular plating of the femur in a series of paediatric patients: a useful alternative to standard lateral techniques. Bone Joint J 2014;96-B:137–42.
87. Oh CW, Shetty GM, Song HR, Kyung HS, Oh JK, Min WK, Lee BW, Park BC. Submuscular plating after distraction osteogenesis in children. J Pediatr Orthop B 2008;17:265–9.
88. Lee SC, Shim JS, Seo SW, Lim KS, Ko KO. The accuracy of current methods in determining the timing of epiphysiodesis. Bone Joint J 2013;95-B:993–1000.

CHAPTER 5
INTRAMEDULLARY NAILING

Introduction
Principle of Splintage
Bone Response to Nailing
    Effect on Circulation
    Side Effects of Reaming
    Reamer–Irrigator–Aspirator
    Bone Healing after Nailing
Nail Design
    Cross-Section
    Nail Diameter
    Curves
    Helical Nail
    Length and Working Length
    Extreme Ends of the Nail
    Supplementary Fixation Devices
    Material
Single and Multiple Nails
Reamed and Non-Reamed Nails
Slotted and Non-Slotted Nails
Interlocking Nail
    Static Locking and Bridging Fixation
    Dynamic Locking
    Poller Screw and biomechanics
        Mechanics of Transmedullary Support Screw
    Antibiotic Impregnated Intramedullary Nail
Dynamization

Closed and Open Nailing
Reaming
Traction Table
    Complications Associated with Traction Table
    Nerve Palsy
    Soft-Tissue Injury
Nail Removal
    Intact Nail with Failed Extraction Device
    Bent Nails
    Removal of Broken Solid Nail
Regional Considerations
    The Femur
        Retrograde Supracondylar Intramedullary Nail
    The Tibia
    The Humerus
    The Radius and Ulna
Elastic Stable Intramedullary Nailing
    Biomechanics
    Corkscrew Phenomenon
    ESIN's Regional Considerations
    The Femur
    The Radius and the Ulna
    The Humerus
    The Tibia

INTRODUCTION

In the 1930s German orthopaedist Gerhard Küntscher invented a metallic intramedullary nail for fixation of femoral fractures. The nail that had a slot could be compressed during insertion in the medullary canal. Once insertion was complete, the nail would expand and grip the endosteal surface of the bone. Küntscher called this 'elastic nailing' and coined the term 'elastic impingement' (radial compliance) to describe its mode of action.

Küntscher performed the first nailing of subtrochanteric fracture in humans in November 1939. In 1950 he developed the technique of medullary reaming and closed insertion of an intramedullary nail without exposing the fracture; this has now become standard practice.

Küntscher believed that the nail imparted fracture stability by radial compliance (Fig. 5.1). Further biomechanical testing has shown that these nails are stable by three-point bending rather than radial compliance.

PRINCIPLE OF SPLINTAGE

A fracture of a long bone can be fixed by internal splintage. Splintage may be defined as a construct in which sliding can occur between the bone and the implant. It provides only relative stability without interfragmentary compression and allows some movement at the fracture site, thus ensuring callus formation.

A nail extends from one end of the bone to the other through the medullary canal and acts as a splint. It allows axial forces to be transmitted to the apposed ends of the bone fragments and prevents angulation, translation and, to some extent, rotatory movement. This is because contact exists between the nail and the bone at the entry point, along the narrow segments of the medullary canal, and at the

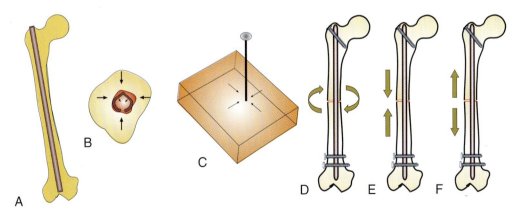

FIGURE 5.1

(**A and B**) Küntscher invented an elastic deformable nail that grips the bone by elastic impingement when introduced in a slightly narrow medullary cavity.[1] (**C**) Comparable mechanical situation is of a nail driven in a block of wood. The wood provides the elastic grip on the nail.[2] Three types of physiological loads act on a nail (**D**) torsion (**E**) compression on the medial side of the nail and (**F**) tension on the lateral aspect of the nail.

cancellous epiphyseal bone on the opposite side. In stable fractures nailing permits early weight bearing. A single nail or a group of nails may be utilized to fix a fracture.

Physiological loading on an intramedullary nail is a combination of torsion, compression and tension (Fig. 5.1D). Bending of the nail under loading creates compressive forces on the concave side of the nail and tension forces on the convex side. When cortical contact is achieved across the facture site, the cortical bone puts up with the loads. When there is no cortical contact, the interlocking screws endure the loads, facedown four-point bending, and may bend or break. Thus, screws should be chosen with the largest root diameter possible; this has led to the use of partially threaded screws, which have a solid body with threads only on the end (Fig. 5.1G).

BONE RESPONSE TO NAILING

Effect on Circulation

The medullary arteries supply the inner two thirds of the cortex, and that the outer third is supplied by the periosteal vasculature via its soft-tissue attachments to the bone. The medullary vessels are disrupted when a fracture occurs, leading to necrosis of approximately 50–70% of the cortex near the fracture site. Intramedullary nailing also damages the endosteal blood supply, resulting in partial cortical necrosis.

The amount of necrosis increases after endosteal reaming, caused either by direct damage to the vascularity of the endosteal surface or by intravasation of marrow elements and fat into the intracortical blood supply, which leads to vessel thrombosis. The endosteal blood supply regenerates around the nail, and the greater the space between the nail and the cortex, the more rapidly this revascularization progresses. The extraosseous periosteal blood supply also increases after nailing and can traverse the outer cortex to revascularize the necrotic endosteum. The regeneration of the nutrient artery itself may not occur for 6 months and is further delayed in the presence of a close-fitting nail.

Side Effects of Reaming

The medullary canal is more like an hourglass than a perfect cylinder. Reaming is an attempt to make the medullary canal of a uniform size to adapt the bone to the nail and thus provide a large contact area between it and the nail (Fig. 5.2). When a single nail is used, it is a common practice to ream the medullary cavity.

Reaming is beneficial as it improves the nail–bone contact area; when the nail is the same size as the reamer, 1 mm of reaming can increase the contact area by 38%[3,5–14]; however, reaming has its side effects. It destroys the medullary circulation causing necrosis of the inner cortex either by direct damage to the vascularity of the endosteal surface or by intravasation of marrow elements and fat into the intracortical blood supply, which leads to vessel thrombosis. Revascularization of the endosteal diaphyseal cortex may take as long as 12 weeks to complete in animal models and probably takes even longer in humans; however, revascularization follows from the periosteal side (Fig. 5.2C). It is completed in a shorter time and may even revascularize the necrotic endosteum. After reaming, periosteal vascular proliferation and hyperaemia occur together with the periosteal new bone formation. The extent of revascularization varies and is related to the extent of the primary damage and the age of the patient: extensive damage and advanced age have a negative effect on revascularization. It may be

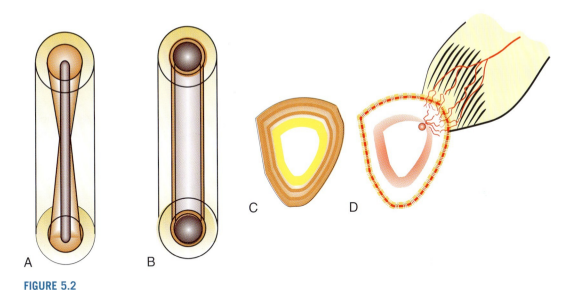

FIGURE 5.2

(**A**) Medullary cavity is not uniform and a nail introduced without reaming is in contact only at its narrowest segment and bending occurs at either end. (**B**) Reaming widens the medullary cavity, lets insertion of a larger diameter nail, improves the length of contact, reduces the working length and increases the stability of the 'tube within a tube'.[1] (**C**) Medullary reaming destroys the medullary circulation; however, the circulation is quickly restored by periosteal arterioles. (**D**) A cross-sectional view of a long bone showing the medullary and periosteal arterioles. Several periosteal arterioles entering the bone cortex through facial attachments remain functional and supply blood to the outer third of the cortex. The periosteal and medullary arterioles anastomose in the cortex and circulation to the inner cortex is quickly restored after reaming.[3]

slowed down or inhibited by the presence of a snug fitting nail or nails in the medullary canal. The delay is most notable where the intramedullary device is in direct contact with the endosteal wall. The time for regeneration of cortical vascularity is shorter in tibias treated with non-reamed intramedullary nailing than in those treated with reamed nailing. The rate at which revascularization occurs may depend on the extent of the reaming performed. Revascularization is delayed or may even fail to occur if the periosteal supply is also excessively damaged.

Heat and pressure are by-products of reaming. Various factors that affect the performance of a reamer are shown in Fig. 5.3A. Hydraulic pressure builds up in the cavity, which far exceeds that of the blood pressure and is independent of the size of the reamer. The reamer simulates a piston-in-a-sleeve; the pressure in the medullary canal changes with quantity of material present in the cavity like blood, blood clots, bone pieces and fat.

The rise in pressure can be restrained by reducing the viscosity of the medullary contents by removing them before starting to ream. A blunt reamer produces high pressure and temperature values and should not be used; a special coating retains sharpness of cutting edges for longer time (Fig. 5.3B and C). Small diameter of the flexible shaft of the reamer keeps the pressure at a low level; a hollow and wide shafted reamer keeps it even lower and facilitates use of thicker guide wire. One-piece shaft-reamer model allows

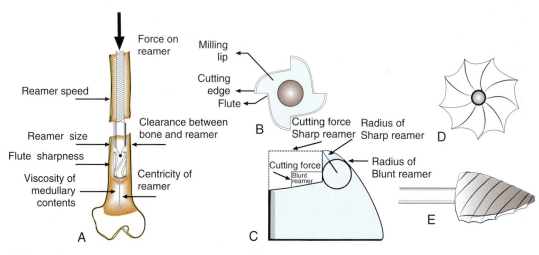

FIGURE 5.3

Factors affecting temperature and pressure generation during medullary reaming. (**A**) Excessive thrust and very high speed of the reamer raise the temperature. A large and a blunt or both reaming heads raise the temperature and pressure. Lower clearance between the reamer head and the bone and presence of high viscosity medullary contents raises the pressure in the medullary canal.[4] (**B**) Functional segments of a medullary reamer. (**C**) The cutting edge of a blunt reamer has a smaller radius and generates lesser cutting force than a sharp reamer. Continued use of a blunt reamer leads to a rise in the temperature and pressure beyond the biological tolerance.[5] (**D and E**) This new reamer design can lower peak intramedullary pressures; it has a narrow reamer shaft, sharp cutting flutes, deep flutes, and a conical shape.[3]

cutting in reverse to help prevent incarceration in a tight canal. It also eliminates repetitive assembly steps, simplifies cleaning and facilitates absolute sterilization.

High intramedullary pressure leads to injection of the medullary fat into the transcortical vessels and to pressure-related fat infiltration into the venous system.

As a result the transcortical vessels close, leading to reduced perfusion of the cortex. Fat infiltration into the venous system may cause fat embolism. The intramedullary pressure also rises when a solid nail is inserted without reaming the cavity.

Use of a cannulated cutter to open the femoral medullary canal provokes a sharp increase in the intramedullary pressure in contrast to its similar use in the tibia (Table 5.1). Insertion of a non-reamed nail in the femur results in the same level of rise in pressure as is observed during insertion of a reamed nail. In the tibia, insertion of a non-reamed nail causes minimal increase in the pressure. Very high pressure levels (up to 600 mmHg), however, are observed when the same nail is introduced briskly and without interruption, as would happen during manual insertion. For this reason it seems safer to insert the non-reamed tibia nail by gentle ram blows rather than by manual force.[6]

A rise in temperature up to 44.6°C has a negative effect on fracture healing since the cell enzymes are damaged by the heat and cannot fulfill their function. The threshold value of heat-induced osteonecrosis is 47°C for an exposure lasting 1 minute. Extruded products of reaming at the fracture site augment callus formation.

Table 5.1 Intramedullary Pressure Changes During Nailing

Activity	Appliance	Femur	Tibia
Opening of medullary cavity	Awl	Insignificant rise	Insignificant rise
	Cannulated cutter	Significant rise	Insignificant rise
Insertion of guide wire	Guide wire	Significant rise	No data available
Insertion of reamer	Fast insertion	Significant rise (much less than in the tibia)	Significant rise (far greater than in the femur)
	Slow insertion	Insignificant rise	Insignificant rise
Insertion of nail	Hollow nail	Minor rise	Minor rise
	Solid nail	Same as reamed (hollow) nail	Significantly lower pressure than reamed (hollow) nail
Inserting distal vent		No change in pressure readings	No data

A decrease in thickness of the cortex decreases the bending and torsional strengths of the bone. However, this biomechanically deleterious effect may be mitigated as additional reaming facilitates introduction of a thicker nail; such a nail offers more bending and torsional rigidity; a nail inserted after reaming provides more stable fixation than one without reaming. Basic physiologic research suggests that intramedullary nailing, either with or without reaming, has measurable local and systemic effects. Insertion of canal-preparing devices and implants into the medullary canal can lead to partial vascular compromise of the endosteal cortex and to venous embolization of fat and other marrow contents. This embolization produces measurable but transient effects on the pulmonary system; however, the clinical effects of the embolization associated with intramedullary manipulations are minimal. Careful surgical technique, including slow and gentle reamer advancement and the use of sharp reamers, can limit the medullary canal pressurization associated with reaming.[6]

Systemic effects of medullary reaming are believed to be the effect of embolization of marrow contents. These marrow contents can be visualized intraoperatively by echocardiography.

It is also possible that canal reaming and nailing of fractures acutely may lead to a so-called second hit and a heightened systemic inflammatory response, while simultaneously leading to the release of IL-10 and suppression of expression. Although it is clear that early stabilization of femoral fractures in trauma patients leads to improved morbidity and mortality, further study is warranted of the immune response generated through reaming and nailing.

Reamer–Irrigator–Aspirator

The 'reamer–irrigator–aspirator' (RIA) is an innovation developed to reduce fat embolism and thermal necrosis that can occur during reaming or nailing of long-bone fractures. The RIA reduces intramedullary pressure and temperature as it sucks out irrigation fluid, bone marrow and bone debris. This material is filtered to remove bone pieces and collected in a closed suction bag. Danckwardt-Lilliestrom, Sturmer and Tammen in 1986, did the original work on irrigation-suction reaming.[8] RIA has a reamer head, a hollow nitinol drive shaft for continuous irrigation and aspiration of reaming debris, a bone particulate filter and closed suction bag.[9] The primary indication for the use of RIA is to effectively size the medullary canal for the acceptance of an intramedullary (IM) implant or prosthesis.[10] It prevents fat embolism and thermal necrosis. The reamed bone fragments and other particles collected during the process are utilized as an ideal autografts in promoting fracture union and for other bone fusions in orthopaedic surgery. It is an effective harvester of multipotential marrow stromal cells also known as mesenchymal stem cells (MSCs) and other osteoprogenitors. It is also useful in debridement of long bones (femur/tibia) for treatment of chronic osteomyelitis. Other indications include stabilization of bilateral femoral fractures in one surgical setting (especially impending pathological fractures) and IM reamed nailing in polytrauma patients with associated chest injury. Reaming the same femur as the non-union site or the opposite number provides autologous bone for grafting.[11] Metabolic bone disease and active metastatic bone disease are specific contraindications to the use of RIA. Significant osteoporosis, advanced age and bleeding disorder are relative contraindications. Meticulous technique, precise entry point and frequent use of fluoroscopy are essential to prevent complications. The most serious potential complication is iatrogenic femur fracture. Eccentric reaming into the anterior cortex, violation of the knee joint and jamming of the RIA device along the canal isthmus might occur. Haematoma formation around the harvest site and considerable blood loss can also occur.

Bone Healing after Nailing

Fixation with a nail of adequate stiffness leads to satisfactory bone healing. If thin and loosely fitting nails are used, delayed union and non-union results. Nail-fixed fractures heal by periosteal callus whereas plate-fixed fractures heal mainly by endosteal callus formation; the mechanical strength of both is similar at 120 days.

NAIL DESIGN

Cross-Section

It is 76 years since Kuntscher first described his intramedullary nail. Many designs were used during the developmental phases that followed. By early 1990s closed, reamed, antegrade intramedullary nailing was established as a standard care for femoral shaft fractures. The cross-sections of nails commonly used at present are shown in Fig. 5.4J–L. The shape, the diameter and the area of the nail determine its bending and torsional strengths. The nails that are currently in use have similar shape and therefore have similar bending stiffness and strength. A circular nail has an area and polar moment of inertia proportional to its diameter (see page 12). Similarly, a square cross-sectional nail has an area and polar moment of inertia proportional to its edge length. Complex cross-sectional shapes need complex calculations to assess their moments of inertia. In simple terms, the further the material is distributed from the principal axis, the greater the moments of inertia.

Shape also plays an important role in the mechanics of the nail–bone interface. A nail with sharp corners or fluted edges resists torsional forces to a greater degree than a smooth-walled nail. The presence of a slot does not reduce the bending stiffness of a nail; however, it does reduce its torsional stiffness. The hollow core of these nails admits a thick and strong guide wire that fills the space almost completely. This ensures that the nail remains centred in the canal and passes smoothly into the distal fragment across the fracture site. Fluting of the nail increases its torsional friction within the medullary cavity. Some nails are designed so that either a portion of or the entire nail is expandable under hydrostatic pressure, thereby allowing the nail to contact the cortex and thus increase its holding power.

NAIL DESIGN

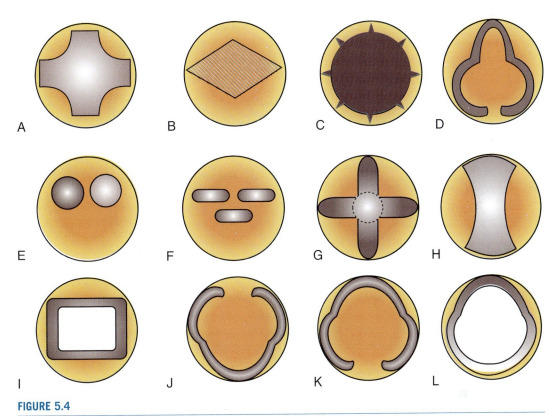

FIGURE 5.4

Cross-sectional shapes of medullary nails used till late 1990s. **(A)** Schneider; **(B)** Hansen-Street or 'diamond'; **(C)** Sampson fluted[2]; **(D)** Küntscher; **(E)** Rush; **(F)** Ender; **(G)** Modny; **(H)** Halloran; **(I)** Huckstep.[13] Cross-section of nails in current use **(J)** AO/ASIF Universal; **(K)** Grosse and Kempf; **(L)** Russell–Taylor.[14]

Nail Diameter

Nail diameter is the most important factor in determining nail strength. The bending stiffness of a nail varies with its diameter: 16 mm nail is 1.5 times as stiff as a 14 mm nail and 2.5 times as stiff as a 12 mm nail. An intramedullary nail of 12 mm diameter and a wall thickness of 2 mm has bending stiffness equal to that of intact femur. The diameter of a nail should always be measured with a circular gauge (Fig. 5.5).

Curves

A nail may be straight, curved or helical.[17] The long bones have curved medullary cavities. A straight nail, if inserted in such a cavity, will bend and produce stresses that may rupture the bone. Nails are contoured to accommodate the curves.

The femur is a curved bone. Its average radius of curvature is 1020 mm. The femoral nail is curved anteroposteriorly to conform to the curvature of the medullary canal (Fig. 5.5B). The nail, when fully inserted, fits snugly and does not produce any untoward stress.

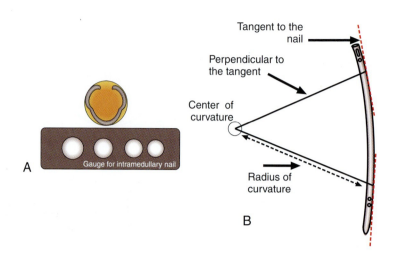

FIGURE 5.5

The calliper gauge is unsuitable to measure the diameter of a triangular medullary nail as it gives a smaller value than the actual. **(A)** A circular gauge measures the diameter accurately.[15] **(B)** Radius of curvature of an intramedullary nail.[16]

An axial force is necessary to insert the nail, as the nail must bend somewhat to fit the curve of the medullary canal. The insertion force is maximal at three quarters of the insertion length and decreases thereafter as the nail straightens out to adapt to the shape of the medullary canal. The insertion force generates hoop stress in the bone. This is a circumferential expansion stress similar to that supported by the hoops of a barrel. The greater the insertion force, the larger the hoop stress. Excessively large hoop stress can split the femur converting a simple, transverse fracture to a comminuted one.

Use of a flexible nail adjusting to the shape of the medullary cavity, overreaming the entry hole by 0.5–1 mm and shorter length of the fracture fragments are some of the factors that reduce the insertion force and the hoop stress.

The most important factor affecting hoop stress, however, is the selection of the point of insertion (Fig. 5.6). If the insertion point is anterior to the central axis of the femur by as little as 6 mm, high hoop stress develops and may lead to bursting of the femur. An excessively posterior insertion point has the same effect. In the medial lateral plane the insertion point should be at the junction of the femoral neck and greater trochanter.

The geometry of the available nails for anterograde insertion in the femur dictate an entry site that is too medial, is far from ideal and is associated with risks and disadvantages (Fig. 5.6). Conventional nail, either straight or arc-of-a-circle requires a medial entry point, at the piriformis fossa, aligned in the anterior–posterior plane within the intramedullary canal. This entry point though well accepted has several disadvantages such as risk to the vascular supply of femoral head, injury to superior gluteal nerve and possibility of fracture of femoral neck.

Helical Nail

A helical nail permits a more lateral entry portal on the femur and is associated with several anatomical advantages over medial entry point.[17] Lateral aspect of the greater trochanter at gluteus medius

NAIL DESIGN

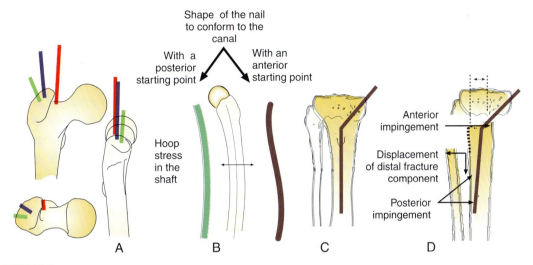

FIGURE 5.6
(A) Distinctive entry points for different femoral nail designs is a critical step in nail insertion. **(B)** The anterior bowing of the femur requires that the proximal insertion point should be posterior to the mid-line of the bone. If the nail is inserted from anterior starting point, deformation is severe and requires excessive insertion force with generation of excessive hoop (expansion) stress that increases the possibility of bursting of the femoral shaft.[18] **(C)** The bend in the tibial nail may cause malposition of the distal fragment. When the bend is superior to the fracture line the nail displaces down the canal. **(D)** When the bend is distal to the fracture line, the nail in effect becomes wider above the bend and may impinge on both the anterior and posterior wall of the canal. At times the nail becomes wedged and further insertion of the nail carries the distal fragment posteriorly and distally.[19]

insertion is the starting point with the helical nail The entry site is safe, does not pose a threat to femoral head's vascular supply, it is far away from superior gluteal nerve and poses no fracture risk, as the bone is softer at the greater trochanter than in the piriformis fossa (Fig. 5.7).

The tibial nail also has a smooth 11° bend in the anteroposterior direction located at the junction of its upper one-third and lower two-third lengths. As the tibial nail is inserted at an angle into the medullary canal, the access canal lies at an angle of 11° to the medullary canal. Only an angled nail can be accommodated in an angled access canal (see Fig. 5.6B).

Length and Working Length

The nail length is considered from three viewpoints:

1. Total nail length
2. Length of nail–bone contact
3. Working length

Total nail length depends purely on anatomical considerations. Too long a nail can protrude at the insertion site causing pain and limitation of motion; too short a nail may compromise the fixation.

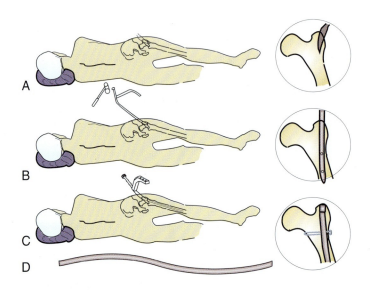

FIGURE 5.7

(**A**) Patient in lateral decubitus; entry portal is being established. The tracing of radiograph shows a curved awl entering the greater trochanter, lateral to insertion of gluteus medius. (**B**) The nail-insertion handle points ventrally. The distal holes in the nail seen in the tracing are orientated in the patient's sagittal plane, at 90° to its correct final position. (**C**) The handle has rotated 90° and lies in the frontal (coronal) plane of the patient. The nail also has rotated 90° during insertion as seen in the tracing. (**D**) A computer generated 'best shape for helical nail' is curved in three dimensions.

The length of nail–bone contact reflects the total surface area contact between the nail and the bone. The larger the contact area, the higher the resistance to motion.

Working length is defined as the length of a nail spanning the fracture site from its distal point of fixation in the proximal fragment to its proximal point of fixation in the distal fragment. A less technical definition states that it is the distance between the two points on either side of the fracture where the bone firmly grips the metal. Thus, working length is the unsupported portion of the nail between the two major bone fragments and reflects the length of nail carrying the majority the load across the fracture site.

The bending stiffness of a nail is inversely proportional to the square of its working length, while the torsional stiffness is inversely proportional to its working length.[7] Shorter working length means stronger fixation.

Working length is affected by various factors. A nail has a shorter working length in bending in fixation of a transverse fracture than in stabilizing a comminuted fracture (Fig. 5.7A and B). Two techniques that modify the working length are medullary reaming and interlocking. Medullary reaming prepares a uniform canal and improves nail–bone fixation towards the fracture, thus reducing the working length. Interlocking screws also modify the working length in torsion by fixing the nail to the bone at specific points. The torsional stability is substantially improved by this technique and is directly related to distance between the two fixation points (Fig. 5.8C and D). Weight bearing with an interlocked nail further improves the nail–bone contact as the nail bends under axial load, reducing the working length and adding to the overall stiffness of the fixation (Fig. 5.8E and F).

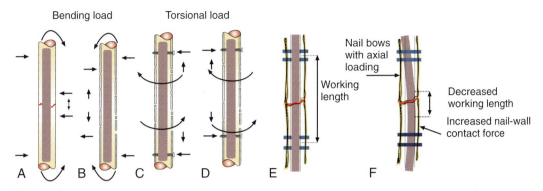

FIGURE 5.8

Working length of a nail. (**A and B**) For bending loads, a nail fixing a transverse fracture has a shorter working length than one fixing a comminuted fracture. (**C and D**) When a nail is fixed to the bone by interlocking screws, the working length for torsional load equals the two definite points of fixation. The torque from distal fragment is transferred through the locking screw into the nail, which is further transmitted to the proximal fragment through the proximal locking screws (**E and F**).[20] With weight bearing, the interlocked nail bows and increases the nail–bone contact near the fracture site. Increased contact force reduces the working length for bending and torsional loads.[18]

The type of load affects the working length. A standard Küntscher nail in the fixation of a transverse fracture has a short and effective working length for the bending load. The same nail offers little resistance to the torsional load and the concept of working length does not apply in this situation.

Extreme Ends of the Nail

The original Küntscher nail had a slot for attachment of an extraction hook in the proximal end. The distal end was tapered to facilitate its insertion in the medullary canal and across the fracture site. The present version of a cannulated locking nail contains a cylindrical proximal end with an internally threaded core to allow firmer attachment of the driver, extractor and target device. Holes for interlocking screws are present towards either end of the nail, minimizing the invasion of the fracture zone and increasing the range of fractures that may be stabilized with this device. A more proximal placement of the interlocking screw holes allows expansion of the indications for nailing to higher fractures, but it also causes the screw to be placed in the femoral neck, with some risk of femoral neck fatigue. A moderately distal placement allows expansion of the indications to more distal fractures, but placing the screws through the wide metaphysis to reach the hole in the nail creates targeting difficulties. Some nails also have slots near the distal end for placement of antirotation wires.

The distal end of the tibial nail is tapered. Such a tip guides the nail in the direction of the medullary canal and prevents inadvertent penetration of the dorsal cortex.

Supplementary Fixation Devices

These are deployed proximal or distal to a fracture site to control rotation and to maintain the bone length. Slot wires, fins and hooks protruding beyond the circumference through special openings in the nail have been used for the purpose. However, single or multiple screws passing through special holes in the nail and taking purchase on both the cortices are popular devices. In most femoral shaft fractures, placement of a single distal screw provides adequate fixation and decreases time spent in targeting. It appears to be unimportant whether this screw is placed in the proximal or the distal screw hole. The use of two screws is generally indicated in infraisthmal fractures to prevent rotation around the nail and flexion as well as extension about a single screw. Two screws are also indicated in severely comminuted femoral fractures, as well as in an unreliable patient refusing to limit weight bearing, and in head-injury patients. Interlocking screws may come loose if they are hammered instead of screwed into position. Hammering causes microfractures of the bone leading to early loosening. Loosening of the screws also occurs in osteoporosis.

An important aspect of nail design involves the area in which the screw holes penetrate the nail. A hole in the body of a nail is a stress riser and a potential site for fatigue failure. Nail failure usually occurs through the screw holes, yet all bending tests comparing various products are conducted on the midshaft of the device. Larger nail diameter and increased wall thickness of the nail in the vicinity of the hole provides increased strength. Cold working of the interlocking holes also helps to increase strength and is especially important in nails with small diameters.

The design of interlocking screws is somewhat more important than nail design. Confining the threads to the distal tip of the screw has been thought to provide additional strength to the screw. Unfortunately, the weakness of the interlocking screw is at the shaft-thread junction, and thus little advantage is gained from a partially threaded screw. Also, this type of screw is less easily inserted than the fully threaded screw and is difficult to extract. Furthermore, the partially threaded screw gains purchase on only one cortex, comes loose more often, and backs out more frequently; thus, its use necessitates the placement of two screws distally. A screw with threads at both ends and unthreaded shaft in between (see Fig. 5.11C) or a fully threaded screw appears to have the more logical design and is easier to use. A more important feature than the threads is the core diameter of the screw. Screw failure is a common complication of locked nails, and a larger core diameter reduces this risk. Materials such as titanium and 22-13-5 stainless steel also improve screw strength.

Material

Nails are made of 316L stainless steel or titanium alloy. The modulus of elasticity of titanium alloy is half that of 316L stainless steel but is similar to that of cortical bone. The stiffness or rigidity of a nail depends both on the material and its design. IM nails with similar designs posses similar ultimate strengths. A single titanium locking screw in femoral shaft fracture is prone to breakage because of higher loading of the screws; use of two distal screws is suggested.

SINGLE AND MULTIPLE NAILS

A single nail is commonly used for intramedullary fixation and is positioned centrally in the medullary canal. The fracture fixation is secured by nail–bone friction and by fixing the ends of the nail to the bone with interlocking screws (Fig. 5.9). The popular nail systems of this type are AO/ASIF, Grosse–Kempf, Klemm–Schennel and Russell–Taylor.

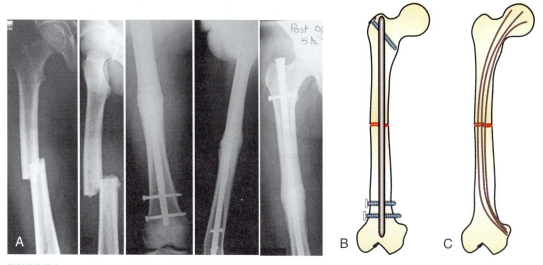

FIGURE 5.9

(A) Radiographs showing intramedullary locked nail for mid-shaft fracture of femur. (B) Single or centromedullary nail fixation of a stable subtrochanteric fracture.[21] (C) Ender nails are effective in fixation of a fracture in osteoporotic bone with wide medullary canal.[2]

In multiple nail fixation several nails of smaller diameter than the standard Küntscher nail are inserted into a non-reamed medullary canal. Fracture fixation is attained by each nail gaining its own three- or four-point fixation with the bone. The Ender and Rush nails are popular examples of this type.

Ender nails are flat, prebent, C-shaped nails and are 4.5 mm in diameter. The leading portion of the nail forms a smooth curve with a blunt bevelled tip; the driving end terminates in a flattened eyelet perpendicular to the curve. The curved shape of the nail provides the three-point fixation in the medullary canal. Multiple nails achieve fixation in multiple planes parallel to the long axis of the bone. Consequently, the fracture fixation is more stable in bending than in rotation.

Rush nails are solid, circular in cross-section and of varying diameter (3–7 mm). They are straight, with a sharp bevelled tip and a hook at the driving end. The hook is driven into the cortex at the end of the procedure. Rush nails are stiffer than Ender nails and must be prebent in order to provide three-point fixation.

Multiple flexible pins can be inserted without a guide wire. They hold well in osteoporotic bones and a snug fit of nails can be obtained in a wide medullary canal. The surgical trauma is minimal as they are inserted from the condylar region through a small entry point and are passed upwards until the sharp tip is in the proximal femur. The greater stiffness makes insertion and manipulation more difficult in Rush nails than in Ender nailing. For similar montages, Rush nails provide increased rigidity and ultimate strength over Ender nails.

Ender and Rush nails are used in treating transverse, short oblique and unicortically comminuted femoral shaft fractures (Fig. 5.9B). Long oblique and bicortically comminuted fractures are unsuitable for treatment by this method because shortening frequently occurs.

REAMED AND NON-REAMED NAILS

Küntscher invented medullary reaming to insert a larger nail and to achieve a stable fixation with improved nail–bone contact length.

Although the terms 'reamed nailing' and 'non-reamed nailing' appear to be mutually exclusive, confusion exists about the use of this terminology, especially with regard to nail diameter. The decision to ream is not strictly related to nail diameter. Some younger patients have very small endosteal canals, and reaming is essential to insert even a 10-mm-diameter nail. In the elderly, the endosteal canals may be very large requiring little or no reaming for insertion of a larger diameter nail.

However, even for non-reamed nailing, reaming of the proximal portion of the femur is necessary so that it will accept the expanded proximal portion of the intramedullary device. In most small-diameter nail designs, the proximal interlocking screw is inserted through an expanded proximal housing constructed to afford extra strength to the coupling of the nail with the proximal interlocking screw. This proximal femoral overreaming is generally required for small-diameter non-reamed nails, but this may also be required to a lesser degree for reamed nails, because the diameter of the shaft of the nail more closely approximates the diameter of the expanded proximal portion of the nail.

'Reamed nailing' is defined as insertion of an intramedullary nail after reaming both the proximal and the distal femoral fracture fragments, with the intent of enlarging the femoral endosteal diameter, especially at the isthmus, so as to permit insertion of a nail with the largest diameter appropriate for the patient. 'Non-reamed nailing' is defined as the insertion of an intramedullary nail without prior canal reaming, specifically across the fracture site (i.e. without intentionally altering the existing diameter of the femoral canal). Therefore, whether to use reamed or non-reamed nailing is a decision that rests on the surgeon concerning the method of preparation of the central portion of the endosteal canal before nail insertion. The terms 'small-diameter nailing' and 'large-diameter nailing' do not denote whether reaming of the canal was part of the nailing procedure.[7]

Reaming simplifies the nailing procedure by creating a smooth medullary canal so that a nail can be inserted with minimal force. Reaming also increases the feasibility of inserting a larger nail than could be introduced without reaming and decreases the chances of splitting the bone during nail insertion. A larger nail offers the possibility of drilling holes through the nail to insert the locking screws. These innovations have made every diaphyseal long bone fracture amenable to intramedullary nailing. A nail introduced after reaming the canal is usually hollow and has a wide diameter (11–14 mm).

Reaming is not mandatory for intramedullary nailing. In the presence of compound fractures and soft tissue trauma, a nail may be inserted without reaming the canal; the nail used in these circumstances is usually thinner (8–10 mm) than the reamed nail. A smaller, solid nail with interlocking provides stability similar to that of a reamed nail. In open fractures, use of a solid nail avoids the large dead space present in a tubular nail where infection could flourish. A non-reamed nail is an alternative to external fixation in open fractures. Reaming is common in femoral nailing while non-reamed nailing is suitable for the tibia, the humerus and the forearm bones.

SLOTTED AND NON-SLOTTED NAILS

The Küntscher nail has a slot that allows compression of the nail during insertion and expansion on final seating to grip the inner cortex of the hollow medullary canal by radial compliance.

A slotted nail is flexible. This flexibility is observed more in torsion than in anteroposterior bending. A flexible nail also tolerates variation in the point of insertion (Table 5.2), thus a nail inserted either from the lateral side of the trochanter or from the piriformis fossa is accommodated in the medullary canal with the same ease.

The concept of interlocking required alterations in the nail slot. Proximal slot closure strengthens the nail to bear the weakening effect of the holes for cross-locking screws. The proximal slot closure also permits instrument attachment for insertion and extraction of the nail and for insertion of proximal locking screws. Nail-mounted proximal locking guides work with precision. The torsional flexibility distorts the distal part of the nail, making it impossible to insert the distal locking screws with proximal nail-mounted guides. Consequently, various methods to insert the distal locking screws – such as the C-arm-mounted targeting device, laser assisted targeting system, radiolucent drill and free-hand technique – were evolved.

Insertion of the distal locking screws through a proximal nail-mounted targeting device is an attractive proposition because it saves substantial operating time. Complete closure of the slot makes this possible as the nail loses its distorting torsional flexibility. The non-slotted nail is more stiff in torsion than in bending; it does not distort on insertion, and proximal as well as distal locking screws can be accurately inserted using a nail-mounted targeting device.

A partially slotted nail is flexible and accommodates some variation in insertion point to a certain extent. A non-slotted nail, being less flexible, must be introduced through a precise point of insertion, failing which there is an increased risk of the bone splitting.

The non-slotted nail–bone construct is more stable than the partially slotted nail–bone fixation in torsion and thus prevents shear stress generation at the fracture site. Absence of shear stress improves fracture healing. Bending rigidity of a nail can be altered by varying the thickness of its wall. Thus, a thicker-walled slotted nail will have similar rigidity to a thinner-walled non-slotted nail. A non-slotted nail can be made in smaller diameter yet have adequate strength. This possibility has led to the development of a non-slotted, non-reamed, locked intramedullary nail which may be solid or cannulated.

Interlocking Nail

The standard non-locked nail is useful in the treatment of simple and minimally comminuted midshaft fractures of femur and tibia; in selected cases early mobility and weight bearing can be achieved.

Table 5.2 Comparison of Slotted and Non-Slotted Nails

Parameter	Slotted nail	Non-slotted nail
Diameter	Larger	Smaller
Wall thickness	Thicker	Thinner
Insertion point	Variation tolerated	Precision mandatory
Stability	Less stable	More stable
Shear stress	More	Less
Stiffness in torsion	Flexible	Rigid (40× slotted nail)
Distal targeting device	Cannot be used	Can be used
Overall performance	Comparable to non-slotted nail	Comparable to slotted nail

However, interlocking nail has made the single non-locking nail, whose only advantages are simplicity and low cost, obsolete. The locked nail is at present a popular implant for diaphyseal fracture fixation.

Static Locking and Bridging Fixation

Screw insertions at the two ends of a nail interlock it with the proximal and the distal fracture fragments. This technique prevents sliding of these fragments along the nail and is called 'static locking' (Fig. 5.10). Interlocking controls both the bone length and the rotation of the fragments but mainly improves the rotational stability of the nail–bone construct. Static locking achieves bridging fixation. In the presence of severe comminution it is undesirable to open the fracture site and handle individual fragments to achieve alignment as further devascularization occurs and the risk of infection increases. In bridging fixation, the implant extends across the zone of soft-tissue injury and fracture but is fixed to the major bone fragments proximal and distal to the injury site.

Although the fracture often appears to be held in distraction by bridging fixation, a favourable environment for periosteal callus formation exists, and healing rather than non-union is the rule. This occurs because the tissues remain viable and the fixation permits limited motion. Static locking is used in fixation of segmental, comminuted, long oblique or spiral fractures, and in stabilization of a fracture with bone loss or in pseudoarthrosis.

Dynamic Locking

When the screws are inserted only at one end of the nail, the fixation is called 'dynamic locking'. This mode of fixation achieves additional rotational control of a fragment with a large medullary canal or of a short epiphyseal–metaphyseal fragment (Fig. 5.10B). The unlocked end of the nail attains fixation in the splinting mode as it snugly fits in the reamed diaphyseal medullary canal (Fig. 5.10C). The bone length is maintained by a stable bone contact, and dynamic locking is effective only when the contact area between the two major fragments is at least 50% of the cortical circumference. Dynamic fixation will fail in the presence of unstable bone contact between the main fragments. When an interlocking

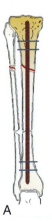
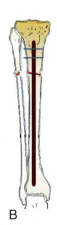
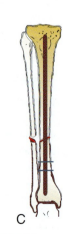

FIGURE 5.10

(A) Static locking: the screws on either sides of the fracture fix the main bone fragments to the nail, preventing their displacement. The fixation is static only with respect to its resistance to shortening and rotation as a limited motion occurs at the fracture site due to minor degree of torsion and elastic bending of the nail leading to healing through callus pathway. (B) Dynamic locking: screws control the rotation of the short proximal fragment. The bone length is maintained by adequate and stable cortical bone contact between the two fracture fragments. (C) Two screws control the motion of the short distal fragment with large medullary canal. The snug fit between the endosteum and the nail in the long proximal fragment prevents rotation of that fragment but permits axial sliding with impaction at the fracture site with loading from the muscle forces and weight bearing.[21]

A   B   C

screw is placed in an oval hole in the nail, some degree of telescopic movement is present, which is beneficial for fracture healing.

Static locking results in predictable fracture healing and there should be a very strong reason not to follow this mode of fixation in a given instance.

Contemporary designs for the femoral nail use two distal transverse cross-locking screws. Proximal fixation is achieved by two inclined or transverse screws or by insertion of screws through the femoral head and neck. In an interlocked nail, the working length in bending and torsion is reduced with axial loading as the nail bends and abuts against the cortex near the fracture, improving the nail–bone contact.

The stability of interlocked nail depends on the diameter of locking screw for a given nail diameter. The holes for locking screws in the intramedullary nail are stress risers; also, the perimeter of the hole may be inadvertently nicked during screw insertion. An increased possibility of fatigue failure of the nail through these holes exists because of these factors. As a rule, nail hole size should not exceed 50% of the nail diameter. The stresses in an interlocked nail increase in a distally located fracture because in this situation the nail is loaded like a cantilever beam (Fig. 5.11). When the femoral fracture site is within 5 cm of the most proximal of the distal locking screws, the peak stresses around that hole may exceed the stress level above which fatigue fracture of the nail may occur. Such a fixation should be additionally protected.

The distal locking screws resist axial and torsional loading and prevent toggling of the nail in an anteroposterior direction in the medullary canal. The amount of this toggle is directly related to the length of the distal femoral fragment and the number and situation of the distal locking screws. Two

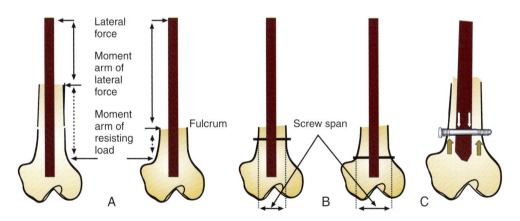

FIGURE 5.11

(A) The stresses in the distal part of the interlocked intramedullary nail increase when the fracture line is closer to the screw hole because the bone support of the nail in bending is decreased, resulting in a smaller moment arm. **(B)** The span (support points) of the screw increases as the interlocking screw is placed farther distally in the femoral condyle. Increased span decreases the strength and stiffness of the screw in resisting four-point bending generated by axial loading through the nail.[18] **(C)** Distal interlocking screw is subjected to four-point loading. When there is poor cortical contact, the interlocking screw bears excessive load and may bend or break. A screw with solid body and threads on either end are easy to use and withstand these loads effectively. The core diameter of the screw is an important element.[3]

distal locking screws should be used when the distal fragment is smaller in length than 60% of the distance between the mid-point of the femoral shaft and the joint line.

The distal interlocking screw is loaded in four-point bending as load is applied during walking. The screw ends are supported by the bone cortices. The unsupported span of the distally placed screw increases with widening of the femoral condyle (Fig. 5.11B). Increased span reduces the stiffness (by the cube of the span) and ultimate strength screw in four-point bending.

The orientation of the proximal locking holes in a non-reamed tibial nail affects the resistance of the nail–bone construct to motion in varus-valgus bending. Parallel orientation (transverse, i.e. 90° to nail axis) of these holes permits medial-lateral translation of the proximal fragment when varus-valgus bending forces are applied as the fragment is able to slide on parallel screw. Oblique (i.e. angled to nail axis, not 90°) orientation of the holes precludes such movement. However, fixation stability is unaffected and both oblique and transverse proximal locking screws show equal axial load to failure. The distal locking screw breakage is pronounced in unreamed tibial nail because the shear forces on the screw are frequently too great especially in more distal fractures where fragments get shorter and shorter. The breakage does not affect clinical outcome. In reamed nailing, screw failures are rare.

The number of locking screw required depends on the fracture location and stability. In stable fractures one distal screw is adequate. The closer the fracture is to the distal locking screw, the less cortical contact the nail has, which leads to increased stress on the locking screw. Additionally, the farther the distal locking screw is from the fracture site, the more rotationally stable the fracture becomes because of friction of the nail within the medullary cavity.[3]

Poller Screw and biomechanics

Poller (German) or Bollard (English) is a strong post made of concrete, metal or wood to prevent cars from entering part of road especially for parking. Blocking (syn. Poller, Bollard) screws were introduced to route an unreamed nail to fix proximal or distal fractures. Now used to centre a guide wire and a reamer by narrowing the canal diameter in metaphyseal region in both reamed and unreamed techniques, devices like a K-wire, a small-fragment screw, a locking bolt or a drill bit function as a provisional guide. Poller screw or blocking screw is a reliable device to obtain satisfactory alignment, improve stability of reduction, avoid malalignment when nailing proximal and distal tibial shaft fractures or in any long bone involving a metaphyseal region. It is critical to gauge medullary canal size and place a blocking screw before commencing reaming; accidental eccentric path may lessen usefulness of the method. The screws should be so placed as to leave adequate space for the reamer and the nail. Besides, a reamer, which may jam against a Poller screw, should be used in incremental steps and its each pass through the screw zone should be watched under fluoroscope. Biomechanical studies suggest that Poller screws can increase the primary stability of distal and proximal metaphyseal fractures after nailing and can be an effective tool to prevent malalignment and/or instability.[22] A posteriorly placed screw prevents anterior angulation, and a laterally placed screw prevents valgus angulation of the fracture (Fig. 5.12A and B). As the nail traverses fracture line, the isthmus serves to properly align the nail in the distal fragments.

Mechanics of Transmedullary Support Screw [24]

Poller screw or blocking screw works on three-point fixation principle as in elastic intramedullary nail or plaster cast for Colles' fracture. A single screw can achieve three-point fixation as long as adequate support exists at two other points of fixation (Fig. 5.13). These supplementary points of fixation may

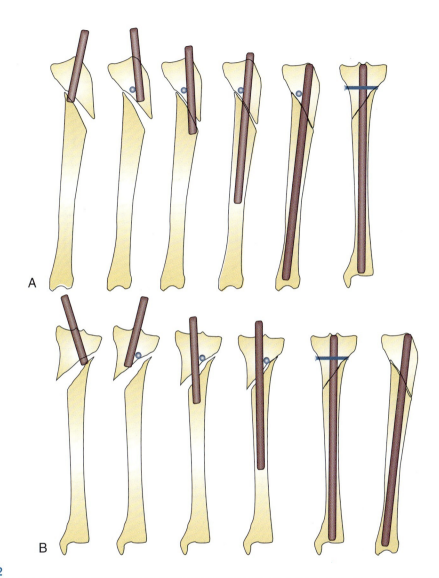

FIGURE 5.12

(A) In a short oblique proximal fragment, a nail consistently exiting posteriorly is prevented by a Poller or blocking screw placed posterior to the central axis in a medial-to-lateral direction. The nail is then passed anterior to the screw and the apex angulation corrects as the nail passes across the fracture site and the fracture is properly reduced after the nail is inserted completely. (B) A laterally exiting nail in a short oblique proximal fragment is guided into the medullary canal by a blocking screw placed lateral to the central axis in an anterior to posterior direction. As the nail is passed medial to the screw, valgus angulation corrects when the nail crosses the fracture line and the fracture is properly reduced after the nails is seated completely.[23]

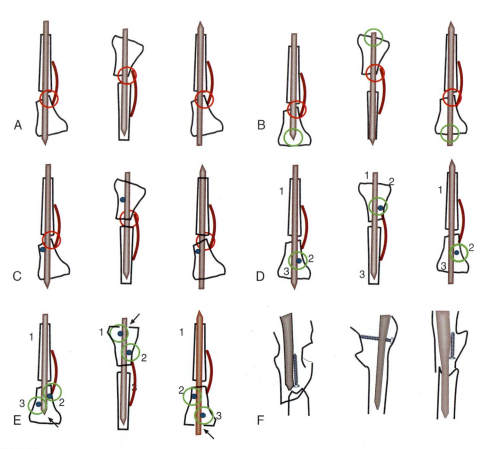

FIGURE 5.13

(A) Malalignment of short fragment follows careless insertion of the nail; red circle highlights the tendency of the nail to make contact with wall of the short segment. **(B)** Soft tissue pull causes malalignment in a well-placed nail. Metaphyseal cortical flare eases malalignment (red circles) even when the nail is located centrally in the distal metaphyseal fragment (green circle). **(C)** Incorrectly placed blocking screw only narrows the medullary canal but does not prevent malalignment because it does not counter soft tissue tension (red circle). Three-point fixation is not established. Interlocking screws do not prevent angular deformity. **(D)** Correctly placed blocking screw on the concave side of the deformity in the short fragment (green circle) achieve three point fixation (numbers) in the medullary canal and counteract the tension band like pull of the soft tissues. **(E)** inadequate distal anchorage of the nail (short nail or poor fixation) or too wide an entry hole (arrows), necessitates a second blocking screw (in the short fragment, on the convex side far from the fracture, close to the tip of the nail) to establish three point fixation. **(F)** Blocking screw principle applied to subtrochanteric fracture. A lateral to medial blocking screw corrected the flexion deformity of the proximal fragment and maintained it till union.[24]

be the point of nail entrance or the cortical wall through isthmus in a long segment, or hold at the nail tip in a short segment. A second blocking screw is needed on the opposite side when fixation provided by supplementary points is insufficient. A transmedullary blocking screw prevents axial displacement caused by imbalanced soft tissues. This three-point arrangement is similar to a tension-band construct that counteracts (neutralize) deforming soft tissue tension. A screw in each plane is necessary when biplanar displacement exists. The interlocking screws through the nail control length and rotation; blocking screws around the nail relieve axial strain in the nailing construct. A transmedullary blocking screw neither blocks anything nor just fills the medullary cavity; it just provides the third point of support on the side of a nail for the short fragment in an intramedullary three-point support system. The term 'transmedullary support screw' is aptly descriptive of synonymous words like 'blocking screw', 'Poller screw', 'Bollard screw'.

Antibiotic Impregnated Intramedullary Nail

Polymethylmethacrylate (PMMA) beads are known to elute antibiotics in the soft tissue. Intramedullary nail impregnated with PMMA is an extension of the same idea (Fig. 5.14). The use of antibiotic eluting nail in eliminating or preventing infection in long bone fractures is common. The main indications are

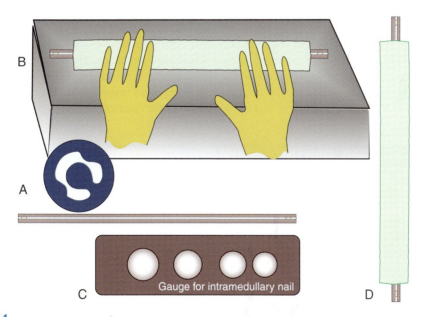

FIGURE 5.14

Antibiotic impregnated intramedullary nail is prepared with 40 g of bone cement and 4 g of antibiotics (usually vancomycin, gentamicin or tobramycin; cefazolin, ciprofloxacin, clindamycin, ticarcillin, teicoplanin, erythromycin/colistin, and cefotaxime may also be used; amphotericin B and C are indicated for fungal infection).[26] **(A and B)** on a non-stick surface soft dough of bone cement is rolled around a 6-mm or 7-mm classic Kuntscher nail with a cloverleaf cross-section. **(C)** A nail gauge is used to achieve uniformity. **(D)** Ready to use antibiotic impregnated intramedullary nail.[26]

(1) treatment of medullary osteomyelitis developed subsequent to nailing; (2) temporarily stabilize the fracture and control pin tract infection secondary to external fixation in polytrauma patients; (3) stabilize the limb in transition from external fixation to locked intramedullary nail (IMN) in a mangled limb. The nail is prepared on the back table during the surgery. Two methods are known. First one uses a 3.5 mm Ender nail and a 40 French chest tube. PMMA is injected in liquid state in the chest tube and Ender nail is inserted in the tube. As the cement sets, the chest tube is cut-off and a nail of 10 mm diameter is ready for use.[25] The other technique uses a 6- to 7-mm thick, straight, cloverleaf Kuntscher nail. PMMA in putty state is wrapped around the nail. The central slot of the nail offers more surface for hold of the cement. A 10 mm nail gauge is used to achieve uniformity and surface smoothness.[26] Antibiotic impregnated intramedullary nail (AIIN) has been shown in studies to be heat stable, with good elution properties from the bone cement and few deleterious effects on bone healing. Smooth surface of AIIN facilitates its insertion through a standard nail entry portal and is easy to remove. AIIN is a useful, easy and low-cost technique to treat IM infection and as a provisional mechanism during the change over from a temporary fixation by an external device to a final fixation. Future development of this technique may include custom-made antibiotic-coated metal nails that may obviate the need for these temporary antibiotic nails.

Dynamization

It is no longer a standard practice to dynamize (weaken) the interlocked nail assembly by removing the locking screws. If healing is progressing normally then there is no need to dynamize. If consolidation is continuing well the removal of the static screw will not improve the quality of the callus.

Dynamization is indicated when there is a risk of development of non-union or in established pseudoarthrosis. The screws are then removed from the longer fragment, maintaining adequate control of the shorter fragment. Premature removal of locking screws may cause shortening, instability and non-union.

CLOSED AND OPEN NAILING

A nail may be inserted by the closed or open method. In the closed method, specialized equipment and fluoroscopy is used to achieve fracture reduction.

The medullary cavity is entered through a small opening distant from the fracture site at the end of the bone. Reaming and nail insertion are accomplished through this portal. The nail should always be introduced 'anterograde', i.e. from one end of the bone; in the femur, for example, it should be introduced anterograde from the piriformis fossa.

Closed anterograde nailing is the method of choice but requires considerable material support and experienced personnel. Percutaneous insertion of the nail eliminates exposure of the fracture site and minimizes soft tissue trauma, maintains periosteal vascular supply and reduces the risk of infection.

In less than ideal operation room conditions, open nailing may be performed. Incarceration of a small comminuted cortical fragment in the medullary cavity and failure to obtain satisfactory reduction are the other two clinical situations when it is necessary to expose the fracture. In the open technique, anterograde reaming and nailing is preferable to the retrograde method. In the retrograde method a nail is introduced into the proximal fragment through the fracture site and brought out at one end of the bone. After reduction, the nail is driven across the fracture and into the distal fragment. Retrograde nailing is tempting but dangerous because there is no control on the point of exit of the nail. In the femur, a nail driven through the fracture can exit on the medial side of the greater trochanter in an intra-articular location and damage the blood supply to the head and neck of the femur. Retrograde nailing should be avoided. The incidence of infection and non-union is, respectively, 6 and 10 times greater in open nailing than in closed nailing.

REAMING

Reaming is an important concept because it can enlarge the medullary canal so that adequate working length can be achieved. The size of the medullary canal limits the size of the nail that can be used; this limits the bending strength of the nail. Reaming facilitates insertion of a nail of larger diameter than could be passed without reaming. Reaming also improves the nail–bone contact, which enhances the rotational stability of the fracture fixation. The process also transforms intramedullary nailing into a smooth simple operation requiring minimal force to insert the nail. If the canal is reamed to a millimetre or two larger diameter than the size of the chosen nail, then the nail easily slides into the medullary canal and its anterior bow is well accommodated without the development of undesirable high stresses near the fracture site, these stresses having the potential to burst open the bone.

The point of entry of the reamer should be precise. A slight deviation may cause eccentric reaming, extensively damaging the canal and compromising the mechanical stability of the construct. Gentle reaming in steps of 0.5 mm minimizes the risk of thermal damage to the bone.

Medullary Reaming – Safe Practices
- Do not use a tourniquet.
- Use a ball-tipped guide wire and check its position by fluoroscopy.
- Start with an end cutting reamer.
- Pay attention to the sound and speed of the reamer. Its slowing and catching is the harbinger of jamming.
- On jamming, withdraw with full power and re-advance. Utilize the ball-tipped guide wire to pull out the reamer.
- Withdraw a flexible reamer only while rotating in a forward direction. Reversing irreparably damages the flexible shaft made from a single coiled wire.
- Stabilize the guide wire during withdrawal.
- Do not grasp a guide wire with bare surgical gloves.
- Check the position of the ball tip after reinsertion.
- Follow the first pass of the reamer across the fracture site under fluoroscopy.
- Stop the motor when crossing the comminuted area with the reamer.
- Ream in 0.5 mm increments and overream up to 2 mm.
- Clean the reamer frequently. Remove bone debris from the reamer flute.
- Discard a blunt reamer.
- Use a metallic skin protector to avoid soft tissue damage.
- Use a high-torque, low-rpm power source for the reamer.

The ball-tipped guide rod is an important instrument; a flexible rod is preferable to a stiff one. The ball tip prevents the reamer from travelling beyond the end of the guide wire and may be used to pull out the jammed reamer. Inability to extract the reamer generally indicates that an infraisthmal fracture has caused a piece of bone to obstruct the intramedullary canal and block the exit of the reamer. A guide rod must then be moved down the canal to push the fragment out of the canal through the fracture site before the reamer can be removed. If the nail fits too tightly during insertion, further reaming or a reduction in nail size is necessary. The nail should advance with each blow of the mallet; if it does not do so, it should be immediately removed before it becomes incarcerated. A large mallet is very helpful in removing incarcerated intramedullary nails. If this is not successful in making a saw slot into the lateral cortex of the femur where the nail tip is incarcerated, it expands the medullary cavity and releases the incarcerated nail.[27]

TRACTION TABLE[28]

Traction table is routinely used in management of femoral fracture fixation. Notwithstanding its familiarity, the patient must be safely positioned on the table to minimize complications. It is challenging to attain symmetric leg length and anatomic rotation; internal malrotation of $>10°$ frequently occurs. Attention to detail may prevent complications. A patient may be placed supine or in lateral decubitus. A radiolucent perineal post is used as fulcrum to apply traction. In supine position the affected extremity is placed into traction in a foot piece or using a femoral or tibial Steinmann pin. The unaffected lower extremity is abducted, and placed into hemilithotomy position; alternatively the healthy extremity can be placed in traction using a well-padded foot piece; counter-traction thus produced eases reduction process and avoids pelvic rotation. Abduction of healthy limb allows space of positioning the C-arm fluoroscope (Fig. 5.15). Nailing may be carried out in lateral decubitus position. The surgical extremity is put in tibial pin traction and the uninjured extremity is stabilized in a foot piece. The extremities are scissored to allow clearance of the C-arm fluoroscope. Safe and suitable patient positioning on a traction table takes time and is not without risks of injury to perineal structures and to the good extremity.

The prime benefit of using a traction table in lower extremity nailing is that it spares an assistant from manual traction, helps indirect fracture reduction and its maintenance by providing consistent traction throughout the procedure. Traction table is often used in fixation of trochanteric, femoral neck, subtrochanteric and femoral shaft fractures. Rarely is this used for tibial shaft nailing.

Complications Associated with Traction Table

Fracture malalignment, neurologic injury, perineal integument and soft-tissue injury, crush syndrome, and well-leg compartment syndrome are well-described complications associated with use of fracture table in femoral fracture fixation. Achieving equal leg length on a traction table is demanding and needs special attention. Internal malrotation $>10°$ is frequent occurrence when traction table is used; the malrotation is less likely when manual traction is used. Use of traction table for an obese patient makes it difficult to gain satisfactory entry point. It is equally hard either to laterally flex the patient's heavy torso or to adduct his injured limb. These manoeuvres are easily accomplished when a radiolucent flat table, free extremity draping and manual traction are

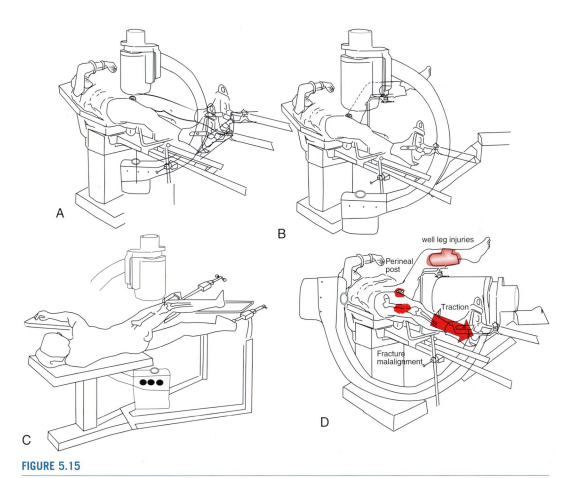

FIGURE 5.15

Patient positioning on a traction table for surgery of femoral fractures. (**A**) The patient in supine position. The fractured extremity is placed in traction, and the healthy extremity is placed into the hemilithotomy position, with the C-arm fluoroscope positioned between them. (**B**) The patient is placed supine with both legs in traction and abduction. The C-arm fluoroscope is placed between the legs. (**C**) The lateral decubitus position. The surgical extremity is placed in traction, and the non-surgical limb is secured to a well-padded leg board. The legs are scissored to allow fluoroscope entry. (**D**) Traction table-related perils in femoral fracture fixation. Use of calf based hemilithotomy placement may cause injury to sciatic and peroneal nerves and compartment syndrome. Severe traction against the perineal post may cause pudendal nerve injury, and damage to the perineal. Incorrect position of the perineal post may also lead to integument and soft-tissue injury and fracture malalignment.

used in the management of subtrochanteric and femoral shaft fractures. It is then easy to gain a straight entry path of the IM nail and prevent fracture malalignment. On a traction table it is difficult to control gravity-induced posterior translation of distal fragment and flexion, adduction and external rotation of the proximal femur fragment induced by pulls of the iliopsoas, adductors and external rotators.

Nerve Palsy

Pudendal, sciatic and common peroneal nerves may be injured on a traction table. Pudendal nerve palsy occurs due to excessive and/or prolonged traction against the perineal post. Erectile dysfunction (ED) is commonly associated with this injury, and the incidence of ED may be as high as 40.5%.[29] It is the magnitude of intraoperative traction, not the duration, correlated with the development of pudendal nerve palsy. Liberal use of intraoperative muscle relaxants expressly decreases the incidence of postoperative ED ($p = 0.02$) as ample muscle relaxation reduces the muscular forces acting on the fracture fragments, which aids in fracture reduction. In majority of instances the injury is transient and resolves within several months. Use of 90° hip–90° knee flexion and straps around the knee and proximal fibula may be the cause of sciatic and common peroneal nerve palsies.

Soft-Tissue Injury

Perineal soft tissue may be damaged due to high pressure exerted by traction force against the perineal post. Malpositioning of the perineal post in the lateral position for shaft fractures causes 10-fold increase in the intramuscular pressure in the medial thigh (Fig. 5.15D). This abnormally high pressure may produce extensive muscle damage akin to crush syndrome and cause renal shutdown. Calf-supported hemilithotomy position of the non-surgical limb causes sharp rise in calf compartment pressure and significantly decreases the mean diastolic blood pressure in the ankle. This combination results in local ischemia, tissue edema and ultimately, acute compartment syndrome.

> **Good Practices**
> Use of traction table for intramedullary nailing of shaft of femur
> - Avoid traction table for obese patients; use radiopaque flat operating table instead
> - Place the perineal post between the genitalia and the contralateral leg
> - Use a well-padded, large-diameter (>10 cm) perineal post
> - Avoid using calf-supported hemilithotomy position for the well leg; instead use heel-supported position
> - Avoid adduction of the surgical leg past neutral
> - Use minimum traction for reduction; use of muscle relaxants reduces the quantum of traction
> - Release traction when surgical time exceeds 120 minutes to prevent perineal soft-tissue injury

NAIL REMOVAL

From the mechanical viewpoint, it is not necessary to remove a nail in a weight-bearing limb and unlike a plate, it may be left indefinitely in the body. Removal initiated by patient request should be delayed for 18 months. Intramedullary devices occasionally induce local changes, which may irritate either the bone or the patient and necessitate removal. Local pain and swelling secondary to backing out of the implant is the other indication for removal; bony union on radiological examination is a prerequisite for such a removal.

NAIL REMOVAL

A sharp angled deformation appearing in the follow-up roentgenogram is a forerunner of appliance failure. A sharply bent device must be removed and replaced, as it has undergone plastic deformation and is very likely to fail with further weight bearing. Bent nails can be removed by forceful straightening and extraction. A nail may fail in predictable patterns when fracture healing is delayed or when non-union occurs. Unlocked nails fail either at the fracture site or through a screw slot. Locked nails fracture at locking hole sites, often at proximal hole of the distal interlocks or by screw breakage.

Nail removal should not be undertaken lightly. Specialized extraction equipment fitting the specific nail must be available. Although removal is usually a straightforward procedure, mismatching equipment, nail breakage, distortion in the bony anatomy preventing removal, and damage to the threads in the proximal end of the nail are common causes of difficulty. It is important to identify the brand of the nail to be removed and have that manufacturer's extraction equipment available. When the implant remains unknown universal extraction equipment set[29] should be available on the back table. To reach a broken implant in presence of bony overgrowth, additional accessories like C-arm image intensifier, curettes, osteotomes and burrs are required. A broken screw extraction set, a vice grip pliers and multiple screwdrivers[30] are useful for removing intact, stripped or broken screws and nails.

Intact Nail with Failed Extraction Device

When one fails to attach extraction device due to damaged threads in nail's proximal end or breaking off of the extraction device, a carbide metal-cutting drill may be used to make hole, slot or channel in the proximal portion of the nail. A hook or a punch may be engaged and nail may be extracted. Femoral head corkscrew may also be engaged in the nail head to extract it.

Bent Nails

A bent nail may be manually straightened and removed. If unable to do so then a small window may be cut at the fracture site exposing the nail. Using specialized drill bit or equipment the nail may be cut through half of its diameter manually straightened and removed from proximal site.[31]

Removal of Broken Solid Nail

It is far more difficult to remove a broken solid nail than a broken cannulated nail. This may be removed from the non-united fracture site. A laparoscopic grasper forces may be used to pick up the solid nail. In another method, the medullary cavity is overdrilled and a circumferential special device is passed over the nail that grasps it and is removed. It is essential to overream the canal, a shortcoming of this technique and other commercially available kits; it may be difficult to pass the sleeve over the fragment; if inadvertently advanced, the fragment may breach the distal joint. A small piece of broken solid nail may be removed by shoehorn technique (Fig. 5-16A).

Many methods that have been used for removing a broken cannulated IM nail are illustrated in Fig. 5.16 B to L. Full weight bearing can commence immediately after the removal of an intramedullary nail, but a return to vigorous sporting activity should be delayed until rehabilitation is achieved.

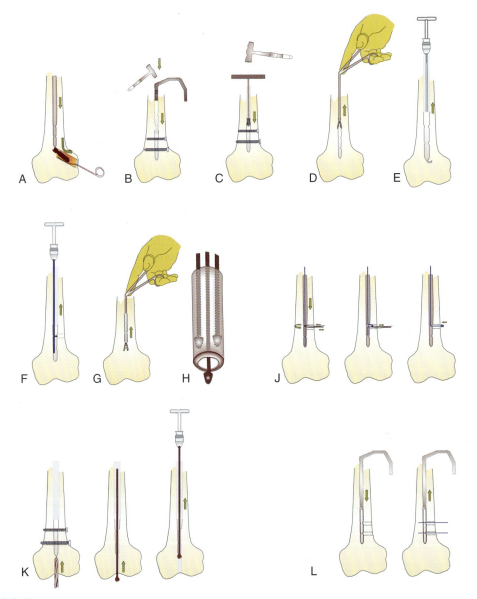

FIGURE 5.16

(**A**) An oblique channel is created in the distal lateral femur. A nail inserted antegrade to push the fragment distally; a Hohmann retractor channels its delivery.[31] (**B**) A smaller nail is impacted inside the retained fragment to pull it out.[32] (**C**) a rigid hand reamer may also be impacted in side the fragment for the same purpose Distal locking screws are removed only after firm impaction has been achieved. (**D**) A laparoscopic force may be used to pick up the loose retained fragment. (**E**) The tip of a stiff wire is shaped like hook to engage the far-end of broken fragment and cull it out. This is the most tried, tested and technically least demanding method that uses readily available items. (**F**) Inserting A thick straight wire and engaging it with a small screw through the interlocking hole may help the effort. (**G**) A rigid sigmoidoscopy grasper is passed through the cannulation in the retained nail and used as a hook to remove the nail. (**H**) Multiple beaded or smooth wires may be impacted in a nail fragment to get a strong grip to pull it out. (**J**) A pliable wire may be passed down the cannulation and snared out; it is then bent several times to fashion a wire ball, which is then used to haul out the fragment. (**K**) A drill hole may be made through the knee to open the far end of the femur. A washer and an olive tipped guide wire are passed retrograde to pull out the retained fragment proximally. (**L**) A larger diameter nail is slid over the retained fragment. Two flexible wires passed through the interlocking holes couple the fragment and oversized nail; both are extracted by attaching a standard nail handle.

REGIONAL CONSIDERATIONS

The Femur

Interlocked intramedullary nailing is the method of choice for the treatment of a fracture of the femur between the subtrochanteric and supracondylar areas (Fig. 5.17). Interlocking improves the stability of the construct. The bending stiffness of the nail–bone construct approaches 70% of the bending stiffness of the intact femur. Interlocked nails are weak in bending in the presence of a cortical gap; the longer the gap, the weaker the construct. The torsional stiffness of the nail–bone construct varies from 3% of the intact femur for slotted nails to 50% of the intact femur for non-slotted tubular nails.

The point of insertion of the nail is of great importance, and any variation may result in bursting open of the shaft (see Fig. 5.6); other factors that reduce this catastrophe are reaming the canal to a larger diameter than the selected nail and use of a flexible nail with curvatures similar to those of the femur. Closed intramedullary nailing with reaming is now a standard practice and the use of unreamed nails is appropriate only in Gustilo grade IIIB and IIIC open femoral fractures and in femoral fractures in patients with multiple injuries, particularly those involving the chest. Avascular necrosis of the head of the femur may occur if the entry point is too far medial and destroys the nutrient vessels.

The angle of the proximal locking screw affects the load capacity of the femoral nail. The more vertical the proximal locking screw, the more likely it is that there is less bone between the screw and the nail, and therefore the higher the chances of failure by push-out of the nail through the trochanter at a lower load. Distal locking screws prevent anteroposterior toggle and should be applied if the distal fragment is shorter than 60% of the length of the femur from the mid-shaft to the joint line. Both proximal and distal locking screws must be in place to prevent torsional deformation. Any compromise may result in malrotation of the distal fragment. Fracture of the distal femur must additionally be protected to prevent fatigue failure of the nail. Distal targeting of the interlocking screws continues to be the most difficult surgical step, and the free-hand technique with a sharp trocar is commonly used. Fluoroscopic visualization of the nail holes needs considerable practice (Fig. 5.18).

A non-locked nail can also fix a femoral fracture with multiple comminution but it is essential to maintain the length of the bone and to control its rotation by means of a short 'antirotation' plate (see Fig. 5.17C). An antirotation plate is also useful in stabilizing a short transverse fragment in the proximal or distal part of the bone.

A combination of nail and cerclage wire is a very effective alternative fixation technique for long spiral and other shaft fractures with a butterfly or large comminuted fragments (see Fig. 7.8).

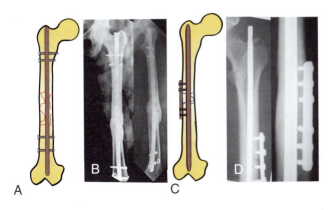

FIGURE 5.17

(**A**) Fixation of a comminuted shaft fracture with a static interlocked nail. (**B**) Radiograph showing a healed mid-shaft fracture of femur with interlocked nail. (**C**) Antirotation plate with a non-locked intramedullary nail. (**D**) Radiograph showing deployment of a antirotation plate and an enlarged view of antirotation plate.

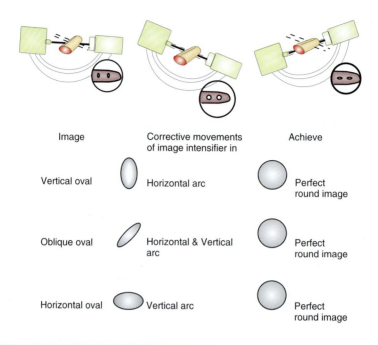

FIGURE 5.18

Image intensifier adjustments to achieve a perfect round image of interlocking hole in free-hand method.[33]

Retrograde Supracondylar Intramedullary Nail

Retrograde nailing is accepted as an excellent method for distal femoral shaft fracture fixation in selected patients. The retrograde supracondylar intramedullary nail is a load-sharing device that does not require the extensive soft-tissue dissection needed for plate application.

A fully cannulated, closed-section, single-piece stainless steel nail with an outer diameter 11, 12 and 13 mm and a wall thickness of 2 mm is available in 150, 200 and 250 mm lengths. It has an 8° apex-anterior bend, 38 mm proximal to the distal end of the nail. Along the length of the nail there are multiple holes for 5.0 mm screws for interlocking that provide flexibility in interlocking screw placement. The first two holes are located at 15 and 30 mm from the driving end. An insertion device is attached to the distal end of the nail, which also acts as an aiming device for interlocking. The entry point and subsequent reaming is aligned with reference only to the condyles, ensuring correct alignment of the condyles with the shaft. The nail is inserted over a guide wire until the distal end lies flush with the cortex of the intercondylar notch (Fig. 5.19). Through the

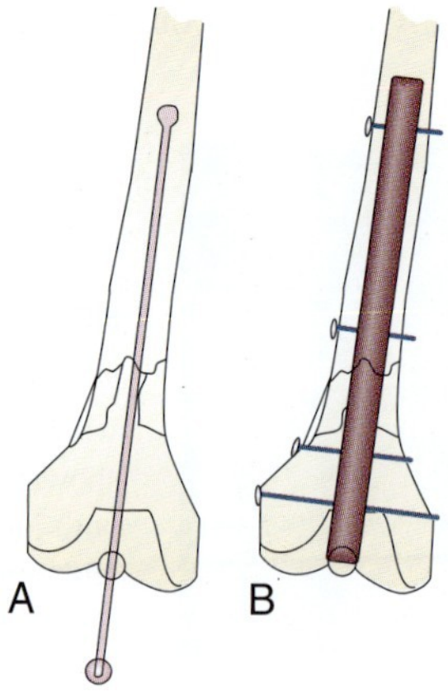

FIGURE 5.19

(A) The intercondylar entry portal is in line with the axis of the femoral canal. (B) Retrograde Intramedullary supracondylar nail in place.[34]

nail-mounted guide, the distal locking screws are placed first, followed by the proximal screws. The stability of fracture fixation is less than that obtained with the blade plate as well as fixed angle screw side plate, and residual instability necessitates caution in initiating postoperative active knee motion. The retrograde nail is indicated in elderly osteopenic patients and in polytrauma patients. Additional applications include the fixation of fractures proximal to total knee arthroplasty and fracture distal to proximal femoral implants. Failure of the nail through the multiple screw holes may occur. Potential complications of use of the retrograde supracondylar nail include stiffness, patellofemoral pain and knee sepsis. With increased use of locking plates, the use of retrograde supracondylar intramedullary nail is diminishing.

The Tibia

Herzog showed that a stiff medullary nail with the cloverleaf design could also be driven into the tibia, provided the nail was bent to 110° to correspond to the proximal tibia and the distal end was narrowed and slightly bent anteriorly; the bends in the tibial nail are named after him.

All fractures of the tibial diaphysis can be stabilized with interlocked nailing. The thickness of the nail should be same or 0.5 mm less than that of the last reamer. As the nail is being inserted, the part still outside the canal should be forcibly pushed towards the femur so that the distal end of the nail is pushed away and does not perforate the posterior cortical wall of the upper third of the tibia. After the tip of the nail has passed down the canal for about 15 cm, the danger of perforation no longer exists, as the nail is then lying parallel to the medullary canal. The nail must advance with every blow of the hammer. Excessive force must not be used. If the nail does not progress, either further reaming or choice of a thinner nail should be considered.

A displaced fracture of the tibia requires special attention. A guide wire with a bent tip is useful to negotiate small displacements (Fig. 5.20 A and B). A fully inserted reaming guide should be in the centre of the distal tibial fragment (Fig. 5.20C). Eccentric reaming may damage the posterior cortex with subsequent perforation of the cortex during the passage of the nail.

In a segmental fracture the intermediate fragment must be stabilized percutaneously with a pointed reduction bone forceps to prevent its rotation and inadvertent stripping of the soft tissue attachments

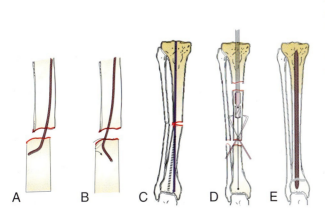

FIGURE 5.20

(**A** and **B**) The curved tip facilitates the passage of a guide wire through the displaced fragments. After reaching the distal fragment the wire is rotated through 180° and then pushed further in. (**C**) The reamer guide must be exactly in the middle of the distal end of tibia. Eccentric position of the guide wire is indicative of an angulation at the fracture site.[15] (**D**) In segmental fractures the intermediate fragment is fixed percutaneously with a pointed reduction forceps to prevent its inadvertent rotation during reaming.[15] (**E**) The nail should perforate the bone scar at the former epiphyseal plate for additional anchorage.

(Fig. 5.20D). The nail should be long enough to perforate the transverse bone scar at the site of the former epiphyseal plate to provide additional stability (Fig. 5.20E).

A thin (8–10 mm) solid or cannulated interlocking nail can be passed without reaming the tibial medullary cavity. Such a procedure is called 'non-reamed nailing' and is useful in open fractures of the tibia. However, non-reamed nailing in the presence of a severely contaminated wound or loss of bone at the fracture site is contraindicated. In the presence of a mild to moderate soft-tissue injury it is a popular practice to ream the tibia up to 10 mm and then insert a biomechanically strong nail.

In the rehabilitation phase, partial weight bearing and dynamization of the construct are recommended to avoid fatigue failure of the thin nail; these measures usually lead to union. 'Exchange nailing', i.e. removal of the thin nail, reaming of the medullary canal and insertion of a thicker nail (11–13 mm), is a viable alternative to bone grafting in the event of delayed union and non-union.

In fractures of the upper third of the tibia, two proximal locking screws are essential. These screws prevent a small proximal fragment from moving during knee flexion. In fixation of a distal fracture a part of the nail beyond the screw holes may have to be cut so as to place the locking screws at the farthest point in the distal fragment to achieve good stability.

Distal locking is always performed first. It is then easy to manipulate the locked distal fragment by moving the insertion handle. Similarly, the handle may be used to apply compression at the fracture site.

The Humerus

The humerus is subjected to large loads (70% of body weight or 10 times the weight of the limb) merely when lifting the arm against gravity. An intramedullary nail is strong enough to resist the prevalent bending loads but is weak in resisting torque (Fig. 5.21A and B). The interlocking technique improves the stability of the nail–bone construct in both loading modes.

In closed nailing of the humerus the fracture site and the radial nerve need not be exposed. This is a major advantage over the plating technique. A fracture, non-union or pathological fracture occurring 3 cm proximal to the olecranon process to within 2 cm of the surgical neck of the humerus can be satisfactorily fixed by interlocked nailing. Small exposure and locked fixation makes anterograde intramedullary nailing of humerus fracture an appealing technique. However, this is associated with high prevalence of residual shoulder disability. Retrograde nailing eliminates postoperative shoulder problems but is technically more demanding. Plate fixation with conventional or locking variety gives predictably good results; minimally invasive plate osteosynthesis (MIPO) techniques promote early healing and give superior cosmetic results.

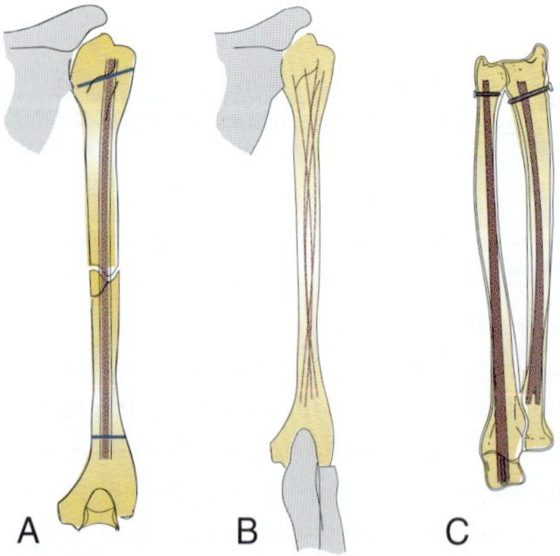

FIGURE 5.21

(A) Interlocked nail for humerus offers adequate bending and torsional rigidity. (B) Stacked nails or Hackenthal pins provide only bending rigidity. (C) Interlocking intramedullary nails for the forearm bones hold a promise but are still under trial.[35]

The Radius and Ulna

The forearm bones resist large bending moments even though they are part of a 'non-weight-bearing' limb. This is due to strong muscle action at the elbow and the wrist. For example, at 30° flexion at the elbow with 110–190 N (23–43 lb) load at the wrist, the biceps generates force up to 1.00–1.48 times body weight, and the joint reaction force at the elbow ranges from 2.7 to 4.1 times body weight. In resisting the bending loads, a radial nail–bone construct is stiffer than the intact bone while an ulnar construct is only 70–80% as stiff as the intact ulna. Nailed forearm bones resist torsional loads poorly.

An intramedullary nail creates a strong construct that is able to resist bending loads but is ineffective in resisting torsional loads.

Intramedullary nails for the forearm bones are available in a variety of cross-sections. Triangular, square or diamond-shaped nails are preferred over smooth round implants because their angled contours firmly engage the circular canal and effectively control rotation. The Sage nail for the radius is prebent to fit the curves of the bone but straight devices also work well. A fixation method other than nailing should be used when the medullary canal is narrower than 3 mm. Fractures of the middle third of the radius and ulna are most suitable for medullary fixation. Although closed forearm bone nailing under fluoroscopy can be performed, only the open nailing method ensures the accurate reduction of the fragments which is essential for a normal range of pronation and supination. In the postoperative period additional immobilization and external support is often needed. Nails with intricate locking devices have been successfully used in small clinical trials (see Fig. 5.19C). A 2008 clinical reports union rate as good as plating, with no periosteal stripping and smaller incision than in plating makes it appealing choice when soft-tissues are tenuous. A brace was required in postoperative period. The authors concluded that the interlocking contoured intramedullary nail system is not superior to plate fixation but can be considered as an alternative to that method for selected diaphyseal fractures of the forearm in adults.[36]

Nailing is a mechanical strategy that at first glance seems biologically destructive, but clinically it works well. Intramedullary nailing is mechanically superior to a plate or external fixation because the location of the nail in the medullary canal assures proper axial alignment, and rotational alignment is guaranteed by interlocking.

ELASTIC STABLE INTRAMEDULLARY NAILING

Elastic stable intramedullary nailing (ESIN) is primary definitive fracture care[37] in paediatric orthopaedic practice. The idea of using relatively low diameter intramedullary nails has been used by Rush and Enders to stabilize long bone fractures, in particular those of the femoral shaft and trochanteric fractures. The method worked by three-point fixation; it failed in adults but worked in children.

The periosteum in children is thick as compared to adult bone. The periosteal blood supply is important for fracture healing and is rarely damaged in a child's fractured bone. Cutting or stripping the periosteum has a deleterious effect on healing in terms of callus formation, speed of healing and bone length. ESIN permits biological healing and callus formation in abundance. Minimal surgical insult to periosteum and closed reduction helps the cause. Elastic nailing permits callus-promoting micromovement at the fracture site. It maintains length, rotation and alignment in both diaphyseal and metaphyseal areas. The healed fractures in children remodel; allowable displacement imprecision should be within remodelling range.

Biomechanics

The elastic nails made of stainless steel or titanium alloy are strong enough to fix children's fractures till healing. ESIN technique is effective only because these fractures heal in half the time taken in adults.

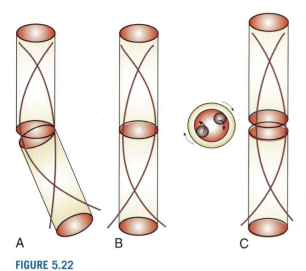

FIGURE 5.22

(**A and B**) Elastic nails when deformed within their elastic limit recoil to steady state and maintain the reduction of a fracture. (**C**) Nails firmly anchored in the starting point and in the distal metaphysis also resist rotational deformity.[38]

Each nail is precurved to achieve three-point fixation. The requisite prebending on a nail should be 3 times the narrowest diameter of the long bone. Often two nails are inserted, similarly prebent and introduced opposite each other to give a balanced fixation that keeps up the correct position (Fig. 5.22). The nail ends are fixed at two points: the entry point and at the far end in the characteristic dense metaphyseal area, universal in children. The nail bent beyond its elastic limit maintains the shape, resists efforts to unbend and creates certain tension in the bone canal. It also resists the tendency to be bent further, thus minimizing the risk of deformation.

Once put into the bone canal, the nail defies angular, compressive and rotational loads; this is attributed to balanced insertion assembly and material's elastic properties. Some surgeons permit the nail to bend during introduction and do not advocate prebending; the nails that are inserted symmetrically effectively perform the same functions, namely maintain length, rotation and axial alignment. The point of maximum curvature of the nail should in the fracture zone; prebending the nail helps to achieve this objective when the fracture is away from the mid-shaft area.

Intact muscle cover of a fractured bone provides certain level of biomechanical stability in ESIN fixation. The method is successful in closed fractures, particularly comminuted ones of the femur and forearm bones. Poor outside support in extensive soft-tissue loss, muscle stripping and grade 3 tibial fractures makes it difficult to use ESIN by itself and further prop up by external fixation or a splint may be necessary. Three nails into single long bone are unnecessary because this unbalances the bipolar matched construct; its use is justified only to resist an excessively external deforming force such as a spastic's muscles.

The choice of elastic nails of titanium alloy or stainless steel is largely a matter of surgeon preference. Stainless steel has higher tensile strength and elastic limit and is stronger than titanium alloy whose modular elasticity and handling properties are complimentary to a child's diaphysis. A stainless steel nail has the strength of a titanium alloy nail, one size larger than itself (e.g. a 2.5 mm stainless steel nail is as strong as a 3 mm titanium elastic nail). The stainless steel is a better choice when medullary canals are disproportionately narrow and are also useful in the management of fractures in a heavier adolescent. One end of commercially obtainable elastic nails is beaked or hooked to facilitate its introduction in the bone canal without hitting the cortex. The nail's outer edge is shaped like a runner of a sledge to facilitate its smooth passage in the medullary cavity (Fig. 5.23). When such a nail is unavailable the tip of the nail must be curved to facilitate its smooth passage through the medullary canal.

Fractures of the metaphysis, or of the transitional area between the metaphysis and diaphysis are more difficult to stabilize by ESIN than of diaphysis. ESIN fixation of a distal diaphyseal or metaphyseal fracture should be fixed by nails entered from the opposite end of the bone; e.g. nails are inserted from supracondylar area of the femur to fix a subtrochanteric fracture; conversely a supracondylar

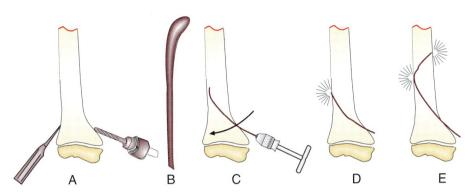

FIGURE 5.23

(**A**) Entry hole for a nail should be a 1 mm larger than the diameter of the chosen nail and may be made with a drill bit or an awl. (**B**) The beak shaped nail is easy to insert and may be used as a reduction tool. (**C**) advancement of the nail using a T-handle. (**D**) The tip of a straight nail must be bent; a straight tip may perforate the opposite cortex while (**E**) a tip bent too long will block the nail's progress in the canal. Elastic stable nails are available in titanium and steel. [39]

fracture is fixed by two nails, one C-shaped and other S-shaped, both introduced from the trochanteric area. The growth plate may have to be perforated to get a firm fixation of a metaphyseal fracture; such perforation is tolerable. However, norms about nail diameter and repeated punctures should be followed. Incorrect positioning of the nail insertions points can have various negative effects. Insertion points that do not lie opposite one another produce differing internal tension and imbalance of the fracture stability and fixation: anterograde nailing of the femur for distal metaphyseal femoral fractures or anterograde and retrograde nailing of the humerus supracondylar fracture and proximal humeral fracture are exceptions. Entry points that are too diaphyseal, damage the musculature during insertion and removal. The nails that are left too long cause severe irritation of the muscle as well as of the skin and may even cause tissue breakdown. Superficial nerves and their branches may be injured during insertion and removal of nails. An injury to the perichondral ring and growth plates may occur at the time of formation of the entry point as well as at nail insertion and may lead to growth arrest.

The nail diameter should be selected to correspond to between 30% and 40% of the narrowest medullary space diameter. Nail diameter is usually 0.4 times the canal diameter. Patients aged 6–8 years require a 3 mm nail for femur fracture fixation; for those aged between 8 and 10 years one requires a thicker nail (3.5 mm) and children older than 10 years need a 4 mm implant. Exceptionally, only one nail is inserted in the radius and in the ulna; both bones are considered as a unit and the nails should occupy 60% of the bony canal. The nails must be of the same thickness and similarly prebent. Nails of differing thicknesses with the same prebent have a different 'restoring force' that pushes the proximal fragment in to a varus or valgus position or cause axial deformity, and eventually leads to functional and cosmetic impairment. This principle is repeatedly ignored. An asymmetrical effect may be desirable when the fracture or soft tissues have a tendency to develop varus or valgus.

The greater the instability of the fracture, the more the inner bracing must be increased. Often there is a lack of internal support. The nails either fail to touch inner cortex or do so very sparingly. Adequate precurving the nail strikingly increases the internal contact pressure and internal support so gained is superior to one obtained from distal and proximal fixation points (Fig. 5.24).

Only correct tensioning of the nails can fulfill the dynamic principles of this method. The circular muscle layers and recoiling force of a prebent nail repetitively restores the normal position of the fracture fragments; symmetrically precurving of both the nails is essential.

Corkscrew Phenomenon

In difficult fracture reduction a surgeon may inadvertently rotate the nail more than 180°, which may lead to coiling of one nail over the other; the coiling reduces internal tension of the nails, they fail to provide axial or rotational stability, and function like a central nail. This is called the 'corkscrew phenomenon'. Once the corkscrew phenomenon is detected, the nail in question must be removed during the same operation and correctly replaced (Fig. 5.23C).

ESIN's Regional Considerations
The Femur

Common complications during femoral nailing are medial wall perforation, failure to catch the proximal fragment and inappropriate nail thickness.

Medial wall Perforation through calcar is avoided by continuous fluoroscopy and timely rotation of the nail. A nail may miss the proximal fragment if images in orthogonal are not obtained. Appropriate nail size is important in ESIN technique.

Preoperative planning for using titanium elastic nails includes measuring the narrowest diameter of the femoral canal and multiplying by a factor if 0.4 to determine the nail size; for example if the minimum canal diameter is 10 mm, two 4.0-mm nails are used.

Ample stability and best possible biomechanics is achieved when nail thickness is 40% of the medullary cavity and both the nails have symmetrical curves and equal thickness (Fig. 5.25). Accuracy in fixation is desirable because any nail replacement or application of hip spica requires a second

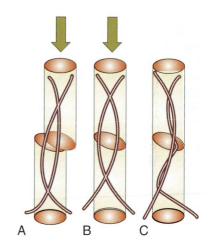

FIGURE 5.24

The greater and more extended the internal contact, the better the stability. **(A)** Loss of reduction due to inadequate internal tension.[38] **(B)** reduction is restored when the nails are adequately prebent. **(C)** Corkscrew phenomenon: multiple turning of nails leads to spiralling of one nail around the other, decrease in stability, and loss of fixation; such a nail must be removed and another inserted to accomplish reduction and stability.[40]

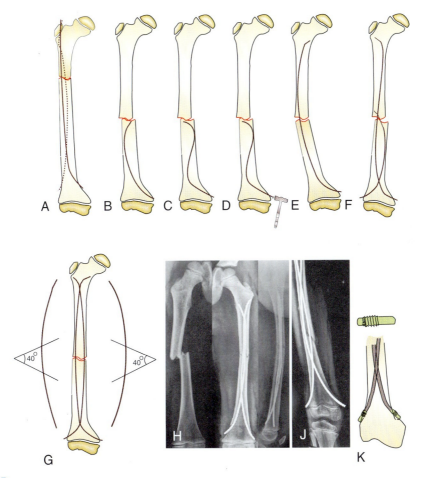

FIGURE 5.25

The advantages of proximal entry include elimination of knee irritation from the nail tip (commonest complaint in children treated with the retrograde technique) and better stability for certain fracture patterns. A disadvantage of proximal entry is the lack of a safe medial and lateral starting point, resulting in unbalanced, asymmetric implants. Also, nail removal sometimes leaves a stress riser in the proximal femur, which is a more difficult area to protect. The transtrochanteric approach is safe and also eliminates the concern about a stress riser but introduces the possibility of trochanteric apophyseal damage, which might lead to coxa valga. Anterograde nailing: (**A**) Transtrochanteric approach; the first nail placed is prebent in a C and second one into an S form. Retrograde nailing[40]: (**B**) nail reaches the fracture level. (**C**) The nail is turned to orient its tip at the opposite fragment. (**D**) The nail is tapped with a mallet across the fracture site. If only the T-handle rotation is used to advance the nail across the fracture site, the nail will often advance into the soft tissues and not into the opposite fracture fragment.[39] (**E**) With one nail inserted a varus deformity presents itself. (**F**) Second nail is introduced and seated at the same level as the first. (**G**) Appropriate rotation of the two nails completes definitive reduction.[39] Nail length is the distance between the proximal and distal physis of the fractured bone. Both the nails are prebent into a C shape; the nails are curved with a mean 40° radius to position the apex of the curve at the level of the fracture. Both the nails are inserted at the same level in the femur. The nails are left lying on the bone and only 1–1.5 cm of the nail is outside the bone distally, and there is no excessive distal bend outwards: this averts skin penetration by nail ends contoured outwards to facilitate retrieval. (**H**) Radiographs showing clinical example of ESIN of femur in a 10-year-old child. (**J**) Prominent nail tip caused repeated skin breakdown. The nail had to be removed after 12 weeks. (**K**) An end cap prevents such complication; end cap is indicated for all unstable fracture patterns. It is applied directly over the nail end by screwing-in action and gets firm hold on the bone by its threads. The end cap widens the insertion hole, which is an advantage in nail removal.[41]

anaesthesia. Skin irritation at the ends of the nail and leg length discrepancy more than 2 cm are frequent complications. Good practices to prevent complications include insertion of nail more proximally from subcutaneous distal femoral physis, to cut the nail smoothly and impact it with a tamp, to bend the protruding nail at a small angle and to avoid full flexion knee exercises before nail removal. End cap prevents the backing out of the nail. The end cap offers a counter-force to the longitudinal forces in the nail and retains the elasticity of the nail. The spring action maintains the stability of the bone–implant interface in the fracture zone. Avascular necrosis of head of femur is extremely rare complication.

The Radius and the Ulna

ESIN is useful technique for 'unstable forearm shaft fracture', i.e. complete shaft fracture of both bones at the same level, with oblique fracture lines and convergent displacement. ESIN consists of ascending nail of the radius and ascending or descending nailing of ulna (Fig. 5.26). The diameter of the nail is two-third of the medullary canal at the midshaft.

When fracture of one bone is displaced and the fracture of the other is minimally displaced or un-displaced, both the bones should be fixed to make possible forearm movements without cast. ESIN method is inappropriate for fractures of the distal third of the shaft or the metaphysis. In this zone, nail should as far as possible be inserted from the dorsal surface, its ends must be prebent to make a contact with the far cortex of the distal fragment (Fig. 5.26B). This will otherwise tilt the distal fragment in the

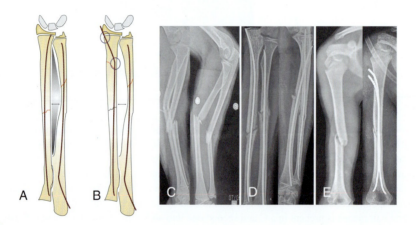

FIGURE 5.26

(A) Unstable forearm shaft fracture is best treated with ESIN in young children. The tips of both nails are turned towards each other to spread the interosseous membrane. Note opposing concavity of the two nails; at the end of the nailing, it is mandatory to rotate the nail 180° to have the concavity of the radial nail towards the ulna. (B) Selection of nails that are too thin, filling less than 60% of the medullary cavity, and lack of correct tensioning of the two nails against one another so that the interosseous membrane is not tensioned appropriately may lead to malunion. ESIN in dia-metaphyseal fractures needs a very distal implantation and prebending of the nail to achieve adequate fixation of the distal fragment.[37] (C and D) radiographs showing fixation of displace diaphyseal fractures of forearm bones (E) radiograph of the humerus showing anterograde insertion, distal to deltoid insertion, for unstable spiral distal metaphyseal fracture. Osteosynthesis stability is proportional to the appropriateness of nail diameter and to the stability of the system with three cortical points.[42]

ulnar direction. A very distal radial shaft fracture may be fixed from a site as far distal as possible but at least 5 mm away from the epiphyseal plate; this entry point will make it possible to contact the far cortex before crossing the fracture line, a prerequisite for stable fixation. Failure to do so leaves the distal fragment fixed only at the entry point and may tilt. A proximal to distal nailing of radius is uncommon because the posterior interosseous nerve is often at risk.

ESIN is definitely the first choice in midshaft and proximal fractures and should be implanted in both bones. ESIN is the preferred method of fixation in all completely displaced unstable forearm fractures, or when there is uncertainty about stability; plates have been replaced by ESIN and used mainly for special reconstructions. Metal is never removed before 4–6 months and refractures are unlikely if its removal is delayed till the fracture is completely consolidated on radiological films.

The Humerus

The ESIN method is indicated in displaced fractures in teenagers in cases of polytrauma or obesity. In principle, humeral nailing is performed in a retrograde manner, monolaterally, only from the lateral side. The distal humerus is exposed and nail entry points are made while watching for the radial nerve; closed insertions are often made too high and endanger the nerve. Two nails are inserted just above the lateral epicondyle on the distal lateral edge of the bone. First is placed with lateral convexity; the other is rotated through 180° to be placed with medial convexity. Posterior nail false passage may injure the radial nerve. Ulnar insertion should be avoided, to spare the ulnar nerve. Stability is enough to lead to healing.

Good Practices

Elastic stable intramedullary nailing
- Choose bigger size nail
- Create a symmetrical construct
- Situate identical curves facing each other
- Achieve maximum curve at the fracture level
- Cross the nails above and below the fracture level
- Avoid corkscrew phenomenon
- Rotate nails to improve imperfect reduction

The Tibia

Children's tibial fractures are usually treated non-surgically. ESIN is used in polytrauma patients or when non-surgical treatment fails to get satisfactory results (Fig. 5.27). For high-grade open fractures or extended comminuted fractures, external fixation remains the gold standard.[43]

The tibia is different from other limb segments being triangular in the cross-section with a dorsal base, and its two sides being aligned diagonally. The planes of the nail are likewise aligned in the diagonal orientation and the tension line is directed dorsally. This arrangement always leads to recurvatum of the tibia when the nails are in normal layout. The recurvatum is counteracted by turning the nail tips in a dorsal direction after definitive placement. Tibia is the only bone where ESIN may lead to non-union, pseudoarthrosis and other complications. Isolated tibial fracture is a case in hand; the fibula

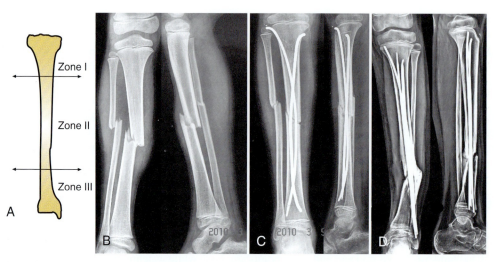

FIGURE 5.27

(A) Indicative zones of tibia. Zone 1: unsuitable. Zone 2: most suitable. Zone 3: suitable with reservations.[40] Because the tibia has a triangular shape, in contrast to cylindrical shape, anatomical stabilization is also difficult. It is necessary to rotate the nail appropriately, depending on the fracture pattern, sometimes with both nails in a valgus orientation to counter the varus force of an intact fibula. Postoperatively, a short leg cast that has been appropriately wedged may be required for 3 weeks. (**B and C**) Radiographs showing a transverse mid-shaft fracture of tibia treated successfully with ESIN. (**D**) Inadequate reduction, incorrect nail insertion points, unequal sizes and numbers of nails lead to angular deformities and non-union in a tibia treated with ESIN.

is often bowed. ESIN fixation often leads to minor distraction at the fracture site and complete reduction does not take place. This treatment can almost be regarded as type of 'pseudoarthrosis model'.[24] Proximal tibial fractures are not treated by ESIN. The tug of the patellar tendon is strong and short segments of nail are unable to counter it. Besides, the distal insertion points damage the tendons.

REFERENCES

1. Schatzker J, Tile M. The rationale of operative fracture care. Berlin: Springer-Verlag; 1987.
2. Mears DC. Materials and orthopaedic surgery. Baltimore: Williams & Wilkins;1979.
3. Bong MR, Kummer FJ, Koval KJ, Egol KA. Intramedullary nailing of the lower extremity: biomechanics and biology. J Am Acad Orthop Surg 2007;15:97–106.
4. Stanwyck TS. Fracture healing and medullary nailing. In: Seligson D, editor. Concepts in intramedullary nailing. Orlando: Grune & Stratton; 1985. p. 27–49.
5. Muller Chr, McIff T, Rahn BA, Pfister U, Weller S. Intramedullary pressure, strain on the diaphysis and increase in cortical temperature when reaming the femoral medullary cavity - a comparison of blunt and sharp reamers. Injury 1993;24(Suppl. 3):32.
6. Heim D, Schlegel U, Perren SM. Intramedullary pressure in reamed and unreamed nailing of the femur and tibia. Injury 1993;24(Suppl. 3):62.

7. Brumback RJ, Virkus WW. Intramedullary nailing of the femur: reamed versus non-reamed. J Am Acad Orthop Surg 2000;8:83–90.
8. Giannoudis PV, Tzioupis C., Green J. Surgical techniques: how I do it? The reamer/irrigator/aspirator (RIA) system. Injury 2009;40:1231–6.
9. The Reamer/Irrigator/Aspirator (RIA) system. Synthes Inc., West Chester, PA.
10. Cox G, Jones E, McGonagle D, Giannoudis PV. Reamer-irrigator-aspirator indications and clinical results: a systematic review. Int Orthop(SICOT) 2011;35:951–6.
11. Quintero AJ, Tarkin IS, Pape H-C. Technical tricks when using the reamer irrigator aspirator technique for autologous bone graft harvesting. J Orthop Trauma 2010;24:42–45.
12. Born CT, Pidgeon T, Taglang G. 75 years of contemporary intramedullary nailing. J Orthop Trauma 2009;23:S1–2.
13. Donald GD, Pope MH. Design of medullary nails. In: Seligson D, editor. Concepts in intramedullary nailing. Orlando: Grune & Stratton; 1985. p. 69–99.
14. Russsell TA, Taylor JC, LaVella DG, Beals NB, Brumfield DL, Durham AF. Mechanical characterization of femoral interlocking medullary nailing systems. J Orthop Trauma 1991;5:332–40.
15. Bohler J. Percutaneous Kuntscher nailing of simple diaphyseal fractures of the tibia. In: Seligson D, editor. Concepts in intramedullary nailing. Orlando: Grune & Stratton; 1985. p. 235–59.
16. Johnson KD. Mechanics of intramedullary nails for femoral fractures. Unfallchirurg 1990;93:506–11.
17. Fernández Dell'Oca. The principle of helical implants. Unusual ideas worth considering. Injury 2002;33: S-A-1–27.
18. Tencer AF, Johnson KD. Biomechanics in orthopaedic trauma: bone fracture and fixation. London: Martin Dunitz; 1994.
19. Henley MB, Meier M, Tencer AF. Influences of some design parameters on the biomechanics of unreamed tibial intramedullary rods. J Orthop Trauma 1993;7:311–19.
20. Browner BD, Mast J, Mendes M. Principles of internal fixation. In: Browner B, editor. Biomechanics of fractures in skeletal trauma-fracture, dislocation and ligamentous injury. Philadelphia: WB Saunders; 1992. p. 243–68.
21. Klemm KW. Interlocking nailing of complex fractures. In: Seligson D, editor. Concepts in intramedullary nailing. Orlando: Grune & Stratton; 1985. p. 293–313.
22. Krettek C, Goesling T, Hankemeier S, Miclau T. The use of Poller screws for metaphyseal tibia and femur fractures treated with small-diameter intramedullary nails. Tech Orthop 2004;18(4):316–23.
23. Ricci WM. Malalignment. In: Ricci WM, editor. Complications in orthopaedics: tibial shaft fractures. Rosemont, IL: American Academy of Orthopaedic Surgeons; 2003. p. 7–14.
24. Stedtfeld H-W, Mittlmeier T, Landgraf P, Ewert A. The logic and clinical applications of blocking screws. J Bone Joint Surg 2004;86-A(Suppl. 2):17–25.
25. Bhadra AK. Roberts CS. Indications for antibiotic cement nails. J Orthop Trauma 2009;23:S26–30.
26. Kulkarni GS, editor. Infected nonunion in long bones – 1. Noida, Delhi, India: Thieme Publisher; 2014. p. 131–63.
27. Winquist RA. Locked femoral nailing. J Am Acad Orthop Surg 1993;1:95–105.
28. Flierl MA, Stahel PF, Hak DJ, Morgan SJ, Smith WR. Traction table–related complications in orthopaedic surgery. J Am Acad Orthop Surg 2010;18:668–75.
29. Uma Surgicals, Mumbai, Maharashtra.
30. Synthes, Paoli PA.
31. Stafford P, Norris BL, Nowotarski PJ. Hardware removal: tips & techniques in revision fracture surgery. Tech Orthop 2003;17(4):522–30.
32. Whalley H, Thomas G, Hull P, Porter K. Surgeon versus metalwork—tips to remove a retained intramedullary nail fragment. Injury 2009;40:783–9.
33. Tanna DD. Interlocking nailing. 2nd ed. New Delhi: Jaypee Brothers Medical Publishers; 2004.

34. Green HD, Seligson D, Henry SL. Intramedullary supracondylar nails. Memphis, TN: Smith & Nephew Richards; 1993.
35. Lefevre C, Le Nen D, Beal D. Intramedullary locking nail of the radius—implant, device, indication. In: International symposium on recent advances in locking nails. Hong Kong: The Hong Kong Orthopaedic Association; 1992. p. 95.
36. Lee YH, Lee SK, Chung MS, Baek GH, Gong HS, Kim KH. Interlocking contoured intramedullary nail fixation for selected diaphyseal fractures of the forearm in adults. J Bone Joint Surg Am 2008;90:1891–8.
37. Schmittenbecher PP. State-of-the-art treatment of forearm shaft fractures. Injury 2004;36:S-A25–34.
38. Hunter JB. The principles of elastic stable intramedullary nailing in children. Injury 2005;36:S-A20–4.
39. Lascombes P, Haumont T, Journeau P. Use and abuse of flexible intramedullary nailing in children and adolescents. J Pediatr Orthop 2006;26:827–34.
40. Slongo TF. Complications and failures of the ESIN technique. Injury 2005;36:S-A78–85.
41. Haas NP, editor. New products from AO Development. Davos Platz: OTK; 2006. p. 16.
42. Sénès FM, Catena N. Intramedullary osteosynthesis for metaphyseal and diaphyseal humeral fractures in developmental age. J Pediatr Orthop B 2012;21(4):300–4.
43. Gicquel P, Giacomelli, M, Basioc B, Karger C, Clavert J. Problems of operative and non-operative treatment and healing in tibial fractures. Injury 2005;36:S-A44–S-A50.

CHAPTER 6

HIP FIXATION

Introduction
Anatomy and Forces Acting on the Hip Joint
Causes of Hip Fracture and Associated Forces
   Hip Protector
Classification of Hip Fractures
Need for Fracture Fixation
Factors Affecting Fracture Fixation
Fixation Devices
   Implication of Fracture Anatomy
   Functional Segments of a Fixation Device
   Sliding Hip Screw
      Supplementary Fixations for SHS
         Antirotation Screw
         Trochanter Supporting Plate
   Modular Sliding Hip Screw
   Locking Plate for Proximal Femur Fractures
   Biaxial Compression Plate
   Intramedullary Sliding Hip Screw
   Multiple Lag Screws
Comparative Features of Fixation devices
   Sliding Hip Screw and Multiple Lag Screw
   Sliding Hip Screw and Intramedullary Sliding Hip Screw
Guide Wire
Traction Table in Fractures of Upper End of Femur
Hip Fracture and Osteoporosis
Regional Considerations
   Acute Pain Control in Hip Fracture
   Technique of Precise Insertion of Lag Screw with a Short Intramedullary Nail
   Extracapsular Fracture
   Intracapsular Fracture
   Implant Removal

INTRODUCTION

Successful treatment of a hip fracture involves understanding of the disruptive forces acting on the fracture line and the constructive ways in which the fixation device should be deployed. Treatment of intertrochanteric fractures is, in fact, applied biomechanics. To achieve an optimal result, important considerations include the physical qualities of the patient's bone, the mechanical basis of the reduction technique and fixation device and biomechanical implications in the postoperative period.

ANATOMY AND FORCES ACTING ON THE HIP JOINT

The intertrochanteric region has a unique anatomy to match its variable function. Normal activities load the hip area with bending torsional and axial forces. These loads are resisted by the large dimension, greater peripheral substance and large cortical surface of the greater trochanter. This region also resists the tension generated by the major muscle groups attached there. At the same time its protrusions act as beam or lever arms for the attached muscles. The intertrochanteric trabecular bone pattern resists the constantly changing combination of forces acting on the hip.

There are large stresses on the head and neck of the femur due to two forces: the abductor muscle force and the hip joint reaction force (Fig. 6.1). The gluteus medius muscle contributes to axial compressive loads along the femoral neck which may be as much as three times the body weight. The weight of the body and the strength of the muscle action together generate forces which act on the hip joint during life. Consequently a hip joint reaction force of equal magnitude and acting in the opposite direction develops.

> **Forces on the hip**
> - Compressive forces generated by gluteus medius
> - Body weight
> - Joint reaction force
> - Bending stress
> - Shear stresses
> - Torque transmitted by the shaft
>
> Neck is offset from shaft – main cause of bending forces.

The hip joint acts like a fulcrum. To be in equilibrium, the joint reaction force must be equal to muscle force plus body weight. The total force acting on the neck of femur may vary from a minimum of body weight up to eight times body weight during fast walking. Bending forces develop in the femoral neck and shaft in response to the forces acting through the head. The femoral neck, which is offset in relation to the shaft of the femur (eccentric column loading, see Fig. 1.16 B), must withstand all these forces. The direction of these forces varies with activity. For practical purposes the resultant load may be taken to lie in the frontal plane at an angle of approximately 15° to the vertical plane, with the forces acting in a medial to lateral direction (Fig. 6.1B).

CAUSES OF HIP FRACTURE AND ASSOCIATED FORCES

On average, a force 10 times of body weight acting along the same angle as the hip resultant load (see above) is required to fracture a preserved human femur. Even then the fracture occurs in the femoral neck and not in the intertrochanteric region which can sustain still greater load.

The forces generated during discordant activities or a fall are considerably higher than those generated during normal ambulation. Failure to absorb energy during a fall, lack of coordination, direct injury to the trochanter and a fall on a hard floor are the usual causes of femoral neck fracture. Subcapital and intertrochanteric fractures presumably occur due to a combination of axial compression, bending, torsion and shear overloads. However, the biomechanical causes of these specific fractures are not clear on clinical or experimental grounds. Two possible fracture mechanisms have been speculated upon. The fact that the fracture rate of the proximal femur relates exponentially to age, suggests that spontaneous fractures occur under nearly physiological overload but are rare. The potential energy that is transformed into kinetic energy during fall is more than 10 times higher than that required to fracture the proximal femur.

Hip Protector

External hip protector, Fig. 6.2, consists of two biodynamically designed oval-shaped shields that disperse the force of the fall, away from the trochanters. These cups are enclosed in special underwear

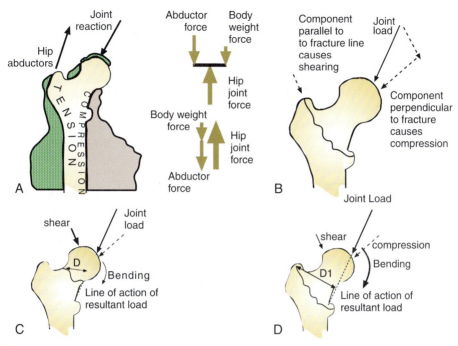

FIGURE 6.1

(A) Stresses generated at the proximal femur due to abductor force and joint reaction force.[1] (B) Loads acting on the trochanteric fracture are parallel and perpendicular to the fracture line and result in shear and compression stresses.[2] (C) In a transcervical fracture, a shear component acts almost parallel to the fracture line. Its effect is to displace the femoral head downwards relative to the femoral shaft. The other component, a compression force, acts perpendicular to the fracture line and compresses the femoral head against the neck of the femur. The bending effect of the joint load is small since the lever arm D is also small and it only tilts the head into a varus position. (D) Similar set of forces act on the intertrochanteric fracture. The bending effect of joint load is greater since the lever arm D1 is longer than D in the previous example. The proximal fragment bends in to varus, compression stresses occur in the medial cortex, and tensile stresses laterally.[3]

and dissipate kinetic energy from an impact on the femur to the soft tissues and muscles anterior and posterior to the bone. External hip protector has been shown to reduce the femoral impact force by 65% and the fracture risk by 53%. To be effective, the device must be consistently worn and requires 10 cm of padding material, which makes it both awkward to put on and awkward to wear.

In a subcapital fracture, the resultant load acting on the head has two major components: compressive and shear (see Fig. 6.1C). The bending moment is a minor load because of the closeness of the line of action of the hip joint load and the fracture line. Compressive loads act perpendicular to the fracture line and impact the femoral head on the neck, increasing the stability at the fracture line. Shear load displaces the head distally in relation to the neck in a direction parallel to the fracture surface; the bending moment component of joint load tilts the femoral head into varus. Compressive overloading often causes an impacted and stable subcapital fracture.

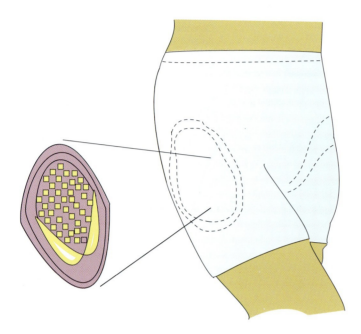

FIGURE 6.2

Hip protector diminishes the impact of the fall, prevents a fracture but is ungainly in appearance and must be worn all the time.[4]

At the intertrochanteric level, the resultant load acting on the fracture also has two major components: compressive and bending (see Fig. 6.1D). The compression is effective if the lateral part of the trochanter is intact. The bending moment is much larger than in a subcapital fracture because of the longer distance between the line of action of the joint loads and the fracture line. The intensity of the bending load is high and in certain cases may reach a maximum of 4000 N, which is much larger than the compressive load. The magnitude of the stress is even greater than the yield stress of a typical hip nail and would result in its failure if all the loads were to be borne only by the implant.

In an undisplaced two-part intertrochanteric fracture the gluteus medius tension is maintained. This contributes to the stability when the fracture is reduced. Frequently, injury separates the greater and lesser trochanters from the intertrochanteric mass. This muscle-release effect of the injury removes the stabilizing effect of the medius tension, tampers with the supportive function of the proximal femur and destroys internal support of the trabeculae. The fracture is then unstable after reduction.

Shear is not a major force, but the axial rotation (torsion) exerted on the femoral shaft during internal and external rotation of the limb is an important factor that could disrupt a fixation.

CLASSIFICATION OF HIP FRACTURES

Many detailed classifications of hip fractures are used in clinical practice. Simplistically, hip fractures may be classified as intracapsular or extracapsular types (Table 6.1).

Intracapsular fractures are further divided into undisplaced and displaced types (Fig. 6.3). Undisplaced, impacted fractures are frequent in the subcapital area and may be treated without attempting to reduce; these

NEED FOR FRACTURE FIXATION

can be fixed in situ. All displaced subcapital and transcervical fractures need to be accurately reduced and securely fixed to ensure healing in order to return to normal activities.

Extracapsular trochanteric fractures are also classified as stable and unstable depending on the degree of comminution; anatomic reduction is desirable, although healing usually occurs. Basal fractures are treated like intracapsular fractures. Subtrochanteric fractures are not discussed here.

Table 6.1 Classification of Hip Fractures

Intracapsular	Extracapsular
Subcapital	Basal
Transverse	Trochanteric
	Subtrochanteric

NEED FOR FRACTURE FIXATION

Hip fractures are complex coupling of fragile patients with fragile bones. An optimal treatment method should address both issues. The accepted treatment for hip fracture is indirect reduction while preserving the correct length, axial and torsional alignment of bone and internal fixation. An additional important goal is preservation of bone viability. A typical patient is an old person who because of the injury is unable to walk, with consequent loss of social and physical independence. Such a patient thus becomes vulnerable and may die from the well-known complications of bed rest in the elderly. The aim of treatment is to minimize the pain and maximize the patient's activities while the fracture is healing. Movement between the bone fragments is painful. Stable reduction and firm fixation eliminates the interfragmentary motion, alleviates the pain, enhances the level of the patient's activity and ensures his or her survival.

If an intertrochanteric fracture is treated by traction, cast immobilization and supported walking, the most likely outcome is a varus deformity of the healed proximal femur. If a hip nail breaks or bends, the result is always a varus at the fracture site. If the fixation device cuts out of a porotic bone of the head–neck fragment, the resultant final position is in varus. The internal fixation device is always resisting a varus-directed load of very high magnitude.

In femoral neck fracture fixation, the shaft and the intact part of the subtrochanteric area act as a buttress and support the load. When the bone supports the load, the implant is spared this task; in hip fixation, a screw thus supports a smaller load at the thread–bone interface. Compressive loads at the fracture site are derived from two sources: physiological forces and compression mechanism of the screw. Interdigitations of fragments and increased friction force due to compression contribute to greater stability and reduce the femoral head and neck's tendency to slide distally and bend to a varus position.

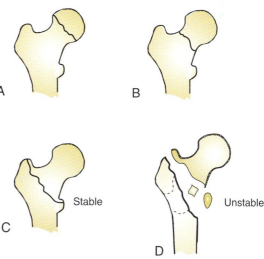

FIGURE 6.3

Classification of hip fractures. Intracapsular fractures: Subcapital (**A**); Transcervical (**B**). Extracapsular fractures: trochanteric fractures Stable (**C**); Unstable (**D**).

FACTORS AFFECTING FRACTURE FIXATION

Success of fracture neck fixation depends on various factors (Fig. 6.4). A hip fracture line, which is more horizontal than vertical, has a better chance of healing. The purchase of a hip screw in the femoral head depends on bone density. There are three parameters of good bone density and all are indicators of the success of a fixation:

1. Singh Index grades 4–6[5]: This radiological parameter is only a rough guide and interobserve bias makes it unreliable; however, it has been used in many currently published series.[6]
   Peripheral quantitative computed tomographic (pQCT) measurement and bone mineral density (BMD) by dual energy X-ray absorptiometry (DEXA) studies are currently the gold standards for assessing bone mass.
2. Cancellous bone density of 1250 CT units[7] and BMD value within ±1 SD.
3. Fixation screw insertion torque of greater than 18.9 Nm.[8]

Factors affecting hip fixation
- Angle of the fracture line
- Bone density
  - Singh Index grades
  - CT units/BMD by DEXA
  - Insertion torque of the fixation screw
- Degree of comminution
- Neck length and neck shaft angle of the femur
- 'Plain film overestimates (by twofold) the degree of comminution'[7]

Hip fixation devices – expectations
- Provide axial compression
- Withstand bending loads
- Resist shear stresses
- Check femoral shaft rotation relative to head and neck

FIXATION DEVICES

Implication of Fracture Anatomy

The pull-out strength of a hip screw is proportional to the square of bone density in the femoral head. The densest spot is at the centre of the head, and a screw should be located there. Other dense spots in the head are in lateral and medial areas, both anteriorly and posteriorly (Fig. 6.4B). Though the best trabeculae are in the centre of the head, there is minimal trabecular support in the middle part of the neck. The additional support of a lateral plate is important in intertrochanteric fracture fixation.

The degree of fracture comminution directly affects the stability. When the comminution of the inferior half of the fracture surface is less than 30% the bone fragments adequately support the load and provide stability. The lesser the comminution, the more resistance is offered to the deforming forces by enhancing compression and shear resistance response. Plain film measurements overestimate the degree of comminution by a factor of two, in contrast to direct measurements of the bone fragments.[7] The length of the femoral neck and neck shaft angle determine the magnitude of bending and shear loads. The higher the values, the larger the loads acting on the fracture site and the less secure the fixation.

Unstable intertrochanteric fracture has four main fragments: the proximal neck, the greater trochanter, the lesser trochanter and the proximal femoral shaft (Fig. 6.5). Analysis of their pattern may help in improving fixation stability. A large posterior and posteromedial void is present; only a fragile lateral

FIXATION DEVICES   245

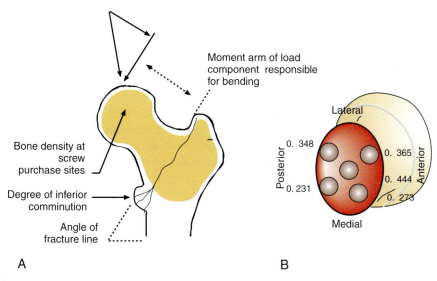

FIGURE 6.4

(**A**) Factors affecting fixation of hip fractures[7]. (**B**) Schematic presentations of bone density in femoral head.[9]

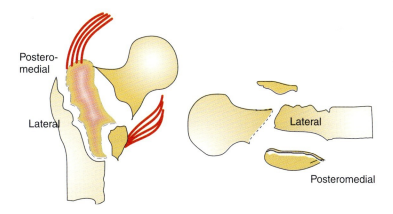

FIGURE 6.5

Four major fracture fragments. Lateral and posteromedial fragments are critical to achieve stability.

wall survives which is an extension of the femoral shaft. With breakage of this frail lateral wall the intertrochanteric fracture resembles a subtrochanteric type; this unnecessary transformation should be prevented. Lateral wall plays a major role in stabilizing and fixing an unstable intertrochanteric fracture, as it serves as a support for axial, rotational and varus stability of the proximal fragment when it interlocks after impaction. Gerard et al.[10] evaluated experimental lateral wall damage and concluded that care should be taken to avoid breaking the lateral wall when drilling at its base during fracture fixation. Lateral wall fracture may occur during or after surgery.

If it occurs, collapse and a long period of disability will follow. This collapse is the main contributor to postoperative morbidity.

In fixation of a hip fracture, bone must support load: the greater this support, the lesser the load on the implant. In a comminuted fracture, stresses on the implant are greater because the bone does not support any load. Similarly, an implant bears more stresses in an intertrochanteric than in an intracapsular fixation because of the greater bending effect of hip joint forces.

Three significant zones along a fixation device are fixation within the femoral head, the mid-segment and the distal fixation either at the lateral trochanteric wall or in the intramedullary canal. An implant's strength to maintain reduction in these three zones is the key to successful healing. Additionally, fixation system should facilitate controlled impaction as the bone resorption progresses. Fracture anatomy, number of fragments and bone quality determine the primary levels of stability which are improved by accurate reduction; fracture compression adds to stability levels. However, bone damage at the fracture site during or after surgery could produce secondary fracture instability.

Functional Segments of a Fixation Device

The proximal section of the implant bestows load-bearing capacity that is reflected in its bending stiffness, load-to-failure and torsional stability. Bending stiffness depends not only on implant's design and material but also on its ability to slide. Increased projected fixation of the implant in the femoral head increases its fixation strength and sliding ability. The type of fixation in the femoral head increases the load-to-failure capability. It has been demonstrated that in uncemented sliding hip screw (SHS) fixation of unstable intertrochanteric fractures, cyclic loading causes irreversible caudal shift and varus tilt of the femoral head; cementing the fixation in the head significantly reduces these irreversible movements. If the fixation in the head is not firm then the bone trabeculae are damaged that leads to secondary instability of the fixation; fixation instability is observed as superior migration or cut-out of the screw through the femoral head.

Midsection on the implant connects the proximal and distal segments and bridges the fracture zone. In this section, the mechanical quality of bending stiffness is tested while providing fracture stability, a biological entity, attesting the biomechanical characteristics of the implant. Cyclic loading and bone remodelling – resorption and formation, further test the implant's integrity. Mid-segment of the implant provides bending stiffness, sliding capability and several axial fixation points. Failure to slide turns a load-sharing implant to a rigid load-bearing implant and may lead to femoral head penetration.

The distal portion of the fixation system must have a secure hold on the proximal shaft. Secondary instability may commence after drilling or reaming.

Fracture of the femoral lateral trochanter cortex and a subtrochanteric fracture may occur during drilling and reaming. Drilling proximal lateral femur with large-sized drill bit may weaken and fracture the lateral wall. In unstable fractures, splintering of the lateral wall of the greater trochanter and its superior migration due to abductor pull thwarts impaction of the neck and trochanteric sections, a prerequisite for fracture compression. Instability and failure in varus lead to non-union. As rule, small-diameter drill bits may be used to preserve integrity of fragile lateral wall.

When pins and screws are used to fix a hip fracture without a lateral plate, it is just the lateral femoral cortex that provides the anchorage; this is effective only till compression is maintained. As and when compression is lost due to resorption of the fracture line, the screw head may move back leading to instability and loss of reduction.

FIXATION DEVICES

Seventy-nine devices are known to have been employed for hip fracture fixation. A few in common use are discussed here.

Sliding Hip Screw

The SHS is a unique implant. It facilitates application of compression across the fracture line at the time of surgery; it also acts as a rail on which axial movement is feasible to achieve impaction of the fracture fragments with the passage of time. It is strong enough to withstand large bending loads and also protects the fixation against disruptive torque transmitted by the shaft in internal or external rotation. 'Dynamic' action of SHS results in reduced incidence of cutout and of penetration of the nail into the hip joint, as opposed to static devices.

The SHS has two major components: a plate with a barrel and a screw.

The screw has a wide shaft with coarse threads at one end. The screw shaft is hollow and narrower than the threaded end. The inside of the opposite end of the shaft has a fine thread, which facilitates application of controlled compression to the fracture; this is achieved by setting a distinctive screw.

Two varieties of lag screws are in use. In the first type the lag screw has a channel that glides over a knob within the plate barrel; the channel permits sliding along the barrel but prevents rotation (Fig. 6.6). The mechanism enhances the rotational stability of the proximal femoral fragment. A non-keyed system cannot prevent screw rotation and jeopardizes rotational stability of the femoral head and neck segment. Use of a keyed SHS system, however, requires that the lag screw be oriented so that the plate can be properly positioned along the femoral shaft.

The second component of an SHS is a bone plate with a barrel attached at an angle. Plate–barrel implants with angles varying between 130° and 150° are obtainable but the one with an angle between 135° and 140° is often used. The screw shaft fits the barrel of the plate and moves freely within it.

The ability of the screw to slide in the barrel is dependent on two factors: the plate–barrel angle and 'screw-in-barrel length'. The optimal plate–barrel angle is a matter for debate. In theory, a sliding device placed at the angle closest to that of the resultant force acting across the hip, optimizes the sliding and eventual impaction of the fracture surfaces (Fig. 6.7). Resultant force in the hip crosses the fracture line at 159° to the neck–shaft angle of the femur. Thus, a 159° plate–barrel angle is ideal in this respect, but it is technically difficult to insert such a plate. Though a screw placed in a barrel at 150° angle, being close to the resultant

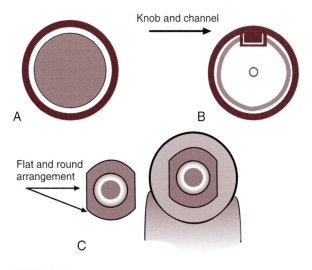

FIGURE 6.6

(**A**) A lag screw-in-barrel mechanism rotates under torsional loads. (**B**) Keyed screw system prevents unwanted rotatory movements. A knob in the barrel and channel in the lag screw and (**C**) Lag screw with two flat sides are prevalent designs.

force, would slide easily, it would also be prone to cut-out of the head. In contrast, a plate–barrel angle of 130° predisposes the screw to more bending load and increases its tendency to jam in the barrel. In actual practice, the plate–barrel angle of 135–140° is preferred.

The ratio of the length of the screw within the barrel to that projecting out of the barrel also affects the ease of sliding (Fig. 6.7B). The longer the length of the screw side of the barrel, the easier the sliding. Optimal sliding results when the tip of the screw shaft is within 1 cm or less of the plate–barrel junction.

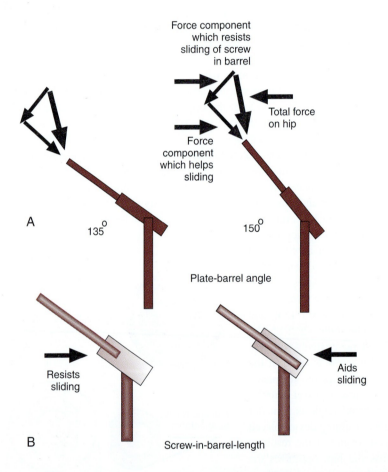

FIGURE 6.7

Factors affecting sliding of a screw in a plate–barrel. Plate–barrel angle alters the proportion of forces acting parallel and perpendicular to the long axis of SHS. **(A)** The parallel component helps sliding while the perpendicular component resists sliding because its bending effect induces friction between the screw shaft and the barrel. The ratio of prosliding to antisliding force, i.e. ratio of parallel to perpendicular force component is about 2 in a 135° SHS and more than 4 in 150° SHS. **(B)** Length of the screw in the barrel changes its sliding freedom. Longer the screw protruding out of the barrel, larger the perpendicular component and higher the friction at the screw–barrel interface and lesser the sliding freedom. It takes more force (1.75 times) to slide a screw when the screw-length outside the barrel is 3.5 times its length within, than a screw that has equal length outside and inside the barrel.[7]

Barrels are available in standard and short lengths. A standard barrel is 38 mm long while a short barrel measures 25 mm. A screw in barrel should be able to slide at least 10 mm to minimize the risk of fixation failure. When a fracture is stabilized with less than 10 mm of available slide, the risk of fixation failure is three times greater than in a fixation with at least 10 mm of available slide. A short-barrel plate is recommended when the length of inserted lag screw is 85 mm or less. In routine practice, screws longer than 85 mm are seldom required. A short barrel is always used in the fixation of a medial displacement osteotomy.

Sliding hip screw – optimum
- Site of screw placement – central
- Angle of plate–barrel – 135–140°
- Screws for side plate – four screws and eight cortices
- Compression – normal bone density

The screw-sliding-in-barrel arrangement permits the fragments to settle towards each other as required, maximizing the stability and improving the contact between the fracture surfaces but precluding varus deformity of the proximal fragment.

If an SHS impacts completely, it loses its sliding capabilities as the screw threads buffet against the barrel. The SHS then acts similarly to an FANP (fixed angle nail plate) and suffers complications common to the latter. Failure to obtain impacted reduction leads to excessive postoperative collapse of the fracture and impaction of the SHS. Excessive collapse of the fracture often occurs in porotic bone. Important dimension of the SHS:

Lag screw		Barrel	
Thread diameter	12.5 mm	Standard barrel	38 mm
Thread length	22 mm	Angle	135, 140, 145, 150
Shaft diameter	8 mm	Short barrel	25 mm
		Angle	135

Recommendations
SHS dimension:
- Thread length: 22 mm
- Standard barrel length: 38 mm
- Recommended sliding length: 25 mm (min 10 mm)
- Total length: 22+38+25 = 85 mm
- The standard barrel should be used with screws 85 mm or longer
- Short barrel for screws 80 mm and shorter

Certain aspects of the insertion technique for an SHS are briefly mentioned. The hip screw is twisted into the head–neck fragment guide over a wire under X-ray control. A special reamer simultaneously cuts the channel for the screw in the head–neck and for the barrel in the shaft. Inadvertent pull-out of the guide wire while withdrawing the special reamer is a frequent event. The guide wire must be replaced precisely in its original position following the technique specific to the instrumentation system being used. Free-hand replacement of the guide wire or insertion of the hip screw without the guide wire may lead to improper placement of the screw and must not be practised. A tap is used to cut the threads in hard cortical and cancellous bone but this step is unnecessary in porotic bone.

The coarse threaded tip of the screw should ideally lie in the central sector of the femoral head in anteroposterior and lateral X-rays. Superior and anterior sector placement is always avoided as the screw is likely to cut-out from these locations (Fig. 6.8). The tip of the screw should lie 5–10 mm under the subchondral bone.

The barrel is installed through a channel in the lateral femoral cortex and the screw shaft freely enters the barrel. The plate should fit the shaft without stress and is attached to it with at least four screws engaging eight cortices. The fracture should be compressed by setting a special small diameter screw in the barrel end of the SHS after fixing the plate. The screw should be twisted to engage the fine threads inside the hollow shaft of the SHS to exert an outward pull. SHS compression screw is 36 mm long and has a hexagonal socket to fit the large hexagonal screwdriver. It is applied to achieve final fracture impaction or to maintain compression achieved intraoperatively. The SHS compresses the fracture surfaces as it is pulled out; the small screw is then removed after achieving adequate impaction. If left in place, it may loosen and cause pain. However, it needs to be left in place to prevent disassociation of the screw from the plate barrel. This infrequent problem results from insufficient contact between the lag screw and plate barrel when either is of shorter length than required. Lack of parallelism between the lag screw and the plate barrel on fluoroscopy, suggests insufficient lag screw–plate barrel engagement. Lag screw–plate barrel disengagement is often associated with unstable fracture patterns and failure to restore the posteromedial buttress. A potential for lag screw disengagement is also evaluated by direct visualization of the lag screw within the plate barrel: when the screw cannot be visualized, a risk of disengagement exists and a compression screw is applied and left in place, not to generate compression, but to hold the screw and barrel together as a unit (Fig. 6.9). In an SHS, compression screw removal is optional: it is left in place in a compression condylar screw (CCS).

Compression should always be applied when the bone density is adequate (Singh Index grade 4-6). The bone shares a higher proportion of the load (almost double) on compression of the SHS as opposed to when compression is not applied. In porotic bone (Singh Index grade 3-1), compression should not be applied because of the risk of stripping out the bone threads and consequent loss of fixation.

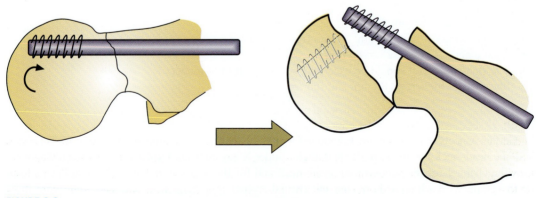

FIGURE 6.8

Anteriorly placed screw is easily pulled out with lateral rotation as very few trabeculae resist this movement.[11]

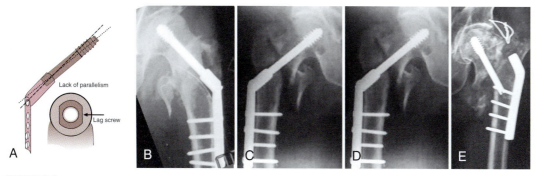

FIGURE 6.9

Insufficient lag screw–plate barrel engagement. (**A**) Lack of parallelism between the lag screw and the plate barrel on fluoroscopy and inadequate visualization of the screw through plate barrel during surgery suggests inadequate lag screw–plate barrel engagement. Both situations allude to high risk of jamming, bending and disengagement of lag screw from the barrel. A compression screw should be applied and left in place to prevent disengagement. Clinical examples of not enough lag screw–plate barrel engagement. (**B**) Compression screw has been left in place and has prevented disengagement. (**C**) The lag screw has failed to slide and has blocked fracture impaction. (**D**) The lag screw has failed to slide and has bent due to cantilevered overload. (**E**) The lag screw has disengaged.

Supplementary Fixations for SHS

Antirotation Screw

In a young strong bone, the proximal fragment may spin while inserting a lag screw, particularly when final seating is executed. The occurrence is more in basicervical fractures. This can be anticipated and prevented. A conventional cancellous screw is inserted as an antirotation screw prior to insertion of an SHS. Before inserting the antirotation screw, two guide wires are passed to avert inadvertent rotation of the proximal fragment. Once the antirotation screw is in place, the SHS is inserted just below it. For ease of insertion in hard bone, drilling and tapping is carried over a longer segment than the length of the intended lag screw.

Sliding hip screw: common causes of complications

- Poor insertion technique
- Non-optimal fracture reduction, ensuing instability, consequent device overloading and failure
- Poor bone quality
- Overloading by patient

Trochanter Supporting Plate

Unstable trochanteric fractures treated with SHS often develop varus deformation of the proximal fragment, with 'cut-out' of the screw and medialization of the distal femoral fragment. The trochanter supporting plate (TSP) reduces the incidence of deformities and associate pain (Fig. 6.10). The plate that is applied on the lateral, tension side of the proximal femur effectively neutralizes the tensile forces during mobilization. TSP's lateral buttressing effect prevents shortening and medialization of the fracture fragments. There is a provision in the plate for placement of an antirotational screw, just above and parallel to the SHS. Screws up to 4.00 mm in diameter and cerclage wires by themselves or in combination are used to fix the trochanteric fragments through the spoon-shaped part of the TSP. The plate does not interfere with sliding of SHS. The laterally placed plate has a low profile and only rarely causes local irritation.

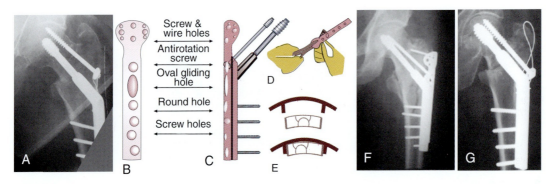

FIGURE 6.10

(A) Antirotation screw in place to prevent inadvertent rotation of the proximal fragment. (B and C) Two profiles of trochanter supporting plate. (D) The plate needs to be moulded before application. (E) It glides over the plate of an SHS. (F) Radiograph of an intertrochanteric fracture fixed deploying a trochanter supporting plate. (G) A wire loop around the fractured greater trochanter maintains its position.

Modular Sliding Hip Screw

A modular SHS for MIPO (minimally invasive plate osteosynthesis) technique is at hand.[13] It has seven components. The lag screws are colour coded and come in lengths from 65 mm to 110 mm, in increments of 5 mm. Barrels are in three sizes and have colour coding, matching the appropriate length of lag screw. A screw locks the barrel to the plate. A compression screw impacts the lag screw. The diaphyseal plate holds the lag screw at an angle of 130°. The bevelled, sharp lower end ensures its smooth and blind insertion. Unidirectional and variable angle locking screws for diaphyseal fixation are a part this technique. The system facilitates MIPO approach, maintains all the characteristics of SHS, and additionally offers stability of locked plating in the diaphyseal zone.

Variable angle SHS system is an extension of the same principle. The plate–barrel angle could be changed to optimize implant-to-bone fit (Fig. 6.11). After insertion of lag screw the suitable blade–plate angle is chosen by manipulation of a setscrew and plate is fixed to the shaft. Setscrew maintains the blade–plate angle throughout the healing period. Variation in blade–plate angle affects the efficacy of the screw-in-barrel sliding.

A single screw and side plate device offer the advantages of a firm fixation on the lateral cortex, a strong and rigid shaft traversing the neck which has weak trabecular support, and achieving consistent central fixation in the femoral head where the strongest trabeculae are situated.

An SHS is often used to fix trochanteric fractures and intracapsular fractures and sometimes to fix a subtrochanteric fracture with a long side plate. Non-union is rare when an SHS is used effectively.

Locking Plate for Proximal Femur Fractures

Locking plates for proximal femur are preshaped and come in right and left versions. The anteversion screws are preset to direct themselves into the femoral neck and head. The two proximal locking screws are inserted at predetermined angles of 95° and 120° and third at 135° at the level of the calcar.

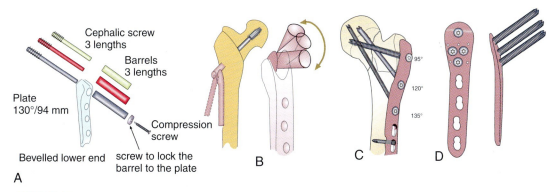

FIGURE 6.11

Implants for proximal femur fracture fixation. **(A)** Modular sliding hip screw.[13] **(B)** Variable angle sliding hip screw. The plate barrel angle can be changed to match individual variation. Two designs of locking plates for proximal femur. **(C)** The three locking head screws are inserted at different predetermined angles; all three screws are in one plane.[15] **(D)** The four proximal locking head screws are distributed in a diamond shape and are inserted at a predetermined angle of 130°.[16]

There are varying numbers of integrated holes that can be used to insert conventional or locked screws in the diaphyseal zone.

Another design is also anatomically preshaped to the metaphyseal zone of the proximal femur and has four proximal threaded round holes for locking screws and are distributed in a diamond shape in the plate.

Percutaneous Compression Plate (Gotfried)[17] is an aerodynamically shaped plate and screws developed with the objective of minimizing surgical trauma and reproducing the walking ability after stable and unstable intertrochanteric hip fracture for an elderly patient with compromised medical conditions (Fig. 6.12). The device permits immediate weight bearing and achieves a statistically significant pain reduction in postoperative phase. Closed fracture reduction to a 135° shaft/neck angle is obtained by traction on a fracture table. A special piece of equipment deals with posterior sag of the fragments (Fig. 6.12B and C). Jigs facilitate introduction of plate and screws. The procedure attributes importance to the integrity of the unbroken lateral fragment of the trochanter which is also the direct extension of the femoral shaft as only remaining buttresses to the more recognized medial and posteromedial fragments. Creating two drill holes of 7.0 mm and 9.3 mm diameters by incremental drilling for compression screws (instead of 16–32 mm drilling required for the screw barrel of more prevalent compression hip screw), preserves integrity of the fragile lateral cortex and provides the best opportunity for osteosynthesis with the proximal part of the fracture complex as well as prevents the collapse of the construct. The double-axis telescoping fixation offers superior rotational stability than a single compression screw. Besides controlled fracture impaction continues till the healing of the fracture.

PcCP device[17] (Efratogo Ltd, Kiryat Bialik, Israel) consists of a plate, with a chisel end that can be inserted through the vastus lateralis muscle up to the lateral femoral cortex and can then glide along the femoral shaft. The surgeon activates two telescoping neck screws to compress the fracture. Controlled fracture impaction ensues as the patient is mobilized during subsequent postoperative ambulation. Three shaft screws are used for distal fixation.

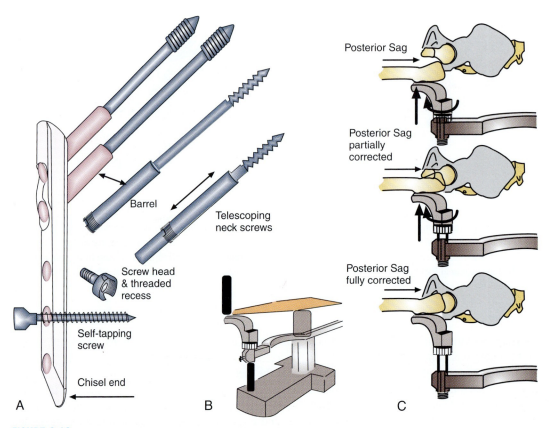

FIGURE 6.12

Gotfried's percutaneous compression-plating device includes a side plate with two neck screws and three cortex screws. An aerodynamically shaped plate (135°, one size) with a chisel end for minimally invasive insertion through soft tissues is connected to the introducer and slid along the femur. Two telescoping compression neck screws (90–140 mm in 10-mm increments) for double-axis fixation have a barrel portion that is screwed into the plate, and a self-tapping screw portion. Three self-tapping screws (31–43 mm in 3-mm increments for distal fixation) for fixation to the shaft of femur. The screw head has a threaded recess and two grooves to facilitate percutaneous insertion and removal. **(A)** Posterior reduction device-PORD (Efratogo Ltd) to achieve and maintain reduction during the surgical procedure as used with a standard orthopaedic operation table. **(B)** PORD is a height-adjustable apparatus with a radiolucent limb support at one end and a standard fixation connector to a fracture table at the other end. Accurate reduction of posterior sagging can be achieved and maintained during the surgical procedure by adjusting the radiolucent section and holding it in desired position by tightening the screw in the housing **(C)**.[18]

Biaxial Compression Plate

The biaxial compression plate (Medoff) permits biaxial sliding, along both the femoral neck and the femoral shaft. A lag screw similar to SHS assembly allows compression along the axis of the femoral neck. The femoral side plate, however, utilizes a coupled pair of sliding components that enable the fracture to impact parallel to the longitudinal axis of the femur (Fig. 6.13). For most intertrochanteric fractures, biaxial dynamization is recommended. A locking setscrew prevents independent sliding of

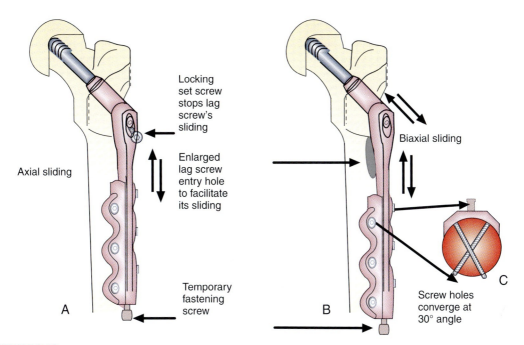

FIGURE 6.13

A locking set screw is used to prevent independent sliding of the lag screw within the plate barrel as in a plain subtrochanteric fracture. When the locking set screw is applied, the plate slides axially on the femoral shaft – uniaxial dynamization. **(A)** If the implant is applied without the locking set screw, sliding takes place along both the femoral shaft and femoral neck. It is necessary to enlarge the distal aspect of the lag screw entry hole by approximately 2.5 cm to prevent the side plate barrel from impinging on the lateral cortex of the distal fragment and obstruct axial sliding. **(B)** The side plate is adjusted while applying so that 1.5–2.0 cm of the plate slide is available; a temporary fastening screw holds the two plate components at desired level during insertion and is removed after the plate holding screws are applied. The anterior and posterior plate-holding screw holes of the side plate are designed to direct the screws to converge at a 30° angle. The anterior screws are applied first and next the posterior ones; rotating the lower limb internally facilitates insertion of posterior screws. Anterior screws are fully tightened only after the posterior ones are inserted. This prevents tilting of the plate anteriorly and causes the posterior row to pull away from the shaft. A four-hole plate is used for an intertrochanteric fracture while a six-hole plate is used for a subtrochanteric fracture.[19]

the lag screw within the plate barrel; when the locking setscrew is applied, the plate slides only axially on the femoral shaft. Uniaxial dynamization is suggested for a plain subtrochanteric fracture.

When opting for biaxial dynamization, it is necessary to distally enlarge the lag screw entry site by approximately 2.5 cm to prevent the impingement of the barrel on the lateral cortex of the distal fragment and obstructing dynamic axial compression (Fig. 6.13B). The Medoff plate is available with only a 135° angle.

Intramedullary Sliding Hip Screw

The intramedullary sliding hip screw (ISHS) has an expanded proximal end with a tunnel for a large diameter, smooth shank lag screw. The intramedullary nail replaces the side plate of the SHS. The increased proximal nail diameter and wall thickness, in combination with screw, design provide greater fixation and stability. The distal end of the nail is fixed to the cortex with two fully threaded screws. The screws statically lock the nail and help in control of rotation and telescoping of the fracture fragments. In delayed union, these 'static' locking screws are removed to 'dynamize' the fixation and stimulate the healing process by removing the load shielding and allowing weight transmission through the fractured bone. An ISHS has the mechanical advantage over an SHS of reducing the distance between the weight-bearing axis and the implant (Fig. 6.14). Implant failure is rare because of the reduced level arm and massive size (17 mm) of its proximal end.

The lag screw withstands the bending moment, which is transferred to the intramedullary nail and counterbalanced by its locking mechanism with the femoral cortex in the medullary canal. Almost the entire load is transferred to the nail and a negligible portion to the medial femoral cortex; an SHS, on the other hand, transfers a large proportion of its load to the medial femoral cortex. The insertion technique, although similar to percutaneous femoral nailing, is more demanding. It is a 'closed' procedure and is less traumatic than insertion of an SHS because of minimal dissection and reduced blood loss. An ISHS is often used for fixation of unstable trochanteric and subtrochanteric fractures. A known

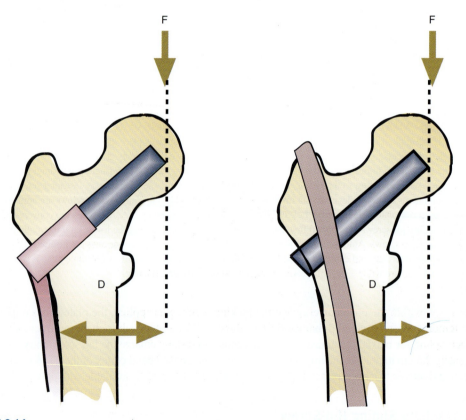

FIGURE 6.14

The deforming force on a device is equivalent to the force F times the distance D and is therefore smaller for an intramedullary nail, where the distance D is shorter.[20]

complication of this implant is fracture of the shaft around the lower end of the nail. Groin and thigh pain on walking are common postoperative complaints following unlocked ISHS fixations, the possible cause of pain being abutment of the distal end of the device against the medullary surface of the bone.

The first design of ISHS suffered complications such as iatrogenic fracture of proximal end and of the shaft, cutting out of neck screw caused by the rotation potential of the head–neck fragment, and thigh pain. A modified version, with longer intramedullary nail than the original design has eliminated many complications and has improved the outcome.[21]

The second design of ISHS has two screws: the lower load bearing 6.5 mm lag screw and a proximal thinner antirotation screw to counter the gyratory (rotational) tendency. The nail's distal tip has been fluted to decrease stress and the distal locking screws have been moved to proximal position to smoothen changes in the construct's stiffness. The design has proved successful for the treatment of unstable intertrochanteric fractures, with a short operating time and minimal blood loss, but is not without complications such as Z-effect (Fig. 6.15).

Experimental data suggest that two screws in osteoporotic femoral head may lead to large stresses in cancellous bone and initiate screw cut-out; data also favour use of single screw nail design for patients with poor bone quality.[23] Continuous cyclic loading causes retroversion, rotation and varus deviation of the head/neck segment; the changes thrust the screw to perforate the bone at the anterior-superior part of the femoral head and its consequential cut-out. A degree of rotation appears in all types of head holding implants. It has been hypothesized that stopping this rotation till the fracture heals would prevent implant cut-out.[24]

The third design, with a single element tackles the problem of cut-out and of stability, both rotational and angular. The refinement is in the introduction of a helical blade for improved load distribution, and

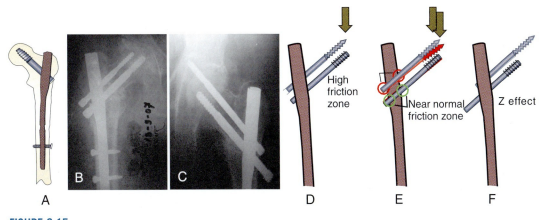

FIGURE 6.15

(**A**) ISHS of first design with modification; the length of the nail is longer than the original. (**B**) Radiograph showing ISHS of the second design. (**C**) The lateral migration of the lag screw and the concomitant medial migration of the antirotation screw causing the Z-effect. (**D**) The origin of this event is dissimilar elastic properties of two screws. Both the screws come under cyclic loading.[22] (**E**) The proximal thinner screw bents easily, jams, fails to slide and cuts out of the head. (**E**) The distal thicker screw is minimally affected, retains its sliding properties, permits impaction of metaphyseal fracture area. (**F**) The Z-effect; proximal screw penetrates the head and distal slides distally.

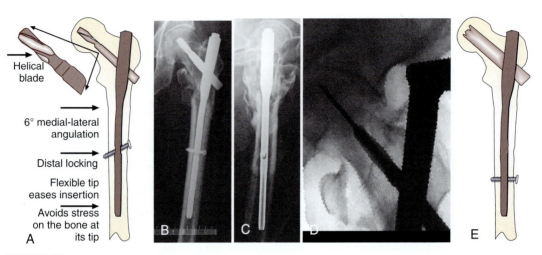

FIGURE 6.16

(**A**) Intramedullary nail with sliding helical blade. Implant is side specific and its angulated shaft facilitates insertion. (**B**) Radiographs showing anteroposterior and (**C**) lateral views of a fracture fixed with the implant.[25] (**D**) Intraoperative radiograph showing wire-guided insertion using a dedicated jig. (**E**) Another ISHS with an I-beam blade that bestows high rotational stability to head–neck fragment.[26]

to offer greater resistance to rotational and angular load values (Fig. 6.16). The helical implant has a small core and its wire-guided insertion requires minimal bone removal in the femoral head and preserves large quantity of surrounding bone. When it is being introduced, the implant's fins compact the cancellous bone around. Once locked, rotation induced cut-outs are prevented or at least delayed because the helical blade prevents rotation of the head–neck fragment. The device has better purchase in the osteoporotic bone. This fact has been biomechanically proven. The implant also permits controlled impaction of the metaphyseal fracture zone.

A variant of the third design is the proximal blade with an I-beam cross-section profile which provides high rotational stability at head–neck fragment and at the blade–nail interface.[25] The lateral end of the blade is angled to finish parallel with the lateral cortex and thus avoid irritation of ilio-tibial tract.

The nail segment of third design has an angle of 6° in the frontal plane to facilitate its positioning at the greater trochanter. It has a curve to match femur's bowing and is available in different lengths to manage intertrochanteric and subtrochanteric fractures. Up to three types of neck–shaft angles are also available.

IMFN Good practices[27]

- Contemplate tip-apex distance (TAD) between <20 mm and <25 mm.
- Use a nail when lateral wall is compromised (reverse oblique fracture and transtrochanteric fracture.
- Deploy a nail to fix unstable fracture; the awesome foursome (Fig. 6.17).
- Install a nail with anterior bow in the elderly; recommended radius of curvature ≤2000 mm.

- Introduce a nail just medial to tip of greater trochanter; this avoids inadvertent enlargement of the entry point, lateral placement of the nail and occasional varus reduction of the proximal fragment.
- Reduce a fracture before reaming; a proximal fracture will not self-align like its diaphyseal counterpart. The nail is not a reduction tool.
- Insert a nail in vertical trajectory; avoid use of heavy mallet for nail insertion. When in difficulty to pass the nail by hand look out for the cause of obstruction like narrow canal or impingement on anterior cortex; inserting starter reamer to recommended depth, overreaming femoral canal by 1 mm, and use of a nail of different specification could overcome the problem.
- Avoid varus angulation of proximal fragment. The tip of the greater trochanter and the centre of the femoral head are coplanar; if the centre of the femoral head is distal to the tip of the grater trochanter, the reduction is in varus; if the centre of the head is proximal to the greater trochanter, the reduction is in valgus.
- Use long nail and lock it for axial and rotational stability.
- Avoid distraction at the fracture site; before locking release the traction and inspect the fracture site under fluoroscope

Multiple Lag Screws

Two to four large, partially threaded cancellous bone screws are used to fix an intracapsular hip fracture. These screws act as lag screws and produce active compression across the fracture site. The compression counteracts the bending and shear forces and uses the compression component of the joint reaction force to improve the stability of the reduction. A single screw is unable to resist the element

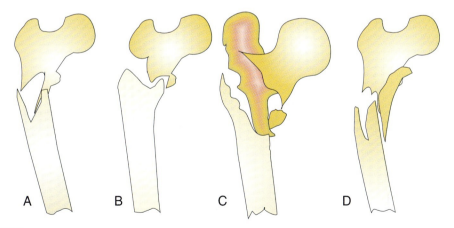

FIGURE 6.17

The four classic unstable intertrochanteric fracture patterns: **(A)** reverse obliquity fracture, **(B)** transtrochanteric fracture, **(C)** four-part fracture with a large posteromedial fragment, **(D)** fracture with subtrochanteric extension. When internally fixed, the bony fragments of these unstable fractures are unable to share the weight-bearing loads, and the load is mainly supported by the internal fixation device; ISHS is the implant of choice.

of torque which although smaller than the bending force, is still large enough to disrupt the fixation (Fig. 6.18). A minimum of two screws is required; usually two to four screws are used. An increase in the number of screws, however, does not result in a proportionate increase in fracture stability. In addition to the factors already mentioned, the lay of the screw in relation to the fracture line (e.g. a screw placed perpendicular to the fracture line produces greatest impaction) affects the fixation.

> **Multiple lag screw fixation**
> - Prevents loss of fracture reduction
> - Prevents posterior and varus migration of the femoral head
> - Maintains bone-on-bone support as the fracture settles by virtue of parallel placement

The densest trabeculae are in the centre of the femoral head and in the subchondral area. With osteoporosis, the trabeculae in the neck area are reduced in number or are absent and there is no support to the shaft of the screw. If all the screws are placed in the middle area of the neck which is devoid of trabeculae, then the screws are supported only at their ends (in the centre of the head medially and on the shaft of the femur laterally).

A screw may lose its ability to slide if the central unsupported part bends when loaded during ambulation. For this reason, at least one screw should be placed as low as possible in the inferior part of the neck so that it may rest for support on the cortical bone. Other screws may be placed in the centre of the femoral head as their shafts may not have any support in the neck segment. The quality of fixation in the head is related more to the points of fixation than it is to the thread type of the screw used for achieving the fixation. The popular technique for an intracapsular fracture fixation is to deploy two to four cannulated cancellous screws parallel to each other along the long axis of the femoral neck. Cannulated screws increase the accuracy of fixation. These screws are inserted over guide wire: jigs are used to precisely deploy guide wires that determine the screw position as well as its length. The guide wire essentially takes the place of a pilot hole used for placing solid screws. Parallel screw placement produces excellent compression by the lag effect of the screws: controlled compression with lag screws is safer in protecting the vascular status of the femoral head.

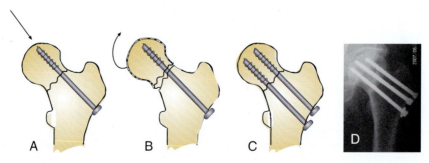

FIGURE 6.18

A single screw resists the bending moment of the joint force (**A**) but fails to resists torque (twisting force) (**B**). At least two screws are required to check the disruptive torque (**C**). (**D**) Radiograph showing a transcervical fracture fixed with three cancellous screws.

(From Radin et al. (1992),[28] redrawn and modified with permission.)

COMPARATIVE FEATURES OF FIXATION DEVICES

The mode of load transfer is different for each device (Fig. 6.19). A few comparable and contrasting features of the four devices are discussed below.

Sliding Hip Screw and Multiple Lag Screw

The fixation strength of both devices is similar. In laboratory testing, the SHS fails by progressive migration of the screw in the femoral head whereas the multiple lag screws (MLS) fail by bending at slightly higher loads, irrespective of their numbers (3, 5 or 7). The SHS screw provides little, if any, torsional stability because it is a single-axis fixation device that inadequately controls torsion, as compared with multiple-axis fixation.[8] The MLS fixation strength does not increase in proportion to an increase in number of lag screws; however, at least two lag screws are mandatory but three screws are preferred for stable fixation.

Sliding Hip Screw and Intramedullary Sliding Hip Screw

An SHS transfers a larger proportion of the bending load to the medial cortex (calcar strain). In contrast, an ISHS supports a far greater proportion of this load and transfers a very small part to the medial

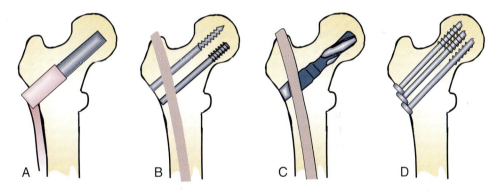

FIGURE 6.19

Different load transfer mechanisms across a femoral neck fracture with four fixation implants. (**A**) SHS helps the fracture components to slide together and impact. The femur partly supports the compressive component of the applied load, as well as resists shear load parallel to the fracture line. The shear component is supported due to impaction, which increases friction at the fracture surface. Also, the bending load is supported by fracture fragment contact in the inferior region of the fracture surface. ISHS bears the applied bending load, which is transferred to the intramedullary nail and is resisted by its contact against the medullary canal of the femoral shaft or its distal locking mechanism. Two designs are in use. (**B**) The first one has a large sliding screw, which is the mainstay of the fixation, and another smaller derotation screw, which is expected to block the rotation of the head–neck fragment. (**C**) The second design has a centrally placed helical blade, which compacts the bone and seeks stability from the packed in bone and squeezed trabeculae. (**D**) Multiple lag screws exert active compression across the fracture site that like SHS fixation transfer axial compressive, shear and bending loads. However, the implants themselves do not transfer load to the femoral cortex.[7]

cortex (calcar strain: SHS 155% of the intact femur, ISHS 7% of the intact femur).[7] The effect of this unloading of medial cortex on fracture healing is unclear at present; however, these different modes of load support and transfer deserve a mention. Use of an ISHS creates the stiffest bone–implant construct. (Stiffness is the resistance of a construct to deformation. The higher the stiffness, the smaller the deformation of the construct, and the smaller the displacement of fracture fragments, giving a more favourable healing milieu.) An ISHS fixed fracture is 76% stiffer in torsion and 37% stiffer in bending than one fixed with an SHS. Similarly, an ISHS fixation is 53% stiffer in torsion and 140% stiffer in bending than an MLS fixation. An ISHS can withstand twice the amount of cyclic load and has a fatigue life three-times longer than that of an SHS. There is an extraordinary rise in use of an ISHS that is not supported by evidence. The increase has occurred in spite of higher incidences of procedure-related complications and no major improvement in functional outcome or patient satisfaction when compared to an SHS.[21]

An evidence based review of literature on ISHS and SHS devices suggest that there are no significant differences in operating room time, blood loss, wound problems, hospital stay, ambulation, functional outcomes, loss of reduction, healing rate, mortality and overall complication rates. The study recommended either an SHS (sliding hip screw) or an ISHS device for stable intertrochanteric fractures and an ISHS device for unstable fractures.[29]

GUIDE WIRE

All these devices use a guide wire for accurate placement. The tip of guide wire is usually threaded. This is done to briefly fix the wire in bone. As a cannulated screw passes over the wire, threaded tip prevents wire's forward motion. The threaded tip also helps fix the wire in overdrilling or tapping procedures. The threads help keep the guide wire in place when a screw needs to be changed.

The junction of the thread and the smooth shaft is a potential weak point. A thread with a uniform root diameter results in a weaker junction with the smooth shaft than a tapered root that starts with the same diameter as the smooth shaft and decreases towards the tip (Fig. 6.20A and B). When a screw is being placed, bending or breakage may occur at this weak junction. A larger guide wire is often marked for direct reading. This is done with etched numerals or with rings or other markings. Direct reading of depth gauge placed along the exposed portion of the guide wire is simple and easy.

The guide wire essentially takes the place of the pilot hole used for placing solid screws. Since the guide wire diameter is always smaller than the root diameter of the screw, there is little chance of overenlarging the 'pilot hole' when inserting a cannulated screw. A cannulated screw is stiffer than a guide wire and takes a straight path as it is being inserted. The passage causes increased stress at a bent section as the wire is straightened when the screw passes over it. Whenever there is difficulty in withdrawing the guide wire after screw placement, the screw is backed out part way, the wire removed, and the screw is advanced again without the guide wire.

Occasionally, a drill bit is used as a guide wire. The length and diameter of the drill bit should be the same as that of the guide wire: it may then be used directly and depth measurements are taken from it. Caution is necessary as the screw is driven over the drill bit. Since bone chips are trapped between the screw and the drill bit, jamming of the screw can occur. The sharp-tipped drill bit is more likely to turn and advance forward than a guide wire with a threaded tip. The tip of a drill bit is monitored with fluoroscopy when it is used as a guide wire. The drill bit is removed after the screw has advanced

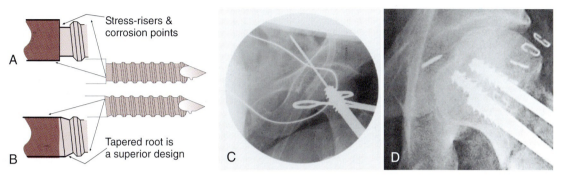

FIGURE 6.20

(A) The junction of the thread and the smooth shaft of a guide wire is a potential weak point because the sharp angles are stress risers and also act as spots where corrosion may start. **(B)** A tapered root that starts with the same diameter as the smooth shaft and decreases towards the tip of the guide wire is a superior design and unlikely to bend or break.[30] **(C)** A guide wire may inadvertently penetrate the hip joint; a bent guide wire is the likely cause; single use of guide wire is recommended. **(D)** The tip of an often used guide wire may break off.

only part way. One example of use of drill bit as guide wire is in fixation of slipped femoral capital epiphysis where the bone is very dense.

TRACTION TABLE IN FRACTURES OF UPPER END OF FEMUR

Use of traction table for fixation of proximal femur fractures has been described as early as in 1927; its use for these fractures is common today as it spares the need of an assistant of providing consistent traction for indirect fracture reduction and its maintenance.

The patient typically lies in supine position and the good limb is held in the fracture table's foot holder. The fracture is first reduced and then the injured leg is fixed in another foot holder. A well-padded post in the perineum prevents undue pressure on the genitalia or the urinary catheter and provides counter traction point. The pelvis should be well supported and remain horizontal.

Position of the perineal post is of significance in the treatment of these fractures. When the perineal post is placed on the injured side, it creates a distraction vector that displaces the fracture fragments (Fig. 6.21); the farther the lateral position of the perineal post, the greater the distraction vector.

Good Surgical Practices
Traction table
- Use well-padded perineal post of 10 cm or larger diameter.
- Place perineal post between genitalia and uninjured side.
- Avoid traction table for obese patients' IM nailing.
- Release traction intermittently when surgical time exceeds 120 minutes.
- Avoid hemilithotomy position for uninjured limb.

CHAPTER 6 HIP FIXATION

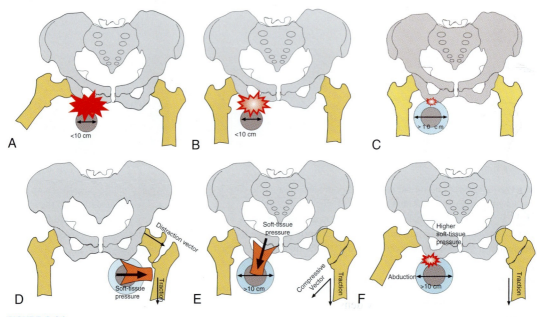

FIGURE 6.21

Perineal post and soft tissue pressure. Size of the post and position of the thigh affects the pressure. A post of 10 cm or smaller diameter exerts a very high pressure. **(A)** Abduction of the ipsilateral thigh increases the tissue pressure. **(B)** A neutral position reduces the pressure to a lower level. **(C)** The pressure drops to a safe level when the diameter of perineal post is more than 10 cm. A perineal post should be well padded and measure more than 10 cm in diameter. Location of perineal post in management of intertrochanteric fracture **(D)**, when located on the injured side resultant vector distracts the fracture. **(E)** The perineal post should be located on the contralateral side; this facilitates the reduction and maintenance of the fracture. **(F)** Placing the uninjured limb in hemilithotomy increases the perineal pressure and may damage the perineal soft tissues and nerves.[31]

In fixation of intertrochanteric femoral fractures, the perineal post should be placed on the uninjured side; this facilitates fracture reduction and maintenance.

The traction table should not be used when dealing with an irreducible variant of intertrochanteric fracture. Clinical picture is of a swelling in front of the hip joint after an injury. Radiographs show a minimally comminuted intertrochanteric fracture with shaft fragment pulled upward by the iliopsoas tendon in anteroposterior view and in front of the head and neck fragment in the lateral view. The lesser trochanter is intact while head and neck fragment has a long spike. The fracture needs to be open reduced on a standard operating table. Three essential steps to obtain reduction are shown in Fig. 6.22.

HIP FRACTURE AND OSTEOPOROSIS

Osteoporosis is loss of bone mass. There is no surgical procedure to improve the quality of tissue. Osteoporosis frequently leads to fracture; hip fractures are common in the elderly population, which has a sizeable incidence of osteoporosis. Osteoporosis renders intertrochanteric fractures unstable. Unstable hip fractures

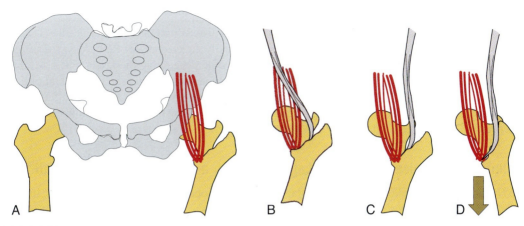

FIGURE 6.22

(A) Irreducible intertrochanteric fracture featuring high riding femoral shaft and an intact lesser trochanter. (B) No traction. Full adduction and external rotation of the thigh to slacken the iliopsoas tendon. (C) A Hohmann retractor placed medial to the shaft to lever out the sunken femoral neck to the front. (D) Traction in abduction and internal rotation completes the reduction.[32] Patients presenting after 2–3 weeks may need tenotomy of iliopsoas.

are frequent, with major posterior and medial cortical comminution and extensive displacement. In osteoporosis, the trabeculae in the head and neck of the femur are reduced in number or are absent (Singh Index grades 3-1), leading to poor screw purchase in the head and inadequate support to the shaft of the screw in the neck segment. The pull-out strength of cortical screws fixing the plate is also diminished. The screws tend to slide more in porotic bone. A hip fracture in porotic bone should not be compressed because of increased risk of stripping the bone threads and consequent loss of fixation. The Singh Index grades are a rough guide to assess the severity of osteoporosis.

In osteoporosis good bony apposition must be obtained so that the load is shared between the implant and the bone. Failure is certain if the device is deployed for fixation rather than to align the bone fragments and share the load.

Hip fracture and osteoporosis

- Disposition to extensive comminution
- Poor screw purchase
- Reduced trabecular support
- Propensity to varus deformity
- Higher implant migration and cut-out rate

REGIONAL CONSIDERATIONS

Acute Pain Control in Hip Fracture

Hip fracture causes severe pain that must be controlled acutely. Use of conventional opioids has limitations and side effects. Fascia Iliaca compartment blockade quickly controls pain and is an effective, low-tech, low-risk, easily learned procedure for surgeons as well as anaesthetist and also may reduce opioid side effects in fragile, elderly patients. The blockade is administered soon after the diagnosis of the fracture and may be done as a bed-side procedure. A line is drawn from the pubic tubercle to the anterior superior iliac spine and is divided in 3 equal sections.[33] The site of injection is marked 1 cm caudal to the junction of the lateral third and medial two-thirds of the line (Fig. 6.23). Femoral pulsations are 1.5 to 2 cm medial to this point. After skin disinfection, an epidural needle (18/20 G Touhy) is used to puncture the skin in sagittal plane at cranially directed angle of 60°; loss of resistance (pop) is felt at two spots: on piercing the fascia lata and while penetrating the fascia iliaca. After the second pop, the needle's angle is reduced to 30° and if no blood is drawn on aspiration, 50 ml of 0.5% Ropivacaine is injected in the compartment.[34] Gentle massage around the site spreads the fluid in the compartment and blocks all the 3 nerves giving complete relief lasting 6–12 hours. The procedure may be repeated till the surgery and also for post-surgery pain relief.

Technique of Precise Insertion of Lag Screw with a Short Intramedullary Nail[36]

The Nishiura technique allows insertion of a lag screw into the optimal position on both planes, inferior half on the anteroposterior (AP) view and exactly central on the true lateral view of the hip. A true lateral view of the hip shows the alignment of the femoral neck axis with that of the femoral shaft. The view is obtained by inclining the image intensifier by 20° from the coronal plane.

The nail is introduced in a standard way and depth of the nail is so adjusted that the guide wire could be inserted in the inferior half of the femoral head on the AP view. The image intensifier is repositioned for the true lateral view. The c-arm and targeting device assembly are so rotated to get a view that shows the aiming rod and the neck of femur are superimposed. In this view the X-ray beam, the targeting device and the femoral neck are on the same plane. A lag screw inserted in this true lateral view will be placed exactly into the centre of the femoral head. A lag screw so inserted can be set forward as closest to articular surfaces as within 5 mm on the AP view without a risk of penetration and tip-apex distance (TAD) under 20 mm could be achieved to eliminate the risk of cut-outs. The technique works with all varieties of intramedullary trochanteric nails (ISHS) but is not applicable for introduction of an SHS.

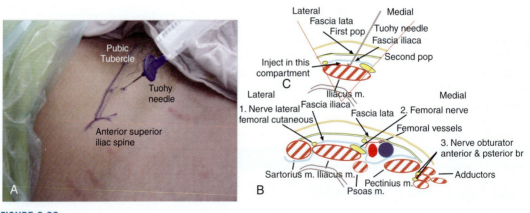

FIGURE 6.23

(A) Facia iliaca compartment block (FICB). The surface markings should always be made in ink as a safeguard. **(B)** Schematic cross-section anatomy of FIC. The block anaesthetizes three nerves: (1) lateral femoral cutaneous, (2) femoral (3) anterior and posterior divisions of Obturator.[35] **(C)** Inset to clarify the location of two 'pops' and the position of the needle inside the compartment.

Reduction and internal fixation is the generally accepted treatment for hip fractures. Use of a fracture table and X-ray control is essential for a successful outcome. The trochanteric area has abundant blood supply and good healing is the rule, as opposed to the subcapital and transcervical area where blood supply is usually suspect and avascular necrosis is frequent. The method of fracture reduction and choice of fixation implant differs with the fracture type.

'Fracture compression' is a tactic executed by a surgeon to compress a fracture; there are no destabilizing torsional and bending forces on the hip joint. 'Fracture impaction' is postsurgical compression, happens passively as a patient is mobilized; the fixation device slides as common activities subject the hip joint to cyclic bending and torsional forces. 'Controlled fracture impaction' also occurs passively; the fixation device has additional capability to control rotation and provides torsional stability. Rotational stability distinguishes between fracture impaction and controlled fracture impaction. Fracture collapse is displacement-impaction of a fracture with a loss of reduction; the distal fragment is medialized but actual impaction does not take place; there may be further damage, like a subtrochanteric extension or lateral wall fracture.

Extracapsular Fracture

The formal displacement osteotomies, namely Dimon–Hughston medial displacement osteotomy, the Sarmiento valgus osteotomy and the Wayne County lateral displacement reduction, that were once popular, are inferior to anatomic reduction for managing load transmission from a biomechanical viewpoint because osteotomies involve a shift in the load-bearing axis and resultant limb shortening. These fixed angle nail plate device stabilized osteotomies, when compared to anatomic fixation with an SHS, were associated with increased mortality, longer hospital stay, higher wound infection rate, increased limb shortening, reduced incidence of return to pre-injury walking ability and more complications of fixation failure. When an SHS is used to fix an unstable intertrochanteric fracture, medial displacement osteotomy does not offer any special advantage and need not be performed: on the contrary limb shortening would almost certainly result. An SHS also permits controlled collapse at the fracture site. Even an (anatomically reduced) unstable fracture may impact spontaneously to a stable and often medially displaced position.

An ISHS fixation is biomechanically similar to an SHS but is technically more demanding than the latter; it takes longer to fix an intertrochanteric fracture with an ISHS than with an SHS. The operating time for an ISHS fixation is same irrespective of the degree of comminution of the fracture whereas SHS fixation time increases with the complexity of the fracture. An ISHS is the implant of choice for the fixation of complex trochanteric fractures in fragile individuals.[37]

Reduction of trochanteric fracture is usually achieved by initial traction to the leg in a semi-abducted and slightly flexed position. After overcoming shortening, the leg is internally rotated. Occasionally open reduction is required. The fracture should ideally be reduced anatomically or in slightly valgus position. Medial bony support is desirable and external rotation and shortening must be eliminated. In a well-reduced fracture, bone shares a substantial load. The SHS is preferred for fixation of the majority of trochanteric fractures.

Fixation failure of pertrochanteric fracture is closely associated with malposition of the lag screw in the femoral head and the highest rates of cut-out occur in the posterior-inferior and in the anterior-superior zones. Baumgaertner et al.[20] have proposed measurement of the TAD as a simple, reproducible method to predict chances of cut-out of the lag screw from the femoral head. The TAD is the sum of the distances from the tip of the lag screw to the apex of the femoral head on anteroposterior and lateral radiographs, after controlling for magnification (Fig. 6.24). TAD is suggested as an intraoperative guide that discourages peripheral and shallow placement, for only if the screw is placed centrally can it be confidently advanced deep enough to achieve a low TAD (<25 mm) without risk of inadvertent penetration of the joint. During surgery after placement of the guide wire but before reaming the neck, TAD is judged by fluoroscopy. On clear anteroposterior and lateral views, after accounting for magnification, the distance between the apex of the femoral head and the tip of the guide wire is estimated. The quality of the fluoroscopy is

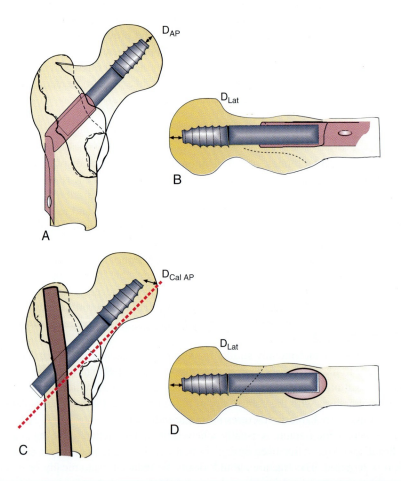

FIGURE 6.24

(**A** and **B**) Tip-apex distance for SHS is the sum of DAP and D Lat, and should always be less than 28 mm. Higher values predict cut-out of lag screw from the head. When the tip-to-apex distance is greater than 45 mm. likelihood of cut-out increases to greater than 60%.[38] Optimal location for tip of an SHS is in the centre of the head in both AP and lateral views. (**C** and **D**) TADcal the tip-apex distance for an ISHS is calculated differently; the reference point is on a line parallel to the calcar. The desirable value for TADcal is <25 mm (range <20 to <25 mm). Optimal location for tip of an ISHS is in the lower quadrant in AP view and in the centre of the head in the lateral view.[39]

(From Kuzyk et al. (2012),[39] redrawn and modified with permission.)

important; it is assumed that the images are perpendicular to the neck and 90° apart. A comparison of the apparent length (or diameter) of the guide wire's threaded tip with its known size gives the amount of fluoroscopic magnification. By and large, TAD will be less than 25 mm when the distance between the tip of the guide wire and the apex of femoral head seems to be less than 1–1.5 times the length of the threaded portion of the guide wire on both views. Regardless of the zone in which the guide wire is placed, if the proposed position results in TAD of greater than 25 mm, reconsideration of the reduction and redirection of the guide wire is called for. In fixation of intertrochanteric fractures with an ISHS a modification, 'calcar referenced tip-apex distance (CalTAD)' may be used. A biomechanical study has suggested that in AP view, 'the closer the lag screw is to the calcar, the greater the axial and torsional stiffness'. The study recommends that while inserting an ISHS for fixing an intertrochanteric fracture, the lag screw on the AP view should lie just above the calcar and in the centre of the femoral neck on the lateral view to reduce CalTAD close to 20 mm.

The routine intraoperative TAD estimation increases the surgeon's awareness of the probability of cut-out of the screw and helps to guide operative decision-making. A robust statistical relationship exists between increasing TAD and implant cut-out rate irrespective of all other variables like the patient's age, the bone quality, the fracture pattern, the reduction stability and the implant angle. TAD measurement is more helpful than any other attempts to describe the location of the screw. Importance of TAD has been restated by a prospective randomized study in 2010; three of their five patients who required revision surgery had a TAD in excess of 25 mm.[21]

Intracapsular Fracture

Undisplaced intracapsular hip fractures – Garden type I, II, impacted and those with angulation on lateral radiographs in subjects older than 70 years and in poor health – are fixed with MLS to prevent displacement, to avoid non-union and to minimize bed rest. The goal of reduction in a displaced intracapsular hip fracture is a position as close as possible to a Garden index of 160/180 (AP/lateral). The Garden index is an expression of the angle of the compression trabeculae on the anteroposterior radiograph over (/) the angle of the compression trabeculae on the lateral radiograph. A perfect anatomic reduction is therefore expressed as 160/180 (Fig. 6.25). On the anteroposterior radiograph, the primary compression trabeculae should ideally be at an angle of 160° to the longitudinal axis of the femoral shaft, whereas on the lateral radiograph, these compression trabeculae should lie in a straight line or 180° with the femoral shaft axis (Fig 6.25). A good reduction has the medial femoral head–neck fragment well supported by the medial neck of the femur. This should be either anatomic or with the head–neck fragment in slight lateral translation in relation to the supporting femoral neck. A slight valgus is acceptable, varus is not. A slight valgus with the superior femoral neck impacted beneath the subchondral bone of the superior femoral head usually provides a very stable configuration. On the lateral view, alignment is again important, with the posterior neck of the distal fragment supporting that of the head–neck fragment.

Adequate trochanteric fracture fixation

- Accurate reduction in AP and lateral X-rays
- Screw position in the head
  - Central or lower sector in AP X-ray
  - Central or posterior sector in lateral X-rays
  - Within 5–10 mm of the joint line
- Plate
  - Four-hole plate to engage eight cortices
  - Short-barrel plate for screw less than 80 mm in length

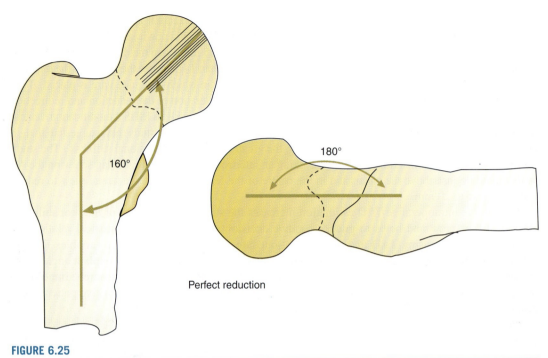

FIGURE 6.25

A perfect anatomic reduction is expressed as 160° anteroposterior/180° lateral which is same as Garden index.

Accurate reduction and stable fixation are essential for successful treatment of an intracapsular fracture. Many reduction techniques are used; this author's choice is the Whitman method.[40] The patient lies supine on the traction table and the uninjured extremity is secured to the footplate. The injured limb is tied in an externally rotated position and abducted to 20°; adequate traction is applied to reclaim a bit longer than normal length. Then, with the surgeon using both hands, the greater trochanter is pushed anteriorly and posteriorly a few times. The extremity is then internally rotated until the patella is internally rotated 20–30°. With one hand, the surgeon now pushes firmly posteriorly on the greater trochanteric area two or three times, and partially releases the traction so that the knee can be gently flexed in the traction 10–15°. This procedure, when practised without modification, gives consistently good reduction. Another useful method of reduction is with traction on a fracture table with the leg in neutral flexion, neutral rotation and 10° of abduction. The leg is then internally rotated as far as possible; then the leg is backed off into a position of 15° of internal rotation. The medial neck spike of the fragment should be well supported by the femoral neck of the femur. In the great majority of fractures without major femoral neck comminution, these manoeuvres yield a satisfactory and stable position. When accurate reduction is not obtainable, open reduction and fixation should be carried out. MLS is the preferred implant for a displaced intracapsular fracture of the hip in adults up to the age of 60 years.

Many clinical studies have proved the superiority of MLS over other devices in fixation of intracapsular fractures. Cannulated cancellous screws are inserted over guide wires. The use of a guide wire ensures accurate screw placement and avoids repeated removal and reinsertion.

Screw positioning is decisive to prevent femoral head migration. The shaft of the distal-most screw rests on the calcar femoris, and its threads fix the inferior femoral head (Fig. 6.26A). For the femoral head to fall into varus, threads of this screw must first cut through the femoral head. In the lateral plane, a second screw is placed to rest on the posterior cortex of the distal fragment at the mid-head level in the anteroposterior plane (Fig. 6.26 B). For posterior head migration to occur, its threads must cut through the head. The inferior screw is placed first, followed by the superior screw. The screws should be tightened simultaneously to apply uniform compression across the fracture and to avoid tipping of the femoral head into varus angulation. In Garden stage I and II fractures, a third screw at the mid-head level on the anteroposterior view and in an anterior position on the lateral view gives additional rotatory stability (Fig. 6.26C). In the Garden stage III and IV fractures, and when neck is comminuted on the posterior surface, a fourth screw superiorly on the anteroposterior view and midline in the lateral view further supplements fixation (Fig. 6.22D). The inverted triangle and diamond patterns of screw placement also fit well into the shape of the femoral neck. The distal screw should neither enter the femoral cortex below the level of the lesser trochanter nor additional holes be made at the level of the lesser trochanter. Since there is no side plate, weakness at this level can lead to a subtrochanteric fracture. Two screw holes at the level of or distal to the lesser trochanter must be used with caution because a crack can propagate between the holes producing iatrogenic fracture.

In summary, three or four parallel cannulated screws placed peripherally around the femoral neck compress the fracture as well as lend excellent rotatory stability. The triangle and diamond patterns adapt well to the different forces applied to the hip in different body positions such as shifting from sitting to standing when the forces generated on the hip are 3 times more than in walking.

An SHS is the second choice for fixation of this fracture. Additional antirotation screw is recommended.

Adequate intracapsular fracture fixation

- Accurate reduction is AP and lateral X-rays.
- Minimum of two screws.
- Screw position in head
  - Central or lower sector in AP X-ray.
  - Central or posterior sector in lateral X-ray.
- Screw placement in neck
  - Parallel: less than 10 angle between two screws.
  - Minimum 4 mm apart.
  - Lowest screw resting on the calcar femoral.
- Washer in porotic bone

Implant Removal

In elderly individuals, hip fracture fixation devices are left in place indefinitely, if there are no complications. However, formation of a painful bursa or local pain over a migrated implant due to collapse of the femoral neck may require plate removal. Implant removal from femoral neck weakens the medial column and the neck may fracture on slight overload or a trivial trauma. When a lag screw or helical blade needs to be removed for mechanical irritation, its shorter replacement should be considered. In patients with severe osteoporosis, (T score >3.5) a planned hip replacement should be thought out.[42] Removal of an SHS assembly becomes an important step in failed fixation of hip fracture. All possible care is taken to avoid further damage to bone during the removal. The SHS plate is removed first. Often there is bone overgrowth over the edge of the plate that needs to be removed. Broken screw removal requires special equipment and can be time consuming.

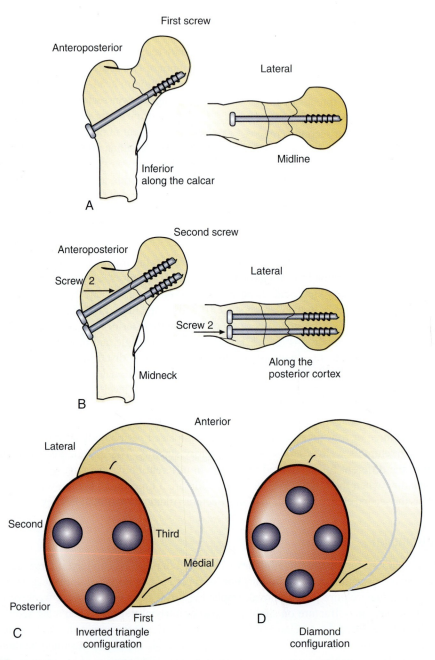

FIGURE 6.26

First screw rests on calcar and prevents varus displacement.[41] **(A)** The second screw rests on the posterior cortex and puts a stop to posterior migration of the head. **(B)** Simultaneous tightening of the screws applies uniform compression and averts tilting of the head in varus. The third screw is placed anteriorly in mid neck to make an inverted triangle configuration. **(C)** In Garden type III and IV fractures a fourth screw is inserted superiorly on the anteroposterior view and midline in the lateral view. **(D)** The triangle and diamond patterns adapt well to the different forces acting on the hip. Fourth screw is recommended when posterior cortex is comminuted.

In young individuals, implants may be removed after radiological union; standard post-removal weight-bearing restrictions apply. In young adults, avascular necrosis of femoral head is known to occur after removal of cancellous screws subsequent to fracture healing.

Lag screw removal is facilitated by use of a specialized wrench that fits over it and a long coupling screw that fits into its female threads. Turning the wrench counter-clockwise and at the same time pulling on it brings out the lag with ease. When these instruments are not available, a large hollow mill is used, which cores out the bone around the threads of the lag screw leaving behind a large void. Before attempting removal of a cancellous screw (cannulated or solid), the screwdriver must be carefully examined. The screwdriver tip must show no signs of wear to ensure a good fit into the hexagonal socket. A system with a hexagonal wrench or screwdriver that converts into a wrench (a rod passing through its handle) is advantageous. Removal of cancellous screw is reduced difficult by bone growing around the head of a large cancellous screw. Bone growth around a round head with an inner recess hexagon is much less of a problem than one with an outer hexagon (Fig. 6.27A). Here the bone

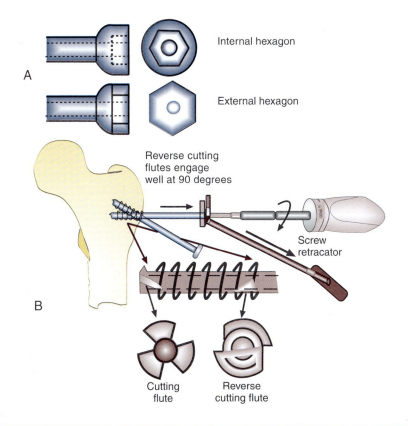

FIGURE 6.27

(A) Screw with a round head and an inner recess hexagon is easier to remove than one with an outer hexagon.
(B) Reverse cutting flutes perform well when a screw retractor brings these at perpendicular to the bone face.[30]

(From Tencer et al. (1996),[30] redrawn and modified with permission.)

must be removed to allow the fitting of the external wrench. It is worthwhile to move a screw over a short arc in clockwise and anticlockwise direction to loosen it. In young individuals who have strong bones, a screw with reverse cutting flutes is useful. The screw cuts its way back through the bone in the femoral neck and the femoral cortex. When the femoral endocortex is reached, the screw is pulled into a position of 90° to the shaft with a screw retractor that fits around the screw neck (Fig. 6.27B), in order to place the reverse cutting flutes at their proper position for screw removal. Reverse cutting flutes do not perform well at oblique angles to the cortex but do function well in this perpendicular position. Not all screws have reverse cutting flutes. Under such circumstances a hollow mill is used to make a tunnel over the screw. The loosened implant is then easily pulled out.

REFERENCES

1. Rybicki EF, Simonen FA, Weis EB, Jr. On the mathematical analysis of stress in the human femur. *J Biomech* 1972;5:203–15.
2. Boyd HB, Anderson LD. Management of unstable trochanteric fractures. Surg Gynecol Obstet 1961; 112:633–8.
3. Gozna ER, Harrington IJ, Evans DC. Biomechanics of musculoskeletal injury. Baltimore: Williams & Wilkins; 1982.
4. Santesso N, Carrasco-Labra A, Brignardello-Petersen R. Hip protectors for preventing hip fractures in older people. Cochrane Database Syst Rev 2014 Mar 31;3:CD001255. doi: 10.1002/14651858.CD001255.
5. Singh M, Nagrath AR, Maini PS. Changes in trabecular pattern of the upper end of the femur as an index of osteoporosis. J Bone Joint Surg 1972;52-A:457–67.
6. Mereddy P, Kamath S, Ramakrishnan M, Malik H, Donnachie N. The AO/ASIF proximal femoral nail anti-rotation (PFNA): a new design for the treatment of unstable proximal femoral fractures. Injury 2009;40:428–32.
7. Tencer AF, Johnson KD. Biomechanics in orthopaedic trauma: bone fracture and fixation. London: Martin Dunitz; 1994.
8. Swiontkowski MF, Harrigton RM, Keller TS, Van Patten PK. Torsion and bending analysis of internal fixation techniques for femoral neck fractures: the role of implant design and bone density. J Orthop Res 1987;5:433–44.
9. Crowell RR, Edwards WT, Hayes WC. Pullout strength of fixation devices in trabecular bone of the femoral head. Transactions of the 31st Orthopaedic Research Society Meeting 1985;10:189.
10. Gerard et al. (1993) as quoted in Gotfried Y. Biomechanical evaluation of the percutaneous compression plating system of hip fractures. J Orthop Trauma 2002;16:644–50.
11. St Clair Strange FG. The hip. London: William Heinemann Medical; 1965.
12. Trochanteric Plate. Paoli, PA: Synthes; 2000.
13. The TRAUMAX® dynamic screw-plate Surfix New Deal SAS Immeuble Séquoia 2 • 97 allée Alexandre Borodine Parc technologique de la Porte des Alpes, 69800 Saint Priest, France.
14. Vary Angle Nail system for hip. Richmond, NJ: Biomet Inc; 1995.
15. Wagner M, Frigg R. Internal fixators. Davos Platz: AO Publishing; 2006. p. 500.
16. Kanghui Medical innovations, China.
17. Gotfried Y. Percutaneous compression plating of intertrochanteric hip fractures. J Orthop Trauma 2000;14:490–5.
18. The PORD™ Device Efratogo Ltd, Kiryat Bialik, Israel.
19. Medoff nail system, Richards Memphis, TN.

20. Parker MJ, Pryor GA. Hip fracture management. London: Blackwell Scientific Publications; 1993.
21. Barton TM, Gleeson R, Topliss C, Greenwood R, Harries WJ, Chesser TJS. A comparison of the long gamma nail with the sliding hip screw for the treatment of AO/OTA 31-A2 fractures of the proximal part of the femur. J Bone Joint Surg Am 2010;92:792–8.
22. Kulkarni SG. Avoiding complication in cephalocondylar nailing for upper femur fractures. Mumbai India: Presented at Traumacon; 2013 August 16.
23. Wang CJ, Brown CJ, Yettram AL. Intramedullary femoral nails: one or two lag screws? A preliminary study. Med Eng Phys 2000;22:613–24.
24. Simmermacher RKJ, Ljungqvistb J, Bail H, Hockertz T, Vochteloo AJH, Ochs U, Werken CVD. The new proximal femoral nail antirotation (PFNAW) in daily practice: results of a multicentre clinical study. Injury 2008;39:932–9.
25. PFN-A, Plot no 118, sector-44 Gurgaon-122002, (Haryana) India: Synthes Medical (P) Ltd.
26. Gehr J, Arnold T, Hilsenbeck F, Friedl W. The gliding nail, a universal implant in the treatment of proximal femur fractures. Eur J Trauma 2006;32:562–8.
27. Haidukewych GJ. Intertrochanteric fractures: ten tips to improve results. J bone Joint Surg 2009;91A:712–19.
28. Radin EL, Rose RM, Blaha JD, Litsky AS. Practical biomechanics for the orthopaedic surgeon. 2nd ed. New York: Churchill Livingstone; 1992.
29. Kaplan K, Miyamoto R, Levine BR, Egol K, Zuckerman JD. Surgical management of hip fractures: an evidence-based review of the literature. II: Intertrochanteric fractures. J Am Acad Orthop Surg 2008;16:665–73
30. Tencer AF, Asnis SE, Harrington RM, Chapman JR. Biomechanics of cannulated and noncannulated screws. In: Asnis SE, Kyle RF, editors. Cannulated screw fixation. New York: Springer-Verlag; 1996.
31. Flierl MA, Stahel PF, Hak DJ, Morgan SJ, Smith WR. Traction table–related complications in orthopaedic surgery. J Am Acad Orthop Surg 2010;18:668–75.
32. Said GZ, Farouk O, Said HGZ. An irreducible variant of intertrochanteric fractures: a technique for open reduction. Injury 2005;36:871–4.
33. Foss NB, Kristensen BB, Bundgaard M, Bak M, Heiring C, Virkelyst C, Sine Hougaard S, Henrik Kehlet H. Fascia iliaca compartment blockade for acute pain control in hip fracture patients. Anesthesiology 2007;106:773–8.
34. Kenkre JS. Personal communication.
35. Range C, Egeler C. Fascia Iliaca compartment block: landmark and ultrasound approach Anaesthesia tutorial of the week 193. Available at: http://www.totw.anaesthesiologists.org; 2010 [accessed 01.01.14].
36. Nishiura T, Nozawa M, Hidenori Morio H. The new technique of precise insertion of lag screw in an operative treatment of trochanteric femoral fractures with a short intramedullary nail. Injury 2009;40:1077–83.
37. Formander P, Thorngren KG, Tornqvist H, Ahrengart L, Lindgren U. Swedish experience with the gamma nail versus sliding hip screw in 209 randomized cases. Int J Orthop Trauma 1994;4:118–22.
38. Baumgaertner MR, Curtin SL, Lindskog DM, Keggi JM. The value of the tip apex distance in predicting failure of fixation of peritrochanteric fractures of the hip. J Bone Joint Surg Am 1995;77:1058–64.
39. Kuzyk PRT, Zdero R, Shah S, Olsen M, Waddell JP, Schemitsch EH. Femoral head lag screw position for cephalomedullary nails: a biomechanical analysis. J Orthop Trauma 2012;26:414–21.
40. Sisk TD. Fractures of hip and pelvis. In: Crenwhaw AH, editor. Campbell's operative orthopaedics. 7th ed. St Louis: CV Mosby; 1987. p. 1750.
41. Asnis SE, Kyle RF. Intracapsular hip fractures. In: Asnis SE, Kyle RF, editors. Cannulated screw fixation. New York: Springer-Verlag; 1996.
42. Seibert FJ, Puchwein P, Lanz Ph, Tanzer K, Clement HP. Femoral neck fracture after removal of PFNA-blade—case report and review of the literature. Injury Extra 2009;40:240–41.

CHAPTER 7

WIRE, CABLE AND PINS

Introduction
Wire
   Size Nomenclature
   Classification of Sutures
   Factors Affecting the Strength of Wire
      Effect of Time
      Twisted Wire
      Kinks and Knots
   Effect on Blood Supply of the Bone
   Methods of Fastening
   Instruments to Handle Wire
   Uses of Wire
Tension Band Wiring
   Introduction
   General Principles
   Regional Considerations
      The Ulna
      The Patella
      The Greater Trochanter of Femur
      The Medical Malleolus
      The Greater Tuberosity of Humerus
      Lateral End of the Clavicle
      Unusual Sites
         Diaphysis of Metacarpal and Metatarsal
         Arthrodesis of the Thumb
         Arthrodesis of the Wrist

Cerclage Wiring
   Regional Application
      The Tibia and Femur
      Patello-Tibial Cerclage
Wire Cables
   Cable Tension-Band Application
Pins
   Use of Kirschner Wire
      Definitive Fixation
      Provisional Fixation
   Regional Considerations
      The Tibial Plateau
      Supracondylar Fracture of the Humerus in Children
      Technique of Pinning
      Technique of Medial Pinning
      Forearm Bones
      Fracture of Radial Head in Children
      The Distal Radius
      Metacarpal and Metatarsal
      Intra-Articular Fracture
      Arthrodesis
      Traction
   Steinmann Pin

INTRODUCTION

Wiring is one of the earliest forms of internal fixation. Wires of brass, iron and silver were used for the purpose. A loop of wire was passed around the fragments or through the drill holes, and the ends were twisted together. Such an arrangement predisposed the fixation to movement between the fragments with resultant irritation and inflammation of the tissues, often leading to infection or non-union.

WIRE

Stainless steel wires are now routinely used for internal fixation of fractures. Wires drawn from other metals, such as pure titanium or its alloys and cobalt–chrome alloy, are also used for the same purpose.

The strength of a wire varies with the material. An 18-gauge wire drawn from cobalt–chrome alloy is stronger than a stainless steel wire of comparable thickness. Multi-filament cable is also used for fixation, since its fatigue sensitivity is higher than that of a mono-filament wire; a stainless steel cable has a fatigue resistance nearly 10 times that of a single stainless steel wire of identical diameter, while a cable of Ti-6Al-4V has a 10-fold improved fatigue resistance over a stainless steel cable. A cable made of coated wires can improve the fatigue-free life by an additional factor of 3. It is interesting to note, however, that only fatigue resistance is improved – the ultimate tensile strengths of single wire and cable are nearly equivalent.

The wires are drawn from the raw material and finished by two processes called annealing and cold working. In annealing, the material is heated to above the temperature of recrystallization, which is about halfway to its melting point. The surface of an annealed wire is of mediocre finish. This wire has greater elongation but possesses a considerably lower tensile strength as compared to that of cold worked wire. Two small lengths of annealed wire can be twisted together (cold working) to fabricate a stronger piece of wire reaching an optimal strength between 4 and 8 turns. Annealed wires are supplied in spool lengths. A metal is cold worked below its temperature of recrystallization. Such wire has a superior surface finish to annealed wire, and has a higher tensile strength. Cold working is an expensive process as it consumes a lot of energy. Cold worked wires are supplied in cut lengths.

Size Nomenclature

The size of the orthopaedic wire, which is supplied in bulk either on spool or in cut lengths, is indicated by a gauge number. By convention the gauge number decreases as the diameter increases. For example, gauge no. 32 represents a thinner wire than gauge no. 18. There are several different systems of gauge nomenclature and all systems use the same gauge numbers, but the diameters differ. Any given gauge number can indicate one of numerous diameters, depending on the system used. Typically a gauge number is based on a constant ratio between diameters of successive gauge numbers with the diameter decreasing as the gauge number increases. In one of the systems the ratio of any diameter to the next smaller is 1.123. Since (1.23) equals 2.0050, diameters differing by six gauge numbers have a ratio of approximately 2. The numbers ordinarily extend from 40 to OOO.

In the United States the American Wire Gauge (AWG) is used, while in Great Britain and Canada the Standard Wire Gauge (SWG) is used. The SWG has larger diameters for comparable gauge numbers than the AWG. Conversion of AWG to metric sizes is shown in Table 7.1.

Table 7.1 Conversion Table for American Wire Gauge Numbers to Metric Measurements[1]

AWG #	Diameter (mm)	Area (mm²)	AWG #	Diameter (mm)	Area (mm²)
0000 (4/0)	11.6840	107.2193	19	0.9116	0.6527
000 (3/0)	10.4049	85.0288	20	0.8118	0.5176
00 (2/0)	9.2658	67.4309	21	0.7229	0.4105
0 (1/0)	8.2515	53.4751	22	0.6438	0.3255
1	7.3481	42.4077	23	0.5733	0.2582
2	6.5437	33.6308	24	0.5106	0.2047
3	5.8273	26.6705	25	0.4547	0.1624
4	5.1894	21.1506	26	0.4049	0.1288
5	4.6213	16.7732	27	0.3606	0.1021
6	4.1154	13.3018	28	0.3211	0.0810
7	3.6649	10.5488	29	0.2859	0.0642
8	3.2636	8.3656	30	0.2546	0.0509
9	2.9064	6.6342	31	0.2268	0.0404
10	2.5882	5.2612	32	0.2019	0.0320
11	2.3048	4.1723	33	0.1798	0.0254
12	2.0525	3.3088	34	0.1601	0.0201
13	1.8278	2.6240	35	0.1426	0.0160
14	1.6277	2.0809	36	0.1270	0.0127
15	1.4495	1.6502	37	0.1131	0.0100
16	1.2908	1.3087	38	0.1007	0.0080
17	1.1495	1.0378	39	0.0897	0.0063
18	1.0237	0.8230	40	0.0799	0.0050

Classification of Sutures

When surgical wire is packaged as a suture material, an entirely different system of calibration is used than for wire. The system employed is also used for other suture materials such as nylon and other synthetics. The size categories range from 12-0 to 10 USP (United States Pharmacopia). The suture material diameter increases as the number increases. The size is based on thousandths of an inch. Originally each size was 0.003 inches larger than the previous one.

It is the metric system of suture size nomenclature that is rational. The size number in this system indicates the suture diameter in millimetres. There are several categories ranging from size no. 0.01 (0.001 mm) to no. 12 (1.2 mm). Equivalent values of different suture materials are shown in Table 7.2.

Factors Affecting the Strength of the Wire

The standard methods of testing the strength of a wire are to measure the tensile strength of a straight wire as well as that of a single knot. The value of a straight pull is always greater than for a knot, with a ratio of about 100:70, i.e. the knot is always weaker, regardless of the type of suture. The strength of a wire varies directly with the square of its diameter.

Table 7.2 Equivalent Values of Different Surgical Sutures and AWG[2]

USP Designation	Collagen Diameter (mm)	Synthetic Absorbable Diameter (mm)	Non-Absorbable Diameter (mm)	American Wire Gauge
11-0			0.01	
10-0	0.02	0.02	0.02	
9-0	0.03	0.03	0.03	
8-0	0.05	0.04	0.04	
7-0	0.07	0.05	0.05	
6-0	0.1	0.07	0.07	38–40
5-0	0.15	0.1	0.1	35–38
4-0	0.2	0.15	0.15	32–34
3-0	0.3	0.2	0.2	29–32
2-0	0.35	0.3	0.3	28
0	0.4	0.35	0.35	26–27
1	0.5	0.4	0.4	25–26
2	0.6	0.5	0.5	23–24
3	0.7	0.6	0.6	22
4	0.8	0.6	0.6	21–22
5		0.7	0.7	20–21
6			0.8	19–20
7				18

Effect of Time

Stainless steel wire maintains its strength over a period of time. Typically, at 6 months it retains its original strength at the time of insertion. But the wire fatigues rapidly when subjected to motion; therefore, it may break and fragment with time.

Twisted Wire

The tensile strength of two single wires increases as they are twisted, and it varies with the tightness of twist (number of twists per inch). It reaches its peak between 4 and 8 turns per inch. The tensile strength then progressively decreases, becoming less than untwisted controls when there are more than 13 turns per inch. A twisted wire is not as strong as a single wire having an equal maximal diameter, because in a twisted wire a portion of the cross-sectional area is empty space.

Kinks and Knots

A square knot weakens the breaking strength of wire by about 30%. In addition, the strength is decreased markedly by repeated bending, kinks or surface defects from instruments. Notches as small as 1% of the diameter of the wire can reduce its fatigue life by 63%.

Effect on Blood Supply of the Bone

It is believed, empirically, that circumferential wire occludes the blood supply of the bone. Specialized investigations have failed to lend support to this belief. Small diameter wires do not cause any damage. Wider bands (0.3–2.5 cm) can produce a ring of devascularized bone; such bands should be avoided or removed early.

Methods of Fastening

Any method of securing the wire ends that is stronger than the yield strength of the wire is satisfactory. The three common methods are as follows:

1. Making a surgical knot
2. Bend-back technique and its variation
3. Twisting the wire

Application of wire
- Twist wire to apply tension and *not* to obtain reduction
- Incorrectly applied wire will
  - break during application
  - break in the primary twist
- Correctly applied wire will
  - untwist
  - break in substance

In principle, a modified square knot can exert the highest compressive force. The modified square knot is made by tightening the first hitch with a wire tightener, then rotating the wire tightener by 180° while maintaining the tension. The second hitch is then tied. In practice, first knot is easily applied and tightened, but it is hard to maintain the wire tension during application of second knot. The knot loosens up in time, and the fixation may fail. Knots hold good only when wire is used to secure soft tissues.

A cerclage wire secured by the bend-back technique (Fig. 7.1) is considerably more stress resistant than one secured by twisting the ends. Such a wire is less likely to break during tightening.

A wire is tightened before application. A single twist is made to maintain the tension in a wire; further twists improve security. A wire when used as a single strand must be twisted to provide stability.

Maximum stability can be obtained if a wire tightener-twister is used; it cannot be achieved with pliers or needle holders – this is critical for long bones. A wire tightener that indicates the amount of tension applied is preferred as it can deliver equal tension on all the wire loops. A wire is most likely to break as it is being tightened, particularly if inadequate tension is applied prior to twisting. A properly tightened wire will gradually untwist rather than break when subjected to stress.

A properly tightened wire may break at some point on its circumference during healing, whereas an improperly tightened wire will break at the basic twist, frequently during or soon after surgery. When multiple wires are used to stabilize a long bone fracture, failure is more likely to occur if the tension varies from one wire to the next.

Equal tension can only be obtained if a wire tightener is used. When many wires are used, they should all be twisted in the same direction, usually clockwise; otherwise it is not possible to remember the direction if further tightening is necessary.

Instruments to Handle Wire

Specialized instruments help in effective handling of the wires. A wire-passer is used to facilitate the passage of the wire around the bone. The wire is threaded in the hollow of the wire-passer and pulled round the bone (Fig. 7.2). Minimal soft tissue trauma and swift action are the advantages of using this instrument.

A wire tightener is used to apply tension to a wire. Gadgets that merely twist the wire without exerting tension do an incomplete job. Wire should be handled by special instruments; needle holders, artery forceps and Kocher forceps are unsuitable for this purpose. Wire holding forceps, wire bending pliers and flat-nosed pliers grip the wire firmly and effectively. A wire tightener that indicates the

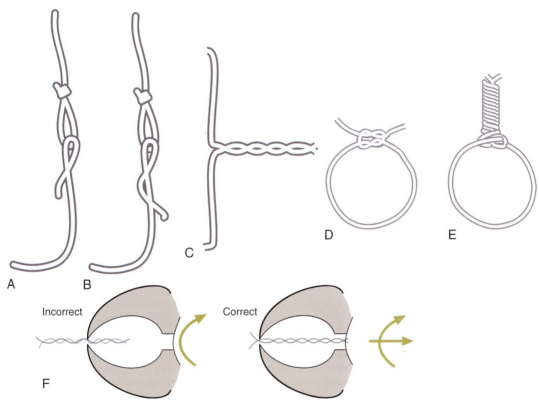

FIGURE 7.1

Methods of joining ends of wire. **(A)** One end of the wire is passed through a loop in the other end and kinked backward fixation: 'bend-back' technique. **(B)** A variation of this technique with one end of the wire passed under itself and against the underlying bone. **(C)** Helical twisting of the wire ends at a high pitch for temporary or definitive fixation.[3] **(D)** Square knot, **(E)** Knot twist, **(F)** Twist a wire; grasp the twist at its base and pulling away from the bone before rotating the pliers. Both limbs must be tightened to obtain symmetrical pressure: two twists in the same limb are of little value.

amount of exerted tension is most useful. A two-arm wire tightener is attached to the wire and the wire loop is controlled while the fragments are manipulated (Fig. 7.2C). The wire is maintained at intersection of the proximal and distal main fragments and butterfly. With correction of rotation and alignment by gentle manipulation of the extremity, the wire is tensioned by spreading the arms of the tightener and twisted until snug. Final adjustments are made and wire is tightened definitively. Because the wire encircles portions of all three fragments, tightening effects the reduction.

Uses of Wire

Wire is particularly useful when firm fixation must be obtained through a small, relatively inaccessible space. Tension band wiring is a technique to achieve maximal fracture stability with the minimum of fixation material. Percutaneous cerclage is a successful method of treatment of a long oblique or a spiral fracture of the tibia.

CHAPTER 7 WIRE, CABLE AND PINS

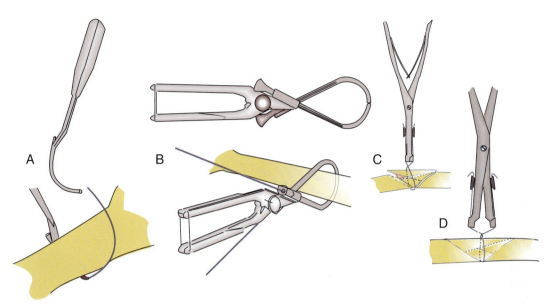

FIGURE 7.2

Two types of wires passers. **(A)** Available in various sizes and curves and is of use in conventional and MIPO methods. **(B)** 'Cerclage passer', designed for MIPO approach; it is used in combination with a cerclage tunneling device and cerclage wire twister (Synthes®, West Chester, PA, USA) for optimum utilization.[4] **(C)** A comminuted fracture with two main and a butterfly fragments is controlled effectively by a cerclage wire passed prior to reduction at the point of junction of three components of the fracture, i.e. the butterfly and the proximal and distal main fragments. **(D)** By spreading the tip of the wire tightener and aligning the limb, the wire tightener may be spun, twisting the wire and effecting a reduction.

Malleable wire of high tensile strength also serves as suture material in tissues other than bone, such as tendon, subcutaneous tissue and skin. A modern use of wire is to reinforce polymethylmethacrylate (PMMA) for immediate stabilization in selected patients with pathological fracture of a long bone due to neoplastic disease. The use of wire significantly increases the strength of PMMA, similar to the steel in reinforced concrete. A wire string of antibiotic impregnated PMMA beads is used to control infection.

Tension band wiring
- Wire must be applied on the tension surface of the bone
- Wire must be pre-stressed (tightened)
- Wire must be strong to withstand tension load
- Strong opposite bone cortex must be present to withstand dynamic compressive loads
- Joint movement must be encouraged to improve congruity and compression

'Wire absorbs the tensile forces, the bone withstands the compressive forces'

TENSION BAND WIRING

Introduction

The basic principle of the tension band has been explained earlier (see Fig. 1.16). The application of this principle permits the use of a minimal amount of a fixation material to obtain excellent fracture stability and immediate functional movements of the contiguous joints. A tensile, fracture-distracting force is generated by normal muscular activities.

The use of a wire for fixation on the tension surface of a fractured bone converts the distracting tensile force into a compressive force. Such a wire is called a 'tension band wire'. Application of a tension band wire ensures that the normal muscle activity will place the fracture lines under compression loading.

General Principles

A tension band must be made of a material that resists tensile forces and can be pre-stressed (tightened). A wire or a cable is frequently utilized as a tension band. The wire is tensioned to apply slight compression to the fracture site, creating a slight gap on the opposite side. When dynamic forces are applied with the contraction of the antagonistic deforming_muscles during normal muscular activity, the tension band resists the tendency for distraction of the opposite sides of the fractured bone and, at the same time, produces uniform compression at the fracture site. In the treatment of fractures of patella and olecranon, the application of a tension band wire achieves dynamic compression during active flexion of the knee and the elbow, respectively.

Let us consider the wiring of the patella fracture in some detail (Fig. 7.3). After an accurate reduction, a tension band wire is tightened (pre-stressed) and fastens together opposing points on the anterior cortex at and around the point of contact. Pre-stressing of the wire produces static compression with gaping of the opposite cortex. The wire must be pre-stressed for the bone to remain loaded in static compression. Flexion of the knee induces dynamic compression and closes the gap in the patella. The tendon force rotates the distal fragment into contact with the proximal fragment because the wire is holding them together.

The larger the tendon force, the greater the compressive force across the fracture surface. It is essential that the cortex on the side opposite the tension band wire is able to withstand the applied compressive loads, or else the wire will be subjected to bending forces, increasing the risk of its breakage. The process is also dependent on the contact at the fulcrum (the anterior cortex) being maintained by the tensioned wire. Loss of bone stock or poor bone quality will allow the development bending stresses leading to wire fatigue and fixation failure. The reaction force and the tendon force both have appreciable components in the same direction, which can only be balanced by a tensile force in the wire.

Thus, the phrase 'tension band' is justified (Fig. 7.3C and D). A similar mechanism with two pieces of hardware connected by a hinge is shown in Fig. 7.3E.

Practically speaking, the tension band wiring can be utilized to fix fractures only in a limited number of locations in the body. The technique can be employed for transverse and comminuted patella fracture, fracture and osteotomy of the femoral greater trochanter, the medial and lateral malleolar fractures, fracture of the grater tuberosity of the humerus (especially where small or osteoporotic fragments are involved), and for fracture of the distal end of the clavicle and of the

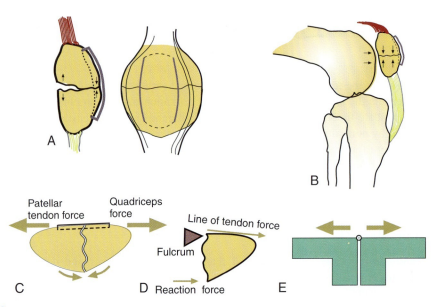

FIGURE 7.3

(**A**) Tightening (pre-stressing) the wire produces static compression on the anterior cortex and opens up the posterior cortex. (**B**) Knee flexion induces dynamic compression and closes the posterior gap. (**C and D**) Intact strong cortex at a distance from the implant is a prerequisite for successful application of the tension band principle. The anterior wire when placed under tension converts the distracting tendon force to compressive force across the posterior cortex. (**E**) The hinge represents the tension band wire.[5]

olecranon process of the ulna. A diaphyseal or metaphyseal fracture with a diaphyseal extension is not amenable to tension band wiring. In this region the lack of cancellous interdigitation in the diaphyseal area prevents adequate resistance to large forces, particularly shear.

A wire, a cable or a non-absorbable suture is used to perform the function of a tension band. Such a wire should have considerable ductility combined with a high yield point and ultimate tensile strength. Usually wires of diameters ranging from 0.4 to 1.5 mm are used. A 1.2-mm wire is used as a tension band chiefly on a bony prominence like the patella and the olecranon that serves as an attachment for muscles and ligaments.

The tension band wire is often applied in a figure-8 fashion around previously inserted, parallel and longitudinally placed Kirschner wires, Steinmann pins or cancellous lag screws. These implants are used as an adjunctive fixation to prevent displacement of the fracture fragments through shearing, translation or rotation. Crossed Kirschner wires are less stable and interfere with interfragmental compression. Movement at the fracture site leads to loosening of the tension band wires and thus to fixation failure. The parallel wires also provide anchorage points around which the tension band wire is placed. Occasionally, the tension band wire may be used without the Kirschner wires, as in the fixation of a transverse fracture of the patella where an irregular fracture line allows perfect reduction by interdigitation of the fracture surfaces (see Fig. 7.5D).

Regional Considerations

The Ulna

Tension band wiring is selectively suitable for locations where the extensor muscle usually provides the major deforming force causing the bending moment at the discontinuity. Wire fixation of the olecranon process of the ulna is an example. After an accurate reduction, a band wire is applied in a figure-8 pattern around two parallel Kirschner wires. Kirschner wires prevent slippage of the tension band wire on the tension surface of the bone with the joint movements. The parallel longitudinal Kirschner wires act as rails along which the bone fragments can slide during dynamic compression exerted in active flexion (Fig. 7.4).

As the triceps force rotates the proximal fragment, the tension band wire, which is on the outermost surface of the olecranon, keeps the two fracture fragments together and maintains the point of contact. The tension band exerts the reactive compression forces across the fracture surface. This is balanced by an equal and opposite tensile force in the wire (Fig. 7.4A).

Tension band wiring is more effective than screw fixation of the olecranon. In a screw fixation the hinge or centre of rotation shifts inwards (Fig. 7.4C) and the outer section of the fracture opens up when the antagonistic muscle forces begin to act. The screw is subjected to bending forces and the rigidity of the screw can only partially prevent the opening up of the outer cortex. These bending stresses on a screw are undesirable and should be avoided, as a screw is likely to bend under heavy loading, leading to failure of the fixation.

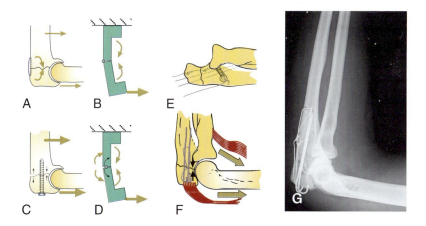

FIGURE 7.4

(**A**) Antagonistic distracting muscle forces are converted to compressive forces by an anchoring wiring on the outermost surface of the ulna. Wire acting as a hinge prevents the separation of the two outer cortices. (**B**) An analogous situation is illustrated by the hardware. (**C**) When a screw is used, the fixation point is not on the outermost surface of the ulna. With the application of the muscle forces the inner cortex is under compression but the outer cortex opens up. Significant bending stresses may damage the screw leading to fixation failure. (**D**) Hardware likeness is representative of the situation.[6] (**E**) The wire passed through the hollow core of a cannulated screw is unlikely to cut through the soft bone. Cannulated screw protects the fixation.[7] (**F**) Parallel Kirschner wires prevent the loss of reduction through shear, rotation and translation. Crossed Kirschner wires are unstable and interfere with interfragmental compression. A wire passed over the Kirschner wire and through the bone is unlikely to slip.[6] (**G**) Radiograph showing application of parallel tension band fixation of olecranon fracture.

In elderly patients with porotic bone the tension band wire may cut through. A practical solution to such a problem is to insert a cannulated screw in the metaphyseal area of the ulna, pass the wire through the screw and tighten in the usual manner (Fig. 7.4E).

Wire prominence is a common patient complaint associated with tension band fixation of the olecranon; it may also lead to skin breakdown and subsequent infection. Wire prominence is usually related to improper Kirschner wire seating at the time of surgery. The tips of the Kirschner wires should be U-bent, shortened and impacted in the bone. A unique non-sliding pin allows the wire to be threaded through an eye in its head so that pin slippage is prevented. Another occasional complication seen with the tension band wire is its cutting out of the distal fragment if the wire is not inserted deep enough below the dorsal cortical surface of the ulna.

The Patella

A patellar fracture can be treated by screw fixation, but tension band wiring is the mechanically sound method of treatment. The patella is a cardinal component in the extension mechanism of the knee. The weight of the leg initiates flexion; the quadriceps musculature produces a counter moment that extends the knee. The quadriceps tension (M1) and patellar tension (M2) produce a force that is equal and opposite (Fig. 7.5). The resultant force (Pf) pushes the patella into the femur. Thus, the patella is subjected to tensile forces on its anterior surface and compression at the patello-femoral articulation.

One should use a technique that converts this massive fracture surface-distracting tensile force into a beneficial compressive force. Only tension band wiring can do this and transfer the massive compressive force to the posterior cortex, which is stronger than the anterior cancellous bone. The alternative method of cancellous screw fixation does produce excellent compression at the fracture site, but it relies on the cancellous bone of the patella for purchase.

Of the two techniques, wiring can withstand greater quadriceps pull than screw fixation. Other methods of fixing the patella are shown in Fig. 7.4B–H.

In the post-operative period after tension band wiring of the patella, active and passive movements of the knee should be performed as flexion of the knee increases the congruity and the compression of the fracture surface.

The Greater Trochanter of Femur

Fracture or osteotomy of the greater trochanter can also be fixed in a similar way using the tension band principle. The antagonistic pull of the glutii and the adductors, using the hip joint as fulcrum, causes a bending moment at the site of discontinuity between the greater trochanter and the femur (Fig. 7.6). Cables have been used at this site, but have been found wanting in stability. Their failure occurs at the crimping stage of application in spite of technically advanced instrumentation.

The Medial Malleolus

Tension band wiring is a suitable option when the malleolar fragment is very small or the bone is porotic, making screw fixation impossible. Two parallel Kirschner wires and a figure-8 wire loop can secure the fracture well (Fig. 7.5B). The tips of the Kirschner wires are bent to make a U and are impacted into the bone.

The Greater Tuberosity of Humerus

In difficult situations, tension band wiring is a good option to achieve fixation. The antagonistic pulls of the supraspinatus and pectoralis major, using the glenohumeral joint as a fulcrum, cause a bending moment

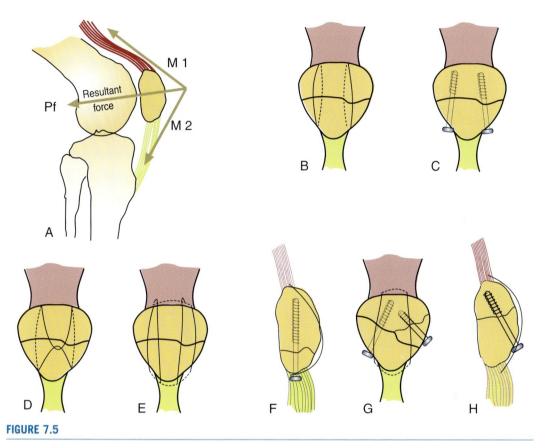

FIGURE 7.5

(A) Tensile forces on the anterior cortex of the patella due to the opposing pull of the quadriceps muscle and the body weight. The resultant force compresses the patella against the femur.[8] Various methods of patellar fixation are **(B)** Magnusson, **(C)** Screw fixation, **(D)** Modified tension band wiring, **(E)** Kirschner wires provide the rotational and lateral stability. Tension band wires for stabilized patellar fracture. **(F)** Tension band wiring protects screw fixation of a small fragment of the lower pole of the patella.[9] **(G and H)** Vertical and oblique fractures are best fixed with screws and protected by a tension band wiring; a tension band wire around quadriceps and patellar tendon cannot compress vertical or oblique fractures.

at the site of discontinuity between the greater tuberosity and the remaining humerus (Fig. 7.6C). Optimal compression is achieved with this method only during functional activity that results in eccentric loading and production of bending moments.

Lateral End of the Clavicle

When indicated, this is an effective method of securing the small fragments (Fig. 7.5D). It is imperative to bend the protruding ends of the Kirschner wires in fixation of the clavicle. The chances of migration of Kirschner wires to vital organs are high and must be considered in this location.

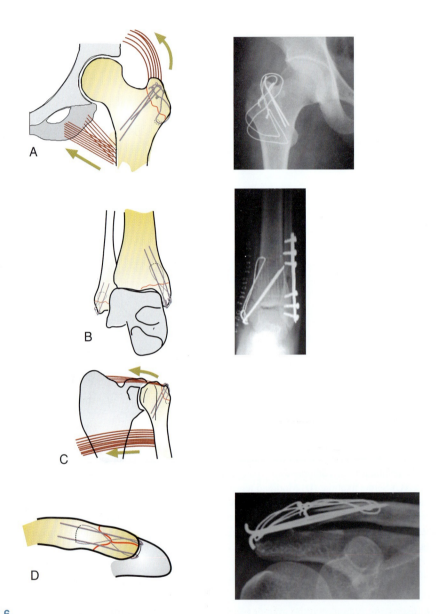

FIGURE 7.6

(A) Tension band wiring of the greater trochanter. Opposing pull of abductors and adductors creates a distracting force, which is converted to a compression force by the tension band. (B) Tension band wiring of the medial and lateral malleoli. (C) Tension band wiring transforms the antagonistic pulls of the pectoralis major and the supraspinatus into a compressive force at the greater tuberosity fracture. (D) The distal clavicular fracture fixed with tension band wiring.[6]

Unusual Sites
Diaphysis of Metacarpal and Metatarsal
As mentioned earlier, tension band wiring is not a suitable method for the diaphyseal fracture, as the cortical interdigitating spicules do not offer good fixation rigidity. The wiring is prone to slippage. In the metacarpals or metatarsals, however, this method can be employed to fix an isolated fracture (Fig. 7.7A).

Arthrodesis of the Thumb
Tension band wiring is a practical solution for achieving arthrodesis of the thumb where the two phalanges are quite small and the bone is porotic (Fig. 7.7B). A bone screw is unlikely to hold. The wire loop absorbs tension forces and provides interfragmental compression.

Arthrodesis of the Wrist
In porotic bone stock, plating is impossible and tension band wiring is a viable alternative (Fig. 7.7C).

CERCLAGE WIRING

The word 'cerclage' wire alludes to surrounding bone fragments and tensioning a wire to hold fragments in alignment. The cerclage wire technique is useful for provisional as well as for definitive stabilization of certain long bone fractures. Temporary cerclage wiring is used to hold a fragment in position until a screw or a plate is applied (Fig. 7.8A). Definitive stabilization of long bone fracture can be achieved by cerclage wiring.

Spiral and oblique fractures longer than 3 inches are suitable for fixation by cerclage wiring (Fig. 7.8B). The fracture must be accurately reduced; an improperly reduced fracture works the wire loose and the fixation fails. A single wire loop always fails; it acts like a fulcrum on which the fragments move. Multiple wire loops are employed. Wires are first applied at the two ends of the fracture to secure the alignment. Additional loops are then placed about a centimetre apart for stability. The wires are evenly tightened.

A cerclage wire may be tightened by either bend-back or helical twisting method (see Fig. 7.1). Specially designed wire tighteners are available for both the modes. Wires are first contoured around the bone, tightened, then adequately twisted; the use of a wire tightener assures best results. 'Failure to purchase a wire tightener is false economy since these devices can apply much more tension than can be achieved by hand.'[10] Research has shown that helical twisting offer better knot security but bend-back cerclage wires produce consistently more tension and fragment stability.[10] A wire cutter of appropriate size is used to trim the excess wires after tightening. The

> **Cerclage wiring**
> - Long spiral fracture, not for short fracture lines
> - Obtain reduction
> - Place wires perpendicular to long axis of bone
> - Adequately spaced multiple wire loops
> - Contour wires around the bone
> - Tension and tighten
>
> *Always*
> - Use a strong wire
> - Use two or more wires
> - Use wire tightener-twister
> - Apply equal tension on all wires – unequal tension leads to early wire breakage
> - Twist in the same direction
> - Support fracture with addition means – never sole means of fracture stabilization

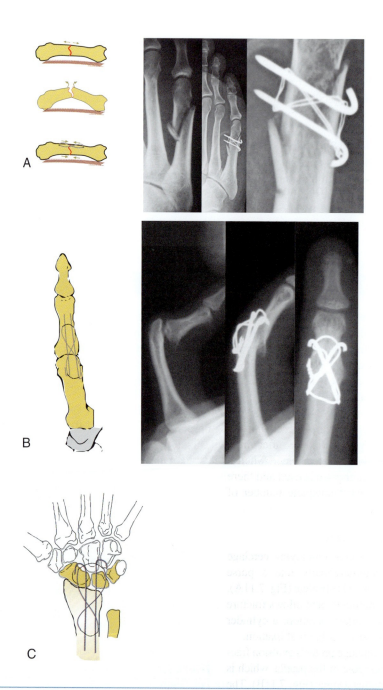

FIGURE 7.7
(A) Exceptional application of the tension band principle to fix a diaphyseal fracture of a small bone. (B) The tension band wiring for arthrodesis of the first metacarpophalangeal joint. (C) The tension band wiring achieves arthrodesis in a porotic wrist where other fixation will not hold.

cut wire tips are bent at right angles to the direction of the wire loops. This step maintains the tension in the wires and avoids soft tissue irritation. The bent wire tip may then be buried in a hole drilled in the bone. Wire removal is not obligatory after bone healing.

Regional Application

The Tibia and Femur

Comminuted fractures of the tibia or femur are successfully treated with an intramedullary nail and cerclage wire (Fig. 7.9). The cerclage wires are applied after accurate reduction. They neutralize the shearing forces and convert them to compression forces. The intramedullary nail is then passed percutaneously to neutralize the bending forces. A plaster cast is not necessary after intramedullary nailing but weight bearing should be delayed for 4 weeks.

Cerclage wires are useful in reducing and maintaining a large wedge fragment or a severely displaced oblique or spiral fracture fragment. These are often used as temporary aid and removed immediately after final fixation; these may be left in place when a locked internal fixator plate is used and there is obstruction to insert adequate number of screws (Fig. 7.10).

Patello-Tibial Cerclage

Patellar fracture fixation employing cerclage wire placed circumferentially like a purse string around the bone is obsolete (Fig. 7.11A). This fixation is inefficient and allows fracture fragment mobility and separation; a cylinder cast must supplement this internal fixation.

Patello-tibial cerclage protects avulsion fracture of the inferior pole of the patella, which is often treated with lag screws (Fig. 7.11B). The tension of the patellar tendon is counteracted with a wire loop passing through the quadriceps tendon and the tibial tuberosity. Over-tightening

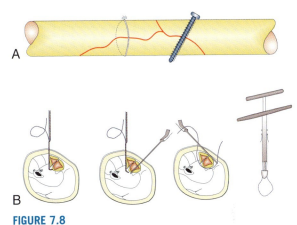

FIGURE 7.8

(A) Temporary cerclage wiring to facilitate lag screw fixation. A comminuted long bone fracture with two main fragments and a butterfly is controlled effectively by a cerclage wire.[3]
(B) The Goetze-Rhinelander-Böhler method of the percutaneous extraperiosteal cerclage wiring for a fracture of the tibia. Application through a minimal surgical exposure causes least damage to the blood supply and reduces the risk of infection. The cerclage wire is introduced through two small stab incisions, one over the anterior and one over the medial border of the tibia by means of a cannulated guide and extraction hook. A wire tightener is used to simultaneously contour and tension the wire around the bone while securing the fixation.[11]

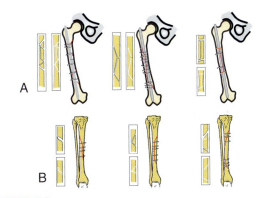

FIGURE 7.9

(A) Intramedullary nail and cerclage wire is a good alternative to interlocked nail in comminuted fracture of femur.[12]
(B) Cerclage wiring of tibial fracture; additional support in cast is essential.

the wire pulls the patella down creating a patella baja and causing chronic patellar pain. A preoperative X-ray of the good knee serves as a guide for normal patellar height. The patello-tibial cerclage wire is removed after the fracture heals, usually in 6–9 weeks. In a soft bone, the cerclage can be anchored distally around a transversely placed bone screw in the tibial spine. In selected cases, reabsorbable 2 mm PDS wires may be used to avoid implant removal.

In short, the uses of cerclage wiring are

- temporary fixation during the plating of long bones,
- reattachment of a fractured or osteotomized greater trochanter,
- as an alternative method when interlocking nailing is not available,
- as an adjunct to intramedullary nailing in the presence of one or more butterfly fragments.

Cerclage wires are also used in conjunction with Ender pins, Zickel nails or other non-locked intramedullary devices for the treatment of unstable femoral or tibial shaft fractures. Fractures about the stem of a femoral prosthesis are commonly treated with multiple cerclage wires as a temporary or definitive fixation. A combination of Kirschner wire and cerclage is helpful in some fractures of the hand and for arthrodesis of an unsalvageable interphalangeal joint. Inappropriate patient selection, poor technique and motion, particularly with delayed union, are the major causes of failure of cerclage wiring.

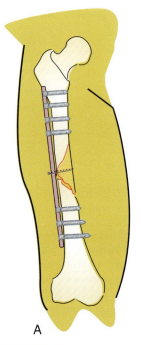
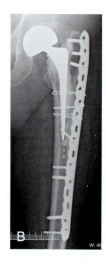

FIGURE 7.10

Severely displaced large wedge fragment may cause a delay in bone healing; a cerclage wire can be used to reduce it. **(A)** In fracture fixation with LIFP, if there is a gap between the bone and the implant such a wire can be left in place. **(B)** Radiograph showing use of cerclage wires in a periprosthetic fracture. Reduction and fixation with wires or cables is preferred in treatment of periprosthetic fractures in elderly because of its nature; it is a low energy trauma with low soft-tissue compromise.

WIRE CABLES

Wire cables are made from high-grade stainless steel. A cable of 1 mm diameter is used for fracture fixation and is certified for long term implantation. Cross-lay cables with easy to grip mat surface finish are recommended for surgical use. The cable that is twisted to right, is made taut for increased strength, has a very low give, takes up little space and is unstressed. Special cutters are used to hack a cable that does not unwind or fray upon cutting. A cable has 49 individual filaments, i.e. seven strands with seven super-fine wires; six of the seven are wound around a core strand (Fig. 7.12). This arrangement makes a cable supple and break resistant. The ISO standard requires a resistance to breakage of 1770 MPa. Cable is available as a 10-m roll, or with ready-made loops in 15, 60 and 120 cm lengths.

Its ends are securely brought together whilst taut using a crimp of very small dimension. Crimp is a type of seal made of high-grade stainless steel that is squeezed into shape. This results in optimal cohesive strength through the interlocking of cable and crimp. The crimp holds the taut cables permanently and firmly together.

A wire cable is pliable, strong and resistant. It does not cut into the living bone. A ready-made wire cable of 15 cm length is particularly suitable for tension banding. With a loop at one end, it is ready to be hooked on a Kirschner wire or a screw (see Fig. 7.15A). With this firm foundation it can easily be pre-stressed, and give a high degree of stability to osteosynthesis. High-density polyethylene sleeve is useful when passing the cable through cancellous bone. The mechanical properties like resistance to fatigue, yielding and breaking strength of a multi-filament cable are superior to that of a mono-filament wire (Table 7.3).

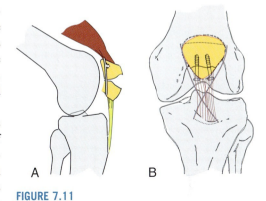

FIGURE 7.11

(A) Cerclage wiring of the patella is ineffective and is seldom used. The fixation is inefficient and allows fragment mobility and separation. (B) The patello-tibial cerclage counteracts the distraction loads on the lower pole of the patella.[9]

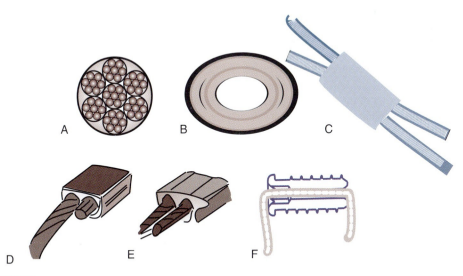

FIGURE 7.12

(A) Classic arrangement of 49 fine wires to make a 1-mm thick cable. Smallest unit has seven slender wires each, six of which are wound around a core strand. The arrangement is repeated to make up the final product that is supple and break resistant. (B) End-on view of oval shape of the crimp; this turns to round after squeezing to lock. (C) Both cables are moulded into one another and pressed into the inner wall of the crimp; their alignment is divergent as the cables are under tension. (D) A crimp of new design with two separate round holes to accommodate cable ends.[13] (E) After crimping, the holes distort to oval shape. (F) High-density polyethylene sleeve through which a cable is passed to protect a soft bone.

Table 7.3 Comparison of Properties of Cable and Wire[14]

Cable as Implant	Wire as Implant
Cable is pliable and strong; no loops and kinks like wire	Wire is rigid
Cable is strong and does not break	Wire often breaks just as one is about to carry out the last twist, one of the most important moments of osteosynthesis
Cable is enormously strain resistant and may be optimally tightened and fixed so that osteosyntheses remain stable and resistant to load	Wire does not tolerate the tension, it tears and goes back into distraction
Cable does not loosen at the crimping site nor does it cut into the living bone	Kinks in a wire straighten out under the slightest muscle tension
Cable-crimp connections are loadable up to at least 600 N	Wire can be given very little pre-tension; it elongates 138%

A cable is used as a cerclage directly on the bone, without squeezing of the soft tissues. Bone can withstand the pressure exerted by the cable. Operator should take all the steps that ensure a cable's tightness after crimping (Fig. 7.13). Innovative uses of cable cerclage are shown in Fig. 7.14.

Cable could also be used for patellar fracture fixation. A load sharing cable is used to partially unload force transmitted to the patella. Since a part of the force carried by the patellar tendon is transferred to a cable placed parallel to the tendon and inserted in bone tunnels in the patella and tibial tubercle, the fracture site and its fixation is partially unloaded (see Figure 7.11B). A cable, when compared to a wire, has significantly increased fatigue resistance to cyclic loading.

Labitzke,[15] a German orthopaedician, in his monograph takes exception to the popular orthopaedic interpretation of tension band principle and emphasizes that the terms static and dynamic compression are incorrect application of the rules of mechanics to operating techniques. Tension bands, irrespective of whether used by engineers or surgeons, are static principle. Structural engineers achieve stability by permanent introduction of high level of forces that opposes and exceeds all the excepted ones. Compression cannot be achieved by means of movement within a system, and movement always means lack of stability and the danger of destruction. Interfragmentary movements are harmful, not 'dynamic' and may lead to distraction. Weber's wire tension banding with Kirschner wires is the best possible application of the principle but has three inadequacies:

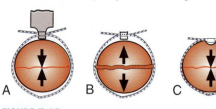

FIGURE 7.13

(A) The crimping device is thick and occupies space when placed directly on bone.[15] (B) A potential gap is left behind that allows movement of the fragments with loss of tension and subsequent loss of fixation. (C) A small hollow, a free space is made with a narrow chisel or bone nibbler in the bone cortex. The thick tip of crimp pliers is accommodated in this depression. The cable remains taught and pre-tensioning is maintained.

- Principle of eccentricity – the banding wires are placed on the surface of patella and eccentrically compress the bone. Eccentric tension bandings are unsuitable osteosynthesis procedures, which both at rest and during movement partially pull apart a fracture of patella or ulna. Because of

ever-present shearing forces, eccentric tension banding tends to lead to the formation of steps and with every movement produces disturbance within the fracture, which can lead to secondary displacement. The term 'dynamic osteosynthesis' is untenable, because the forces freed during movement are destructive; there is also no stimulus to promote healing.
- Use of wires as tension band. Labitzke mathematically and mechanically proves that wire elongates easily when put under tension.
- Failure to use two stabilizing Kirschner wires.

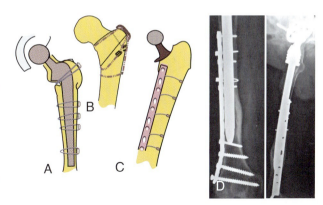

FIGURE 7.14
(**A**) Cable is used as prophylactic banding in revision surgery, (**B**) to reattach greater trochanter,[16] and (**C**) to stabilize fractures. (**D**) Radiographs showing use of cable in a periprosthetic fracture.

New Principle of Bilateral Cable Tension Banding Operation

The biomechanics of tension banding has to be revised because the 'eccentric-dynamic' model has too many disadvantages for bone healing. It is unjustified to continue to use wire tension banding in the prevalent forms because all its variants lack pressure, do not resist muscle pulls and their results are not optimal.

The bilateral cable tension banding is a constructive compression principle. Tension-resistant wire cables pull fractured fragments so firmly together that a stable pressure osteosynthesis develops. Exercises or other manoeuvres to promote healing are unnecessary.

Two longitudinal Kirschner wires are necessary in every instance. Static interfragmentary compression is produced by permanently acting cable tension bandings that are attached to Kirschner wires and firmly grasp the patella laterally (Fig 7.15).

As majority of the quadriceps tendon fibres pass through the anterior sector of the patella, the resultant force of the tension banding advantageously runs through the anterior center of the fracture.

It is re-emphasized that optimally positioned Kirschner wires (Fig. 7.16) at least of 2 mm thickness are necessary on every occasion to anchor cables for applying tension, neutralize large shearing and bending forces, and stabilize fragments through additional pinning.

Bilateral cable tension banding osteosynthesis procedures achieve high stability in patella fractures; according to Labitzke, 'There is no indication for primary patellectomy'.

Eccentric tension banding methods produce trivial pressure on extensor side and pull the facture apart near the joint surface. Transverse and flexion forces are poorly absorbed. Isometric triceps activity reduces pressure on the extensor side and increases pressure ventrally. Isotonic triceps activity with the mere function of creating movement does not alter the basic tension of the banding and fracture crevice gapes. A step develops and the joint surfaces become incongruous.

Fixation of proximal ulna and olecranon fractures by two lateral cable tension bands is also recommended on biomechanical principles. Two intramedullary Kirschner wires are laid parallel in the center of the ulna and temporarily support the reduction. Two lateral cables are stretched between these

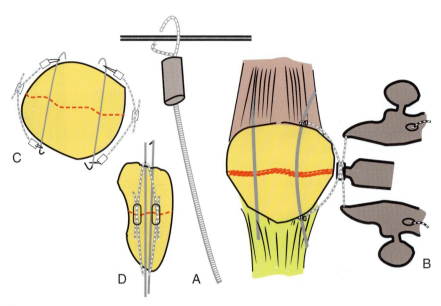

FIGURE 7.15

(**A**) Ready-made cable loop passed around a Kirschner wire makes a sound foundation for applying tension. (**B**) Ten-degree bowing of two ends of a Kirschner wires is a visual indicator of adequate tension on the cable. (**C**) Bilateral cable tension band. Both ends of the Kirschner wires are shortened and first bent ventrally and are then turned medially so that the cables cannot slip off. The cable tension bands are laterally placed and exert high compression force. (**D**) Tracings of X-ray films show well compressed fracture and accurately reduced articular surface.

wires and an anchor screw or plastic sleeve passing transversely through the ulna shaft (Fig. 7.17). The arrangement produces high static compression over the entire fracture area, neutralizes distracting forces of the triceps and biceps as well as shearing, bending and turning moments that may arise.

PINS

A surgical pin is a thin straight wire possessing remarkable resistance to bending. Martin Kirschner (1879–1942), a surgeon from Heidelberg, was the first to use thin wires (0.7 mm chromium-plated steel piano wire) for applying traction in fracture management.[17] He modified a Steinmann pin to apply skeletal traction because Steinmann pin often caused considerable local damage. Kirschner also developed a device to put thin wires under tension to achieve more stability, a principle now being used in ring fixators. Kirschner never approved of these wires to fix a fracture; Otto Lowe (1932) was first to describe their use for fracture fragment stabilization.[10] The terms Kirschner wire and pins are used interchangeably here.

The tip of the Kirschner wire is sharp enough to facilitate insertion in the bone. Two common designs are a diamond point that has two bevelled surfaces and a trocar point with three cutting edges (Fig. 7.18). The trocar point is better suited for insertion in hard cortical bone.

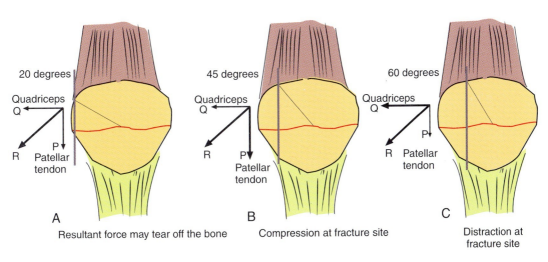

FIGURE 7.16

The search for finest position for Kirschner (K) wire.[15] (**A**) K-wire is passed at the point where a 20° line from the center of patella crosses its rim. The pressure force P is stronger than the transverse force Q but the lateral cushioning of the bone is too thin and there is possibility of pulling out of K-wire. (**B**) The best position of the K-wires is the point where a 45° line from the center of patella crosses its rim. At this point the pressure force P developing form the resultant for R is the same size as the transverse force Q. The lateral cushioning of the bone is thick enough to prevent any pullout. (**C**) When the K-wire is passed at the point where a 60° line from the center of patella crosses its rim, the pressure force P developing from the resultant force R is too small compared to the transverse force Q.

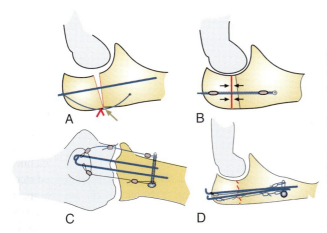

FIGURE 7.17

(**A**) Force applied from beyond the middle of the cross-section of ulna, like eccentric tension banding, produces slight pressure but pulls apart the joint surface and a gap, step and joint incongruity develops; the larger the eccentric pre-tensioning the larger the gap the joint surface. (**B**) Bilateral cable tension band produces high static compression across the fracture line. No gaps are seen. (**C and D**) Tracings of X-ray films show implant position in bilateral cable tension banding.

Often both ends of the pin are sharp, thus a pin can be inserted either in retrograde or antegrade directions across the fracture surfaces. Kirschner wire may have a smooth or a threaded surface. Threaded pins have superior holding power in the bone and are less likely to migrate, but they are also difficult to insert and harder to remove. The thread does not improve the bending stiffness of the pin. Smooth pins are easy to handle. The stiffness of the pin is related to the fourth power of its root

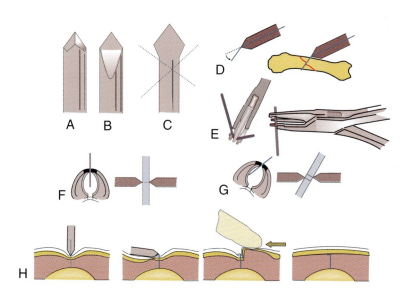

FIGURE 7.18

End of Kirschner wire or Steinmann pin with **(A)** a trocar point and **(B)** a diamond point.[3] **(C)** A variant of a diamond point design creates a hole larger than the diameter of the pin. A wire with such a point should not be used. **(D)** A metal tube with flanged end is an effective instrument to bend a Kirschner wire. **(E)** A specialized plier with one split jaw precisely bends a pin to 90° at a pre-selected point.[18] **(F)** Proper method of cutting a pin. The jaws should meet at the same level on opposite sides of the pin. **(G)** An oblique cut can be made (to produce a point on the pin) by placing the jaws in the same position, but rotating the pin cutter on the pin a plane perpendicular to the previous cut. Incorrect, but commonly used, method of cutting a pin.[11] A rotational force results, which in trabecular bone or thin cortical bone may be sufficient to cause a fracture. **(H)** Bending, cutting and sinking the K-wire under the skin.[19]

diameter. A smooth pin therefore has higher bending stiffness than a threaded pin of the same diameter, as the root diameter of a threaded pin is smaller than that of a smooth pin.

Use of Kirschner Wire

Pins are versatile and are often useful for internal fixation. A pin has a relatively small diameter and is inserted through the soft tissue and bone with relatively little trauma. Kirschner wires are placed in bone either by hand with a Jacob's Chuck or at low speed with a power drill. Hand-driving of K-wires can be done with a twisting, circular motion of the chuck much as one would drive a screw. Alternatively, a back and forth motion of the wrist with pressure applied down the chuck will also advance the implant. A power drill is not essential for Kirschner wire placement; however, one with a quick locking and release mechanism saves substantial time and is also useful for its insertion through dense bone such as in the olecranon or calcaneus. The soft tissues tend to wind round the Kirschner wire during insertion and must always be protected. Various types of guides are in use: a telescoping guide attached to the drill, or an external guide with a handle is an everyday device.

Definitive Fixation

Whenever a Kirschner wire is used for definitive fixation, the end of the pin should be cut a centimetre under the skin and should be bent and sunk under the skin; a long one will protrude through the skin, either due to the pressure from within or from outside. If a wire is cut too close to the bone, it is difficult to locate it at the time of removal. The jaws of a wire cutter are always placed at right angles to the wire. If they are placed at any other angle, a twisting force develops while snapping the wire. This force is transferred to the bone and as a result unintentional fracture can occur in a small bone, particularly in the cancellous area (see Fig. 7.18D and E). A sharp point at the pin tip can be fabricated by making an oblique cut and then rotating the pin to make the second oblique cut. The free end of the wire must always be bent with an instrument (see Fig. 7.18F). The bending force, if transmitted to the bone, can cause an inadvertent fracture; gripping and stabilizing the pin during bending prevent this complication. There is a genuine danger of migration of a straight pin into the bone or into the soft tissues; a pin is known to travel a long distance across the soft tissue planes. When using a pin around the shoulder, it is imperative that the tip be bent.

A pin enclosed in a plaster cast should not touch the cast but move freely inside. There is considerable movement between the cast and the bone due to the presence and the thickness of the soft tissues. If a pin touches the plaster, forces are transferred to the bone, leading to pin loosening and loss of fixation. A pin must be removed after it has served its purpose.

Provisional Fixation

Kirschner wires are useful for provisional fixation of a comminuted fracture. They assist in accurate placement of the fragments and implants, especially the plates and the screws. Multiple wires may be inserted without any additional trauma. When provisional stability has been achieved, X-ray pictures may be made to visualize the strength and weakness of the construct.

Planning is essential while inserting Kirschner wires for provisional fixation. Pins are introduced in such a way that they do not obstruct the final placement of the definitive implants (Fig. 7.19). For example, wires are passed parallel to each other in the same direction in which the lag screw is to be introduced so that there is no obstruction to compression of the fracture with the lag screw.

Regional Considerations

The Tibial Plateau

Kirschner wire clusters are used to support the cartilage and subchondral bone after a localized depression of the tibial plateau has been corrected by elevation and bone grafting. The extent of the stiffness produced by the pins is dependent on the pattern in which they are applied (Fig. 7.20). Two pins placed at an angle from the same insertion point provide minimal stiffness. A grid pattern constructed with four to six pins offers the most effective support. The best stiffness thus produced is less than 30% of the intact

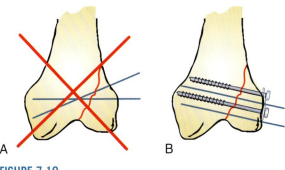

FIGURE 7.19

(A) Kirschner wires placed at an angle for temporary fixation obstruct screw placement and application of compression. (B) Parallel Kirschner wires facilitate the same.

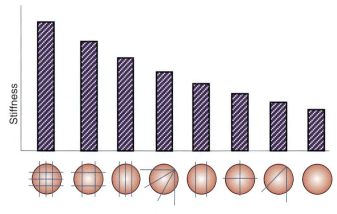

FIGURE 7.20

A comparison of stiffness provided by various Kirschner wire configurations used to support a depressed region of the tibial plateau (not to scale).[20]

bone, which is still significantly better than that contributed by the bone grafting alone.

Supracondylar Fracture of the Humerus in Children

Kirschner wire is used for the definitive fixation of a displaced (Gartland type 2 or 3) supracondylar fracture in a child. Surgical treatment of supracondylar humeral fracture has reduced the problems of venous outflow obstruction and consequential complications. Putting pins in a small bone that is surrounded by a fat swollen soft-tissue envelop is difficult and may damage neurovascular structures due to errant pin placement. Although elbow flexion maximizes soft-tissue management but it is not a mechanically stable position. The total stability of the fracture depends on the placement of pins in a strong position to prevent displacement of the fragments. Pin placement is the key to success of maintenance of the skeletal alignment and recovery of function. The stability depends on three factors that are under surgeon's control:

1. Size of the pin
2. The number and distance between the pins along the line of fracture
3. The pins placement on both sides of the fracture

Pins may be placed as crossed pins or lateral pins. Visual indicators for safe pin placement are applied after reducing the fracture. In the lateral view, obtained by manoeuvring the image intensifier till the teardrop is seen on the end of the bone, a K-wire is placed over the arm to bisect the bone along its long axis (Fig. 7.21). A line is the applied and extended to the medial side of the arm across the end of the arm. In anteroposterior view, the medial and lateral columns are found and the K-wire is placed along the desired trajectory of the pin. A line is then drawn on the arm to give a visual prompt and it is extended to bisect the line previously drawn along the long axis of the arm. Such visual cues allow better hand-eye coordination for the inexperienced and occasional stabilizer of elbow fractures.

Currently lateral-only pinning technique is in vogue for almost all supracondylar fractures; it has been proven biomechanically to be of equivalent strength to a cross-pinning construct (Fig. 7.22). In a severely swollen elbow a potential risk to ulnar nerve exists in medial pin insertion method. However, there are definite indications for applying a medial pin:

1. Fractures with medial obliquity
2. High supracondylar fractures (meta-diaphyseal fractures)
3. Very Low supracondylar fractures
4. Fractures with medial comminution

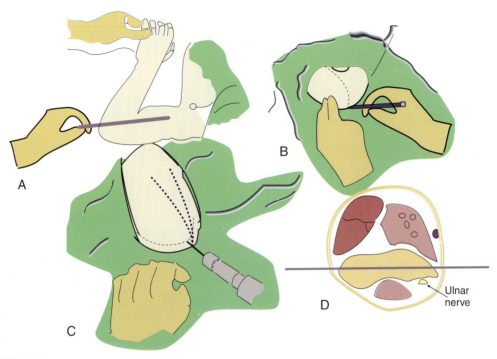

FIGURE 7.21

(**A**) Supracondylar fracture of humerus is accurately reduced and secured by elbow hyperflexion. (**B**) A line drawn on medial and lateral side of arm along the humeral plane. (**C**) Further lines are drawn and pins are deployed along lines that intersects the planes. (**D**) Pin must be placed anterior to the ulnar nerve.[21]

Technique of Pinning

Achieve reduction by applying traction, pressure on olecranon, and maintain elbow flexion; confirm reduction on fluoroscopy in Jones AP, lateral and column views. Jones view of the distal Humerus is axial AP view of a hyperflexed elbow.[22] Back of the hyperflexed elbow lies flat on the surface; forearm is pronated when displacement was postero-medial or supinated for postero-lateral displacement. Internal or external rotation of the arm through a 20° arc helps to visualize the columns.

Using the visual landmarks discussed above, a proximally directed wire is passed from the lateral cortex through the center of the olecranon fossa to exit on the medial side. This wire is inserted from slightly anterior to posterior direction in the coronal plane as seen in the lateral view. The passage through the olecranon fossa creates a very stable construct because the wire has a 'quadri-cortical' hold in the bone. A well-spaced second lateral wire is placed parallel or divergent to the first one. A third wire is needed when instability persists; it may be inserted from lateral or medial side. The accuracy of reduction and position of wires is checked on fluoroscopy in flexion and extension employing anteroposterior, lateral and two oblique views. Lastly, the wires are trimmed.

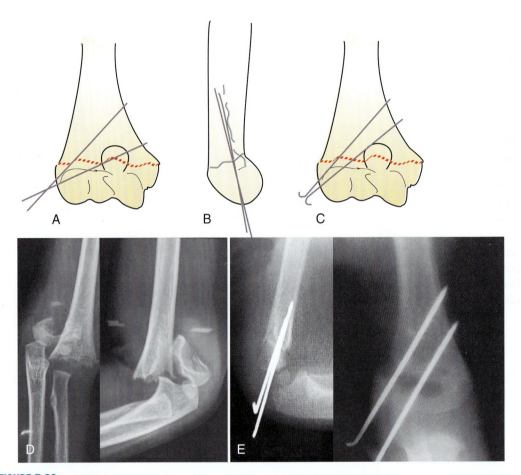

FIGURE 7.22

(**A**) Divergent pin placement. The more medially placed pin is penetrating the olecranon fossa. (**B**) In the lateral view, the pin should be centered, which ensures the proximal fixation is in bone. (**C**) The pin entry points are too close to each other and may function as a point of rotation leading to loss of reduction. (**D**) Radiographs of a displaced supracondylar fracture in a child. (**E**) Closed reduced and stabilized by percutaneous pinning.

Technique of Medial Pinning

A lateral pin is inserted first to achieve a level of stability. The elbow is semi-extended to protect the ulnar nerve. It is prudent to make a small incision (0.5–1 cm) over the medial epicondyle, retract the soft tissues and the ulnar nerve, and then place the medial wire under vision. The wires should cross in the proximal segment at an angle of around 40–50°. Pins are bent and trimmed outside the skin. Soft padded strong slab is applied for comfort on the posterior aspect for 2 weeks. The K-wires are removed at 4 weeks after surgery; children regain range of motion in a few months, and physical therapy is unnecessary.

Forearm Bones

The Kirschner wire is an unsuitable implant to fix forearm bone fractures as it fails to control the rotational alignment and maintains the axial alignment only to a limited extent. External support in a plaster cast is mandatory; non-union is frequent.

In exceptional circumstances, its use for fixing forearm bone fractures in children provides primary definitive fracture care; however, plaster cast should be used for additional support. Three patterns of deployment are known (Fig. 7.23).

Fracture of Radial Head in Children

A Kirschner wire of 1.2–2.5 mm diameter is gently contoured and its last 3 cm are sharply bent (Fig. 7.24). Two centimetres proximal to radial physis, the cortex is penetrated by a bone awl or a drill bit, the prepared pin is introduced into the medullary canal and is directed cephalad along the long axis of the bone. It is pushed upwards till its point engages the inferior aspect of the fracture elevating

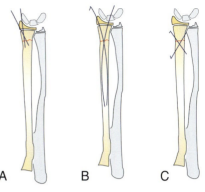

FIGURE 7.23

(**A**) Trans-epiphyseal K-wire fixation with penetration of opposite cortex in transition zone. (**B**) Intramedullary. (**C**) Cross-wires in metaphyseal zone.[23]

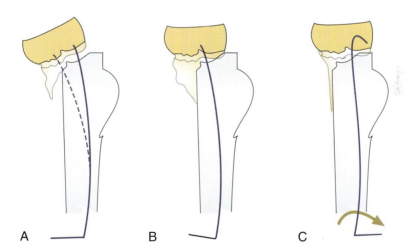

FIGURE 7.24

Closed reduction of radial head fracture. (**A**) A pre-bent Kirschner pin introduced in the medullary canal at a point 2 cm proximal to the epiphysis and engages the fractured surface of the radial head. (**B**) Cephalad movement of the Kirschner pin elevates the head and pushes towards the lateral condyle of the Humerus; the condyle prevents over-correction. The lateral periosteal sleeve acts as check-rein against medial displacement. (**C**) The final seating is achieved by rotating the pin to overcome residual lateral shift. Wire is left in the bone and limb is protected in a splint for two weeks.[24]

and repositioning it under the lateral condyle. Once the tilt has been corrected, a lateral shift of a few millimetres often remains and its correction is achieved by turning the pin around its long axis through 180° that its point faces inwards. This shifts the radial head medially and reduces it. The tension produced in the intact periosteum on the lateral side prevents its medial over correction. The lower metaphyseal end of the pin is cut and skin closed. It is difficult to reach the epiphysis with the point of the wire if the tilt is more than 80°; however, it is always possible to obtain partial reduction of the head by direct manipulation, by digital pressure or by an external pin.

The Distal Radius

Fracture of the distal radius is the commonest fracture of the upper extremity. Till late 1960s this fracture was considered benign, and conservative treatment was the rule. The population involved was elderly and malunion was a frequent occurrence. Over the years, however, a growing number of young males, manual workers and sport enthusiasts have suffered high-velocity injuries, often with complex wrist fracture. Conservative treatment of the fracture in the younger population leads to malunion with consequent pain and disability.

The goal of treatment of distal radius fracture should be to obtain and maintain an anatomic reduction; the former is easy but difficult to maintain, and loss of reduction after conservative treatment is common. The displacement is not correlated with the type of immobilization but with the initial displacement and dorsal comminution. Cast immobilization does not prevent finger movements. The contraction of the flexor tendons transmits compression forces along the axis of the forearm and the carpus abuts on the distal radius, resulting in its proximal migration and. shortening. Furthermore, a non-displaced fracture is not always stable. One must always look for dorsal comminution and anticipate a secondary displacement. Biomechanical studies confirm that malunion affects the function of the wrist; the complication is poorly tolerated and requires treatment.

Percutaneous pinning is an effective technique in maintaining the reduction of an unstable extra-articular fracture or an unstable, moderately displaced intra-articular fracture. It is also useful in obtaining and maintaining the reduction of grossly displaced intra-articular fragments and is frequently used in combination with external fixation. Relative contraindications to percutaneous pinning include osteoporosis and severe comminution.

Biomechanical studies of pin fixation support the use of a minimum of three pins for fixation of a distal radial fragment. Although four-pin configurations provide the greatest stability, these may be utilized selectively, as the patient is subjected to additional risk (Fig. 7.25). Whenever the ulna is engaged, the construct provides superior resistance to fracture displacement. The pins that cross the radial fracture provide greater stability. The proximal trans-ulnar radial pin is safe and avoids damage to the distal radial joint.

Al Kapandji of France observed that a Kirschner wire yields because of its flexibility and allows the distal fragment to move out of position. The movement continues until the wire rests against the inferior edge of the proximal fragment and cannot bend any further (Fig. 7.26A and B). He has suggested an 'intrafocal pinning' technique. Kirschner wires are inserted directly in the fracture line after a manual reduction; secondary displacement of the distal fragment is then impossible due to the close contact of the distal fragment and the pins. The pin then acts as an abutment (buttress) pin (Fig. 7.26C–G).

A stable fixation requires three pins at precise locations: the first pin is inserted between the tendons of the extensor carpi radialis and the extensor pollicis brevis; the second is placed posterolaterally close to Lister's tubercle, avoiding the extensor pollicis longus; the third is introduced posteromedially,

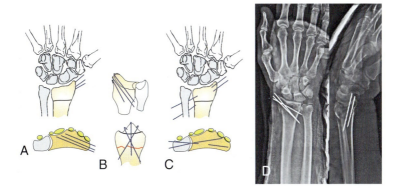

FIGURE 7.25

Stable wiring configurations for the distal radial fracture. (**A**) Three radial pins. (**B**) In a modified technique to enhance stability three pins are placed from radial styloid process towards and through the dorsal, volar, and ulnar cortices of the proximal fracture fragment: additional rotational stability is achieved by bending and counterblowing these in the styloid process.[25] (**C**) Two dorsal radial pins with one proximal and one distal trans-ulnar pin.[26] (**D**) Radiographs showing application of three stabilizing pins.

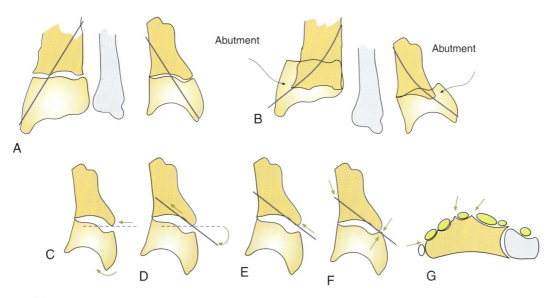

FIGURE 7.26

Kapandji technique. (**A**) The pin is located far away from the edge of the proximal fragment. (**B**) It bends until it is firmly stopped by the edge of the proximal fragment; the reduction is lost. (**C**) The stages of intrafocal pinning: C to G. (**C**) The fracture is reduced and the wire is introduced first perpendicularly into the fracture gap. (**D**) It is then moved obliquely, until it touches the far cortex, (**E**) the wire is then drilled into the far cortex. (**F**) Further dorsal displacement is prevented by the wire. Two more wires are inserted from the dorsal surface (see text).[27]

passing between the extensor digitorum tendons and the extensor carpi ulnaris tendon. Additional cast immobilization is not necessary, allowing immediate rehabilitation and, therefore, a better functional result.

Great care should be taken in every case to choose the treatment that suits the real functional needs of the patient, rather than automatically pursuing a perfect radiological result using over-aggressive treatment.

Metacarpal and Metatarsal

Fractures of metacarpals, metatarsals and phalanges are successfully treated by a Kirschner wire fixation, as the overall length of the bone is short and subsequent load on the fracture is modest. Definitive fixation achieved by the Kirschner wire is weaker than that achieved by a dorsal compression plate or an external fixator; however, wiring has some advantages. The Kirschner wire fixation can be performed percutaneously, inflicting minimal surgical trauma, i.e. without opening the fracture site or stripping the periosteum. Fig. 7.27 illustrates various K-wire fixation techniques for fixation of metacarpal fractures.

Patankar[29] has described an easy and inexpensive technique to stabilize a spiral or comminuted fracture of metacarpal with locked K-wires (Fig. 7.28).

In a transverse fracture of a metacarpal or metatarsal, bending generates mainly shear load at the fracture line. The transverse metacarpal or metatarsal ligaments limit the torsional load, which is of a lesser

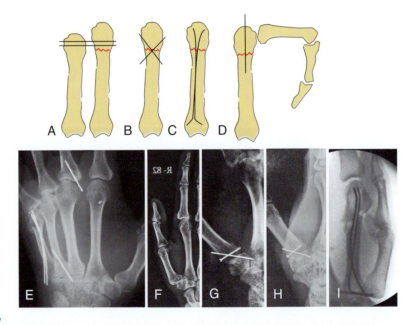

FIGURE 7.27

Pin fixation techniques for metacarpal fractures.[28] (**A**) Transfixion pinning, (**B**) cross K-wire, (**C**) 'bouquet' antegrade intramedullary technique to fix a stable metacarpal fracture. (**D**) Retrograde intramedullary wiring. (**E**) K-wire fixation of multiple fractures in hand. (**F, G, H**) Bennett fracture stabilized with a screw and a K-wire. (**I**) Locked antegrade intramedullary K-wires for unstable metacarpal fracture.

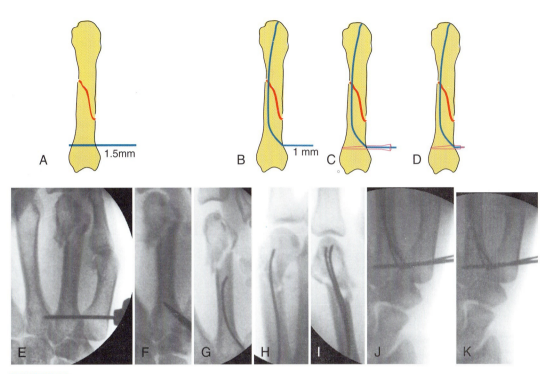

FIGURE 7.28

Locked antegrade intramedullary K-wire for unstable metacarpal fracture-Patankar method.[29] **(A and E)** Entry hole crafted on the dorso-lateral cortex using a 1.5-mm K-wire; additional hole is created in the far cortex to facilitate locking of the K-wire. **(B, E, F, G, H and I)** After fracture reduction, stabilization is achieved by inserting a 1-mm thick, blunt, pre-bent wire along the medullary cavity into the distal subchondral bone. **(C and J)** K-wire is bent to 90° and 16 G additionally beveled hypodermic needle is advanced over it to engage the hole in the far cortex. **(D and K)** The wire and needle are cut together; crimping of the hollow needle prevents wire's migration.

magnitude. Wires placed at 90° to each other in a cross pattern control the shear at a transverse fracture line. Four crossed wires best stabilize transverse fracture of a small bone; two wires, even of a larger diameter (1 mm), do not provide the same degree of stiffness. Four longitudinally placed wires provide the next most stable construct. Other configurations are weaker than these two (Fig. 7.29A and B).

In an oblique fracture line, the shear and torsional loads are in play in equal strength and are well controlled by the parallel wires introduced at a right angle to the fracture line. In an oblique fracture, orientating the pins perpendicular to the fracture line effectively resists shear and torsion (Fig. 7.29C). Longitudinally placed wires poorly stabilize oblique fractures.

In brief, four crossed Kirschner wires for a transverse fracture line and three parallel and perpendicular wires for an oblique fracture line will provide the best stability.

Displaced fracture of neck of fifth metacarpal is difficult to manage. The reduction is effectively controlled by inserting two to three wires to fan out in the head. This arrangement is also known as bouquet technique (Fig. 7.29D).

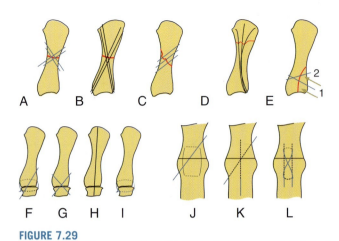

FIGURE 7.29

(A) Four crossed wires produce strongest fixation of a transverse fracture of a small bone. (B) The longitudinally placed wires resist torsion poorly since they are nearly parallel to the long axis of the bone, which is also the axis of torsional force. The wires are anchored in the cortex to resist loads. (C) Three wires of 1 mm diameter placed parallel provide strongest fixation stiffness in oblique fractures.[30] (D) Bouquet technique. Two to three wires are fanned out in the head to control reduction.[31] (E) Kirschner wire fixation of an intra-articular phalangeal fracture: first wire is inserted at right angles to the fracture line: the second, inserted at an angle, maintains the applied compression and precludes the loss of reduction.[3] Different fixation methods to fuse the trapeziometacarpal joint.[32] (F) Tension band, (G) crossed Kirschner wires, (H) cup and cone and (I) cerclage wiring. Patterns of Kirschner wire fixation of an interphalangeal joint: J–L. (J) Oblique Kirschner wire with a cerclage wire on the dorsal aspect, (K) one oblique and one longitudinal Kirschner wire and (L) two longitudinal cross-wires with a dorsal wire loop.[33]

Intra-Articular Fracture

Kirschner wires can effectively stabilize an intra-articular fracture in a small bone as the destabilizing load on the fracture line is small (Fig. 7.29E). First, a Kirschner wire is inserted at right angles to the fracture plane. The fracture fragments are then manually compressed with a forceps, and a second Kirschner wire is introduced obliquely to stop redisplacement and maintain the compression.

Arthrodesis

Four alternative methods are available to fuse the trapeziometacarpal joint (Fig. 7.29F–I). Tension band fixation of this joint for arthrodesis is strongest in resisting compression, tension, toggle and torsion loads. Cerclage wiring is a close second in all respects. Cup and cone and crossed Kirschner wiring come distant third and fourth, respectively. Fusion of an interphalangeal joint can be performed by three different methods (Fig. 7.29J–L). Two longitudinal Kirschner wires with a dorsal figure-8 wire loop provide the strongest stabilization against anterior–posterior bending and torsional loads.

Kirschner wires are routinely removed when they have served their purpose. In children duration is after 3–4 weeks while in adults they are removed after a period of 4–6 weeks.

Traction

Application of axial tension improves the bending stiffness of a Kirschner wire. Tensioning stiffens a small diameter K-wire and then it can then withstand high bending loads. A 1.6 mm Kirschner wire can withstand a traction weight of 22 kg at the lower end of the femur without cutting through the bone. Kirschner wires may be used in any of the common sites for skeletal traction. Kirschner had designed a traction stirrup that caused many problems. The wire was tightened and solidly fixed to the stirrup; every movement of the limb that changed the direction of the traction forces caused pivoting of the stirrup and moved the wire in the bone. Kirschner wire, being thin in diameter than a Steinmann pin, exerts more pressure on the bone. Persistent movement and higher pressure predispose to loosening and infection. Kirschner wire is now seldom used for traction.

Steinmann Pin

Fritz Steinmann (1870–1933), a surgeon in Bern, Switzerland, introduced pins for skeletal traction (1908).[34] A similar effort in the year 1903 by an Italian orthopaedic surgeon, Allessander Codivilla, is less recognized. The pins were driven transversely through the skin and into the bone and were then used as anchor points to provide traction to the fracture in bed-ridden patients.

Steinmann pins are made in diameters from 3 to 6 mm and in lengths from 150 to 300 mm. The pointed end is usually of the trocar or diamond point design but tips with a small niche are also availave point has a positive rake angle that cuts the bone rather than scraping it, as occurs with the trocar or diamond tips. Flutes facilitate removal of chips from the hole made in the bone. Less heat is generated when a pin with niche point is used than one with a trocar point or a diamond tip. However, pre-drilling with the appropriate drill bit is recommended before pin insertion.

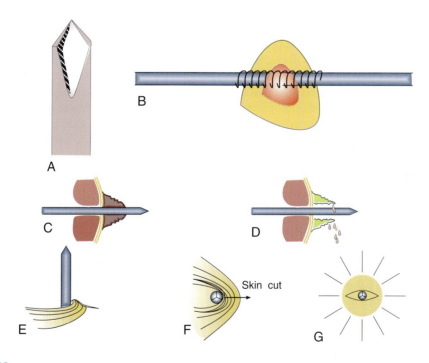

FIGURE 7.30

(**A**) Steinmann pin with cove (niche) point.[3]. (**B**) Partly threaded pin provides firm fixation in the bone. (**C and D**) The pin exit holes in the skin should be sealed with adhesive dressing like tinct. benz. co. as it bonds well to the pin and the skin and prevents movement between them. Non-adhesive dressings allow such movement to take place, leading to ulceration, infection and pin loosening. (**E and F**) If the skin is puckered on one side, a slough results. (**G**) Skin incision equalizes the tension and prevents its necrosis.[35]

Steinmann pin insertion
- Always pre-drill a hole with a sharp drill bit.
- Use a power drill. A hand drill or T-handle induces a wobble factor and makes an oval hole that predisposes to loosening.
- The Steinmann pin tip cuts poorly. Direct insertion into dense bone with power may cause bone necrosis due to excessive heat production.
- Make liberal skin cuts around the pin exits. Make the long axis parallel to the line of the pull.
- Never pierce the skin with the pin tip. This leads to sinus formation as the dermis is pushed inside the wound.
- Use a drill sleeve to protect the soft tissue.
- Cover the sharp end of the pin to protect the patient and attending personnel.
- Ensure that no tension exists on the skin after traction is applied; if necessary make additional cuts to relax the skin and prevent its necrosis.

The shaft of the Steinmann pin is smooth or threaded. Threading of the pin facilitates fixation within a bone so that infection, otherwise facilitated by metal–bone motion, is prevented.

Steinmann pins that are partly threaded in the central section are easy to introduce and are as effective as fully threaded Steinmann pins (Fig. 7.30B). As the thread diameter is 0.5 mm larger than the pin, the threaded segment is as strong as the rest of the pin.

Common sites for applying skeletal traction are the upper end of tibia, lower end of femur, lower end of tibia, calcaneus and olecranon. In children, damage to the epiphysis must be avoided.

Steinmann pin incorporation in a cast can maintain length and rotation in a long bone fracture. One or two Steinmann pins are inserted above and below the fracture. After reduction the limb is supported in a plaster cast incorporating the Steinmann pin (pin and plaster technique). The stability of this construct is not very satisfactory. The plaster breaks down at pin inclusion sites. The grip of the plaster on the pin loosens in time, leading to the movements of the pin. Then plaster weight and relative movement between the limb and cast lead to pin loosening and pin tract reaction. Pin and plaster technique is a viable alternative when external fixation is not available.

Steinmann pins are mainly used for traction through the femur, tibia (proximal or distal end) or os calcis. Traction is best applied with a Böhler stirrup or bow, which fits over the pin ends. Special pulleys with bearings are available and are useful when applying balanced traction. The design of the clamps holding the pin is such that the movement of the stirrup does not rotate the Steinmann pin and lead to its loosening because the bearings on the stirrup clamps allow free rotary movements on the pin.

REFERENCES

1. AWG to mm conversion chart. Accessed 2014 December 10, 10.58 pm. Available at: http://www.rapidtables.com/calc/wire/awg-to-mm.htm.
2. Surgical suture. Accessed 2014 December 10, 10.40 pm. Available at: http://en.wikipedia.org/wiki/Surgical_suture.
3. Gershuni DH. Principles of wire and pin fixation. In: Chapman MW, Madison M, editors. Operative orthopaedics. 2nd ed. Philadelphia: JB Lippincott; 1983. p. 329–38.

4. Synthes (USA), 2011 West Chester, PA, USA.
5. Radin EL, Rose RM, Blaha JD, Litsky AS. Practical biomechanics for the orthopaedic surgeon. 2nd ed. New York: Churchill Livingstone; 1992.
6. Browner BD, Mast J, Mendes M. Principles of internal fixation. In: Browner B, editor. Biomechanics of fractures in skeletal trauma - fracture, dislocation and ligamentous injury. Philadelphia: WB Saunders; 1992. p. 243–68.
7. Hertel R. Technique of osteosynthesis. In: Rowley DI, Clift B, editors. Skeletal trauma in old age. London: Chapman Hall; 1994. p. 63.
8. Hungerford DS, Barry M. Biomechanics of the patellofemoral joint. Clin Ortho 1979;144:9–15.
9. Banjamin JJ, Bried J, Dohm M, McMurtry M. Biomechanical evaluation of various forms of fixation of transverse patellar fractures. J Orthop Trauma 1987;1:219–22.
10. Harasen G. Orthopedic hardware and equipment for the beginner: part 1: pins and wires. Can Vet J 2011;52(9):1025–6.
11. Albright JA, Johnson TR, Saha S. Principles of internal fixation. In: Ghista DN, Roaf R, editors. Orthopaedics mechanics: procedures and devices. London: Academic Press; 1978. p. 124–222.
12. Tscherne H, Haas N, Krettek C. Intramedullary nailing combined with cerclage wiring in the treatment of fractures of the femoral shaft. Clinic Ortho 1986;212:63.
13. Acumed 5885 NW Cornelius Pass Road Hillsboro, OR.
14. Giannoudis PV, Kanakaris NK, Tsiridis E. Principles of internal fixation and selection of implants for periprosthetic femoral fractures. Injury 2007;38(6):669–87.
15. Labitzke R. Manual of cable osteosynthesis. Berlin: Springer; 2000.
16. Thakur NA, Crisco JJ, Moore DC, Froehlich JA, Limbird RS, Bliss JM. An improved method for cable grip fixation of the greater trochanter after trochanteric slide osteotomy. J Arthroplasty 2010;25(2):319–24.
17. Martin Kirschner. Available at: http://en.wikipedia.org/wiki/Martin_Kirschner. Accessed 2014 December 18, 11.39 pm.
18. Uma surgicals Pvt Ltd, Bombay Central, Mumbai.
19. Jupiter JC. (2000) Hand fractures: assessment and concepts of surgical management. In: Thomas P. Rüedi, William M. Murphy, eds. AO Principles of Fracture Management, Volume 1. AO Publishing Davos Platz. p. 385.
20. Beris AE, Glisson RR, Seaber AV, Urbaniak JR. Load tolerance of tibial plateau depressions reinforced with a cluster of K-wires. Transactions of the 34th Orthopaedic Research Society Meeting 1988;13:301.
21. Reynolds RAK, Jackson H. Concepts of treatment in supracondylar humeral fractures. Injury 2005;36: S-A51–6.
22. Jones KG. Percutaneous pin fixation of fractures of the lower end of the humerus. Clin Orthop Relat Res 1967;50:53–69.
23. Schmittenbecher PP. State-of-the-art treatment of forearm shaft fractures. Injury 2004;36:S-A25–34.
24. Metaizeau JP. Reduction and osteosynthesis of radial neck fractures in children by centromedullary pinning. Injury 2005;36:S-A 75–7.
25. Habernek H, Weinstabl R, Fialka C, Schmid L. Unstable distal radius fractures treated by modified Kirschner wire pinning: anatomic considerations, technique, and results. The Journal of Trauma 1994;36(1):83–88.
26. Graham TJ, Louis DS. Biomechanical aspects of percutaneous for distal radial fractures. In: Saffar P, Cooney WP, III, editors. Fractures of the distal radius. London: Martin Dunitz; 1995. p. 28–35.
27. Kapandji A. Treatment of non-articular distal radial fractures by intrafocal pinning with arum pins. In: Saffar P, Cooney WP, III, editors. Fractures of the distal radius. London: Martin Dunitz; 1995. p. 71–83.
28. Weinstein LP, Hanel DP. Metacarpal fractures. J Am Soc Surg Hand 2002;2:4.
29. Agashe MV, Phadke S, Agashe VM, Patankar H. A new technique of locked, flexible intramedullary nailing of spiral and comminuted fractures of the metacarpals: a series of 21 cases. Hand (NY) 2011;6(4):408–15.
30. Viegas SF, Ferren EL, Self J, Tencer AF. Comparative mechanical properties of various Kirschner wire configurations in transverse and oblique phalangeal fractures. J Hand Surg 1988;13A:246–55.

31. Foucher G. "Bouquet" osteosynthesis in metacarpal neck fractures: a series of 66 patients. J Hand Surg 1995;20A:S86–90.
32. Stokel EA, Tencer AF, Driscoll HL, Trumble TE. A biomechanical comparison of four methods of fixation of the trapeziometacarpal joint. J Hand Surg 1994;19(1):86–92.
33. Kovach JC, Werner FW, Palmer AK, Greenkay S, Murphy DJ. Biomechanical analysis of internal fixation techniques for proximal interphalangeal joint arthrodesis. J Hand Surg 1986;11A:562–6.
34. History of surgery. Available at: http://www.historyofsurgery.co.uk/Web%20 Pages/0482.htm. Accessed 2014 December 19, 5.56 am.
35. Charnley J. The closed treatment of common fractures. Edinburgh: E & S Livingstone; 1970.

CHAPTER 8

EXTERNAL FIXATORS

Introduction
Classification
  Pin fixator
  Ring Fixator
Pin Fixator
  Components
    Pin
    Tip
    Thread
    Core
    Shaft
  Clamp
  Central Body
  Compression–Distraction System
Frames
  Unilateral Frame
    Unilateral Biplanar Frame
  Bilateral Uniplanar Frame
  Bilateral Biplanar Frame
  Modular Frame
Mechanical Properties of External Fixators
  Number of Pins
  Pin Diameter
  Distance between Bone and Support Column
  Pin–Clamp Interface
  Pin–Bone Interface
  Preloading
Ring Fixators
  Rings
    Half-Ring
    Arches

Ring Connections
  Bolts and Nuts
    Bolts
    Nuts
  Rods and Plates
    Rods
  Threaded Sockets and Bushings
  Supports, Posts and Half-Hinges
  Washers
  Wrenches
Frame Assemblage
  General
  Ring Inclination
  Space between Skin and Ring
  Ring Position at FON Sites
  Ring Orientation
  Wire Positioning on the Same Ring
  Wire with Stopper
  Wire Tensioning
  Wire Fixation
  Guide Wire
  Pulling or Traction Wire
Schanz Screws or Half-Pins
Hinges
  Hinge Function
Fracture Healing with External Fixation
  Unilateral Uniplanar versus Bilateral Biplanar Frame
  Unilateral Uniplanar Frame with Varying Rigidity
  Effect of Fracture Type on Its Healing in External Fixation

Use of Minimal Internal Fixation
Compression versus No Compression under
   External Fixation
Constant Rigid versus Dynamic Compression
   under External Fixation
Plate Fixation versus External Fixation
Dynamization
Reverse Dynamization
Bone Grafting in External Fixation
Frame Construction
Infection and Pin Loosening
   Pin-Related Causes
   Soft Tissue-Related Causes
   Surgeon-Related Causes
Bone Regeneration with External Fixator
External Fixator, What Next?
Removal of an External Fixator

Regional Considerations
The Tibia
   Periarticular Fractures
The Femur
The Radius and Ulna
The Wrist and Hand
The Humerus
The Pelvis
Polytraumatized Patient
Use in Children
The Developing Countries and External Fixation
War, Natural Catastrophe and External Fixation

INTRODUCTION

In the management of limb injuries, external skeletal fixation and wide variety of its applications now has a firm place in the armamentarium of techniques available to the trauma surgeon. External fixation is a method of immobilizing fractures by means of pins passed through the skin and bone. External fixation of fractures is perhaps a misnomer in that the fixation is achieved by staunch pins traversing the bony fragments at right angles to the long axis of the bone. In some situations these pins pierce the limb completely, while in others penetration is from one side. In either case the protruding pins are joined outside the limb by a rigid scaffolding, of which many different designs exist. It is this external scaffolding that lends the name to the method.

In external fixation, a minimum of metal exists inside the tissues. The fracture elements are at will realigned, distracted or compressed. The wound area is well exposed, local lavage, flushing, dressing and surgical procedures are easy and convenient and cause minimal discomfort to the patient. Efficient stabilization of the fracture segment facilitates limb elevation and early movements of adjacent joints. Patients remain mobile and hospitalization time is reduced.

Malgaigne (Paris, 1849), in an attempt to avoid metal implantation in bone, which then frequently caused 'hospital gangrene', devised adjustable metal hooks that pierced the skin to hold the fracture fragments together. The hooks were withdrawn after early fracture healing. The modern external fixator has evolved to its present state from this primitive stage.

CLASSIFICATION

The two main types of external fixators are pin fixators and ring fixators (Fig. 8.1).

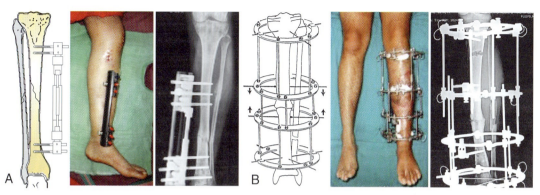

FIGURE 8.1

(A) Pin fixator[1]. (B) Ring fixator.[2]

Pin Fixator

Pin fixators are excellent for routine work. These are applied quickly to stabilize most diaphyseal fractures. Wound access is adequate for management of soft tissue injuries.

The pin fixator has many disadvantages. The fracture needs to be reduced before constructing the frame. The presence of a fixed bar, remote from the axis of the bone, limits the adjustability of the frame to control angulatory and rotatory deformities, though the presence of a joint between the pin clusters does overcome the problem to some extent. The pin fixator is a cantilevered system and does not allow axial loading at the fracture site like a ring fixator. There is a high incidence of delayed union or non-union unless the fixator is modified or early bone grafting is carried out. Angulatory deformities may occur in bone segment transport and limb lengthening procedures. A unilateral fixator needs to be improvised while crossing joints such as the ankle or in the stabilization of pelvic fractures, and is less than ideal in these situations. The frames are not suitable for progressive correction of deformities.

Ring Fixator

In this mode of external fixation, the frames have a major place in the treatment of problems requiring complex reconstruction. These frames replicate the structure of a long tubular bone and are somewhat like an exoskeleton (Fig. 8.1B). The bone is stabilized by tensioned wires acting like an elastic band. The frames give sufficient stability for even the most complicated diaphyseal fracture. Fracture healing is better than in a pin fixator, as weight bearing produces micro-movements that favour faster healing. Multiplane deformity correction, both in bone and in soft tissue, can be performed while using these frames.

Ring fixators also have a few disadvantages: they are heavy and cumbersome. It is a time-consuming procedure to plan and construct a frame. Poor access to the soft tissues makes other surgical procedures difficult. There is a risk of neurovascular damage as the pins and wires traverse the entire thickness of the limb. From a practical viewpoint, thin tensioned wires predispose to low levels of pin tract infection. Oedema is a commoner occurrence in ring frames than in unilateral frames.

Ring fixators are excellent for progressive deformity correction, limb lengthening and management of non-union, but are too elaborate for routine limb injuries.

Following sections describe pin and ring fixators in some detail.

PIN FIXATOR

Components

A pin fixator is made up of many building blocks, each with individual biomechanical and clinical characteristics (Fig. 8.2). In general terms these are described under five headings:

- bone screws or pins for attachment to the bone
- clamps
- couplings
- central body
- compression–distraction system

Pin (Synonyms: Schanz Screw, Half-pin)

The stabilizing hold on a bone segment is obtained through a specialized bone pin that does not pass much beyond the far cortex. The pin has threads at one end and a rounded tip at the other. It is self-tapping and at times self-drilling and is available in 3–6 mm diameter.

The half-pin is the mainstay of the external fixator. It is a modified cortical screw. It does not exert interfragmental compression like a cortical screw and is used only as a holdfast. It does not have a head, and the shaft is very long. It is stronger than the cortical screw. The inner diameter (core diameter) of the pin is slightly larger than the inner diameter of a corresponding cortical screw, e.g. 3.4 mm instead of 3.2 mm for a 4.5-mm screw. This increase in diameter improves the torsional and bending strength of the pin.

A Steinmann pin that passes through the bone is also used in external fixation. It is available with a threaded central section in 3, 4 and 5 mm diameters. The threads grip the bone and prevent loosening.

The external fixation pin is described under four headings: tip, thread, core and shaft.

Tip

The triangular tip cuts its own thread in a bone (Fig. 8.3A). A pilot hole is drilled before inserting the pin. A variety of pin tips are in use (Fig. 8.3B).

Thread

The threads take hold in the bone and provide a secure purchase.

The cutting threads of the pin initiate the bone thread formation; sizing threads bring these up to the

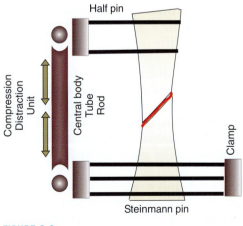

FIGURE 8.2

Basic components of external fixator.[1]

required shape and size. For good bone thread formation it is imperative that the cutting edges of the pin thread should extend up to the first sizing thread. Depending on the length of the threaded portion, a pin may have a hold in one or both cortices.

The external fixation pin with a short thread engages only in the distal cortex. Such a pin crossing the near cortex as a solid bar offers greater stiffness than a pin with a long thread engaging both cortices. The stiffness of the short threaded pin depends on the diameter of its shaft, which is thicker than the core diameter of the thread. A 4.5-mm pin with short threads anchoring only in the far cortex gives a more rigid system than a 5.0-mm pin with long threads engaging both the cortices (Fig. 8.4A).

Core

Core diameter affects the strength of a pin; the torsional strength of a pin varies with the cube of its core diameter. Doubling the core diameter of a screw increases its capability of withstanding torque by a factor of 8. Its tensile strength changes by the square of its diameter.

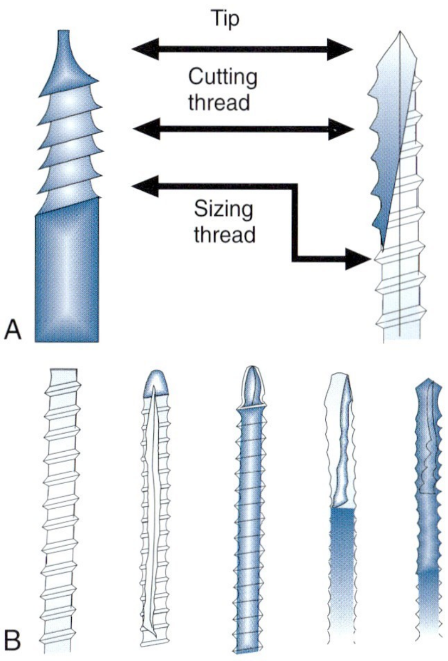

Shaft

The shaft is the strongest part of the pin. It is considerably more rigid than the threaded portion of the pin, since rigidity is proportionate to the diameter. The shaft is used to fasten the pin to the clamp.

FIGURE 8.3
(**A**) Details of half-pin tip. (**B**) Five types of half-pins.[3]

Clamp

The clamp provides the connection between the pins and other components of the fixator. These are of two types (Fig. 8.5). An individual pin is fastened to the frame by a single pin–tube articulation. The second type of clamp can hold a group of pins together and attach them to the main frame. Both permit multiplanar adjustment of the pin-tube interface and can cope with variations in the number of pins and the distance between them; they can also be positioned at variable distances from the skin.

A few clamp designs require special couplings, which connect the clamp and central body.

Central Body

The central body, a connecting rod or a tube is the main structure of the fixator. It is manufactured from materials as varied as stainless steel, titanium, plastic and carbon fibre-reinforced resin. Modular systems employ rods or tubes and a variety of tube-to-tube articulations that interconnect the pins or pin groups. Increasing the number of the rods affects the rigidity of the frame. Many designs with large single connecting rods are also available.

318   CHAPTER 8   EXTERNAL FIXATORS

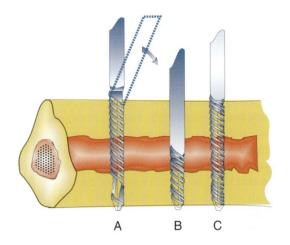

FIGURE 8.4

(**A**) A pin with threads that take hold on both cortices may deform as the stiffness depends on diameter of the engaging part, the thread, which has smaller diameter than the shaft of the pin (**B**). When the shaft occupies the near cortex (**C**), the pin has greater stiffness. In a pin with gradual taper over the entire threaded length, the threads in the proximal cortex have the same diameter and hence same stiffness as the shaft of the screw.[4]

Compression–Distraction System

The compression–distraction assembly can be fixed to the main structure in special circumstances. These devices are useful to apply compression at the fracture surface or for bone segment transport.

FRAMES

The three-dimensional structure built with the components of a fixator system is called a fixator frame, construct or fixator configuration. Pin fixators may be applied in several configurations (Table 8.1).

In a uniplanar fixator frame all the pins are in a single plane. Schanz screws (half-pins) are employed to construct a unilateral uniplanar frame (Fig. 8.6A). When Steinmann pins are used the fixator configuration is termed bilateral uniplanar (Fig. 8.6B). Schanz screws are inserted in two planes in the construction of a unilateral biplanar frame (Fig. 8.6C), while a combination of Steinmann pins and Schanz screws is employed in creating a bilateral biplanar construct (Fig. 8.6D).

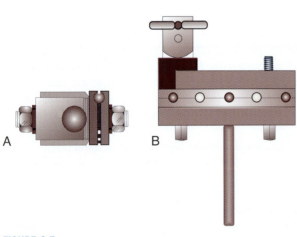

FIGURE 8.5

Two types of clamps. (**A**) Single pin clamp.[5] (**B**) Multiple pins clamp.[6]

Unilateral Frame

A unilateral uniplanar frame is simple to construct and is best-suited stabilization in regions where the local topography, anatomy and functional considerations make the erection of a double frame or of a triangulated assembly inadvisable or impossible (Fig. 8.7A). This assembly has stood the test of time and is popular. The stiffness of this frame in the sagittal plane is higher than in a bilateral uniplanar. The increased stiffness neutralizes most bending forces that tend to cause displacement of the fragments. During the construction of the frame 'safe corridors' should be followed in all the limb segments to ensure the safety of the soft tissues. These safe soft tissue corridors for pin insertion are determined by anatomical considerations. Study of the limb cross-section helps in selecting safe areas for pin insertion to prevent injury to neurovascular structures and to avoid impalement of muscles and tendons. When there is no impalement of muscles or tendons, the associated joints maintain their function during the treatment period and after removal of the fixator. Fewer skin entry holes reduce the possibility of bacterial contamination and the number of scars. The frame is an almost purpose-made configuration for tibia fractures. Walking is greatly facilitated and the patient can squat or sit cross-legged. The anatomic restrictions of application of the frame are minimal and it may be used for complete fracture treatment in external fixation. The frame is useful in stabilizing fractures of the humeral shaft, the ulna and the radius. If there is a clinical indication for external fixation of the femur, the unilateral uniplanar frame is the one most frequently used. In the lower extremity, the stability achieved by the unilateral uniplanar frame is usually sufficient.

In general, the unilateral uniplanar frame is useful in the management of open fractures. Although freedom of pin placement exists, there is almost no possibility of improving the reduction alignment once the frame is completed. Another disadvantage of this frame is vulnerability of the anterior tibial crest; should infection occur the strongest portion of the tibia could be severely damaged.

Table 8.1 External Fixation Frames – Classification

Type	Frame
1	Unilateral
1A	Unilateral uniplanar
1B	Unilateral biplanar
2	Bilateral
2A	Bilateral uniplanar
2B	Bilateral biplanar (3D)
3	Modular

Unilateral Biplanar Frame

This frame is the most stable of the unilateral frames and is well-suited for the treatment of tibial fractures since a large surface of that bone is subcutaneous. Pins are inserted at various positions without going through muscles, tendons, nerves or vessels. This frame is an elegant way to achieve an extremely stable fixation of the tibia while retaining freedom of pin placement. A unilateral biplanar frame is useful for prolonged application of the fixator in the presence of bone loss or severe soft tissue damage (Fig. 8-7B).

Bilateral Uniplanar Frame

This frame, too, finds its chief application in fractures of the tibia. In the presence of sufficient bone contact, as in a transverse or short oblique fracture or in an osteotomy, axial compression may be employed by preloading the Steinmann pins of the proximal and distal fragments towards the fracture (Fig. 8.8A). Since a long

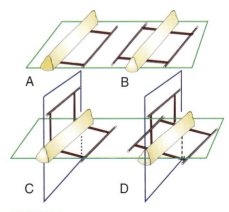

FIGURE 8.6

External fixator frame designs. (**A**) Unilateral uniplanar. (**B**) Bilateral uniplanar. (**C**) Unilateral biplanar. (**D**) and Bilateral biplanar.[4]

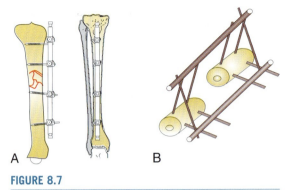

FIGURE 8.7

(A) Unilateral uniplanar frame. (B) Unilateral biplanar frame increases stability for long term fixation.[5]

oblique or spiral fracture has a tendency to slide, it is best to achieve interfragmentary compression with one or two lag screws. Depending on the stability produced by the lag screws, the bilateral uniplanar frame is either applied with axial compression or used simply to neutralize bending and shearing forces (Fig. 8.8B). In the presence of a bone defect or severe comminution, one cannot apply compression for fear of producing shortening. The stability of this frame is improved by prestressing the Steinmann pins within each main fragment.

The symmetry of the bilateral uniplanar assembly offers certain mechanical advantages over the unilateral uniplanar frame. It almost completely eliminates lateral movements of the fragments and it allows for uniform distribution of stresses on the cortices and the external structure of the frame. However, when the assembly does not provide conditions of perfect pin alignment, irregularities in the distribution of stresses result, with consequent over-stressing of the bone. This may lead to the deformation of the pin entry hole and the reduction of the pin's grip on the bone itself. Moreover, the good degree of stability offered by the bilateral frame is often reduced over time as a result of abnormal stresses to which the bone is subjected. The skin is exposed to two possible sources of bacterial contamination and double the number scars are left upon removal. Furthermore, as the pin bridges a bilateral frame it is faced with applicational restriction on limbs as a result of

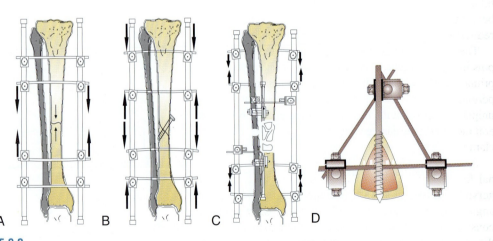

FIGURE 8.8

(A) Bilateral uniplanar frame. Pin preloading in different clinical conditions. (B) Bilateral biplanar construct. Pins are preloaded in each main fragment.[5]

the anatomic configuration of the various segments. A transverse pin can safely be passed only at limited places and, in fact, should be used only for lesions of the leg and the supracondylar region of the femur.

Once popular, this frame has many anatomical, clinical and mechanical disadvantages. A bilateral uniplanar frame is considerably weaker than a unilateral sagittal frame in the sagittal plane, where most of the clinically relevant stresses apply. The transfixing pin may damage nerves and vessels. Impalement of muscles and tendons obstructs the normal function of the joints. Access to the wound is difficult, and the frame is cumbersome to wear and a source of discomfort to the patient.

Bilateral Biplanar Frame

This frame is indicated mainly in the tibia, occasionally in the distal femur, and very rarely in the region of the elbow. It offers greater torsional stability than other frames, with only a few additional pins. The frame is useful in the presence of a large bony defect and in achieving arthrodesis of the knee and of the elbow (Fig. 8.8C and D).

This configuration neutralizes the bending moments in the ventro-dorsal or sagittal plane, which is of great advantage in the post-operative mobilization of the lower extremity after arthrodesis of the knee joint.

Modular Frame

The unilateral uniplanar frame requires pins to be placed in a particular order and does not allow any variation to accommodate soft tissue conditions nor does it permit secondary correction without new pin placement. In a modular frame, which is a modification of the unilateral uniplanar frame, the pins may be inserted as local condition demand. The pins, usually two in each segment, are connected to a short tube with a pin–tube clamp (Fig. 8.9A and B). A third tube and tube-to-tube clamps are used to connect the short tubes in two bone segments. All the tubes can be rotated in relation to each other and fixed in any relative position to improve the fracture reduction.

The modular frame gives unprecedented freedom of pin placement and permits the positioning of pins in different planes according to the anatomy and the nature of soft tissue damage. In the event of primary malalignment, loosening the tube-to-tube clamps permits readjustment of the fragments. A standard unilateral uniplanar configuration can easily be converted to a unilateral modular three-tube frame by applying two tube-to-tube clamps.

An example of the usefulness of this frame is the external fixation of the humerus, where damage to the radial nerve is avoided by applying the pins in two planes at right angles to each other (Fig. 8.9C). A modular frame can be constructed quickly with tube-to-tube clamps to stabilize the pelvis in a polytraumatized patient (Fig. 8.9D). The frame is frequently used in treatment of open tibial fractures (Fig. 8.9E).

Modular frame – advantages

- Total pin placement freedom
- Increased fracture reduction possibility
- Secure fixation
- Easy dynamization
- Quick pin addition or removal
- Applicable in segmental fracture and joint injuries
- Stable for bone segment transportation

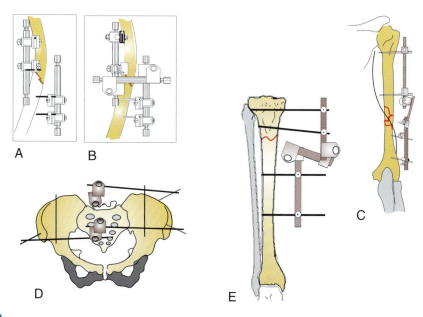

FIGURE 8.9

(**A** and **B**) Modular frame. (Schematic representation[7] redrawn and modified with permission.) (**C**) Application to humerus (**D**) Stabilization of pelvis (**E**).[8] Reduction and stabilization in tibia (**F**).[9]

MECHANICAL PROPERTIES OF EXTERNAL FIXATORS

The aim of application of external fixation is to achieve an environment conducive to fracture and soft tissue healing. It is important to consider the engineering characteristics of the fixation system to be used so that a frame with the appropriate geometrical configuration may be chosen to match the biomechanical and biological demands. Some beneficial factors are known, while there are grey areas as far as the optimal stiffness is concerned. The option is always available in any configuration to change the stiffness of the fixation during the progress of treatment.

Pin fixators are commonly applied in the five patterns. Any change in the particulars of a given frame type changes its stiffness. The important factors influencing stiffness are the number of pins used, the pin diameter and the distance from the bone to the support column of the fixator (Fig. 8.10). Pin separation distance and the stiffness of the support column also influence overall fixator stiffness. The pin–bone interface, and pin–clamp and tube–clamp junctions play an additional role because clamp slippage or pin loosening leads to the bone fragments.

Number of Pins

The greater the number of the pins, the better is the stability. The number of pins, however, is governed by anatomical and clinical situation. A minimum of two pins per segment in the tibia and three per

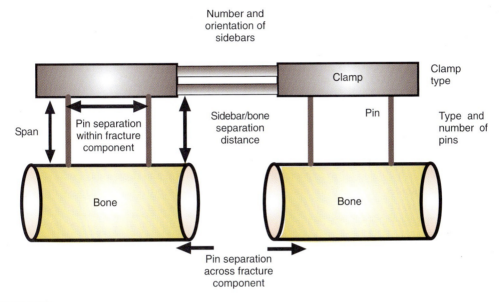

FIGURE 8.10

Factors influencing the stiffness of the frame[10] and stability of the fracture fixation.[11]

segment in the femur are essential. Increasing the pin separation distance across the fracture decreases the rigidity of the frame. An increase in the pin to pin distance in a bone segment increases the bending stiffness of the frame. The bending stiffness of a frame decreases as the pins are moved out of alignment; the torsional stiffness of the frame is increased by a factor of 280 with a pin angle of 90° compared to 0° (all pins aligned).

In summary, external fixator stiffness increases with an increase in

- Pin number and diameter
- Pin separation distance in a bone segment
- Pin insertion angle
- Rod number and diameter

External fixator stiffness decreases with an increase in:

- Pin separation distance across the fracture
- Rod–bone distance

Pin Diameter

Two pin diameters are considered. The optimal outer thread diameter for tibial and femoral pins is between 4.5 and 5.5 mm, and for radial and ulnar pins it is 3.5 mm. The metacarpals and metatarsals can take 2.5-mm pins. The inner or core diameter of an external fixation pin is usually slightly greater than the core diameter of the comparable cortical bone screw, e.g. the core diameter of a 4.5-mm pin is 3.4 mm instead of 3 mm. The core diameter determines the torsional and bending strength of an external fixation pin. The difference between the outer (thread) and inner (core) diameter or thread depth determines the anchorage of the external fixator pin. A short threaded pin with a hold on the distal cortex is stronger than a fully threaded pin.

Distance between Bone and Support Column

The closer the pin clamp can be to the pin–bone interface, and the minimal the pin span, the more rigid the fixation will be for any given configuration. The optimal distance between the rod and the bone appears to be 4 cm, which also allows space for soft tissue swelling and dressings.

Increasing the number of rods from one to two substantially improves the stiffness of the frame. The stiffness of the rod is directly related to its cross-sectional moment of inertia. Stiffness of the rod influences overall fixator stiffness. A change in the side bar configuration also changes the stiffness of the frame; Fig. 8.11 shows the effect of these changes.

Pin–bone interface – stress-reducing factors

- Pin
  - Large diameter
  - High modulus material
  - Multiple pin cluster
  - Reduced span
  - Preloading
- Fixator
  - Two-plane fixation construct
- Patient
  - Reduced weight bearing

Pin–Clamp Interface

Pin–clamp interface slippage is the commonest cause of loss of stiffness of a frame.

Pin–clamp slippage is prevented by regular and periodic tightening of the pin clamps to maintain adequate grip. This is done in the clinic or, in suitable cases, by the patient.

Pin–Bone Interface

The pin–bone interface is the Achilles heel of external fixation. Biomechanically, there seems to be a race between the gradually increasing load-carrying capacity of a healing bone and failure of the pin–bone interface. Under various loading modes, pins are primarily subjected to bending. In stable fractures, axial dynamization of an external fixator restores cortical contact and decreases the pin–bone stresses.

In an unstable fracture, stresses on the pins can approach a very high level and thus they may break. This can be prevented in a number of ways. Large-diameter pins made of high modulus material are less prone to bending. Small pin span also reduces bending of the pin. Bending stresses are minimized when multiple pins are applied in a cluster at critical fixation points. Preloading of a pin substantially reduces the bending stresses. A high level of stress and poor local hygiene predispose to pin tract infection and subsequent loosening. Application of a two-plane fixator substantially reduces stresses on the pins.

The stresses at the pin–bone interface can be reduced easily by the prevention or reduction of weight bearing, but this may not best meet the biological needs of the fracture. A compromise has to be made between the provision of the necessary mechanical stimulus for healing the fracture tissue and

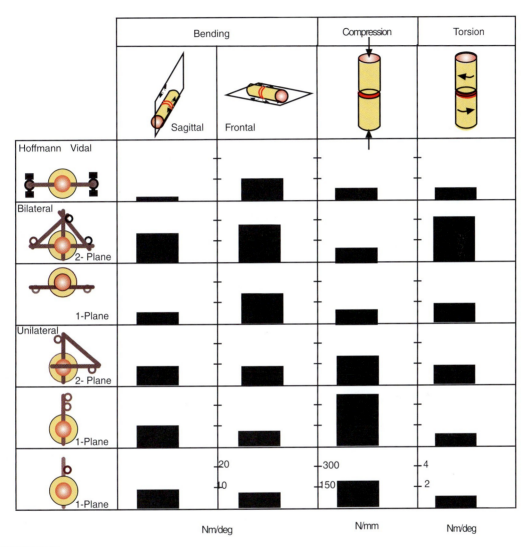

FIGURE 8.11

Changes in the side bar configuration changes the overall stiffness of the construct.[12]

the need to minimize the stresses at the bone–screw interface; achieving this balance is a constant challenge.

Undoubtedly, surgical pin insertion technique must also play important role in the uneventful performance of the pin–bone interface. If the pin insertion technique is inadequate (such as eccentric location of the pins or thermal necrosis of bone tissue due to the use of a blunt drill bit), loosening and failure at the pin–bone interface can be predicted.

Preloading

In external fixation the potential for relative movement between the pin and the bone is high because the pin is not preloaded (tensioned) as in internal fixation. Preload is a static force of sufficient magnitude applied to an implant to overcome all dynamic and muscular contraction forces and to maintain uninterrupted pin–bone contact. Lack of tension at the pin–bone interface leads to micro-motion, which in turn induces loosening of the pin in the bone. If pin loosening is to be avoided, the pin must abut firmly against the cortex.

The accompanying figure depicts the mechanical conditions associated with a pin–bone interface. It shows a longitudinal section through the bone and the pin, assuming that the dimension of the pin fits exactly one of the holes within the cortical bone (Fig. 8.12A). A bending load from right to left (Fig. 8.12B) will load the left contact surface, and the more proximal (left) and the more distal (right) will undergo different loading conditions. The bone at the left contact surface will be compressed and elastically deformed. The pin may move slightly to the left and a gap would appear at the right contact surface. A displacement in the contact area is very small (a few micrometres) but compared to the size of the tissue cells such displacement may be very large.

The biological process that leads to pin loosening is visualized in Fig. 8.12C. Osteoclasts initiate bone resorption that starts at the periosteal or endosteal surface and progresses along the pin. Eventually, the two processes merge and result in complete loosening of the pin. The bone resorption removes only about a tenth of a millimetre of bone around the pin, but the pin will loosen even with this minimal resorption.

Fig. 8.12D shows how preloading the pins from right to left along the long axis of the bone at insertion prevents micro-motion at the interface. An additional functional load from right to left along the long axis of the bone increases compression at the left contact surface and further opens the gap at the right. A functional load to the right reduces compression and reduces the gap but to a very small extent. Such a bending preload, or preload along the long axis of the bone has limited effectiveness because it stabilizes only one of the interfaces. The interface at the opposite surface of the pin will gape and move, though with relatively little strain due to the increased distance between the surfaces. The best

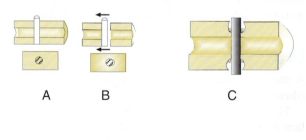

A   B   C

FIGURE 8.12

Pin–bone interface. (**A**) Pin precisely fits the bone. (**B**) Bending load produces different deformation on two surfaces of the hole. (**C**) Pin loosening mechanism. (**D**) Axial preloading of the pin. (**E**) Radial preloading. (**F**) Optimal pin-pilot hole mismatch is 0.1 mm, see text.[13]

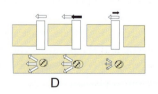

D

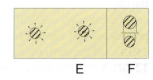

E   F

method to preload the interface is a radial press fit. This is achieved by inserting a pin that is larger in diameter than the predrilled hole – a designed misfit.

Fig. 8.12E shows that the entire surface of the pin within the cortex is radially preloaded. Additional functional load increased compression on one side and reduces it on the other side. This additional load only affects the applied preload and intermittent gaping does not occur.

It is obvious that too small a preload will not stabilize adequately. How much radial misfit can the bone tolerate? The optimal misfit is 0.1 mm (Fig. 8.12F). A mismatch of more than 0.3 mm results in permanent mechanical damage, instability and consequent micro-motion-induced bone resorption. To prevent pin loosening, an external fixation pin that will preload radially by a mismatch of up to 0.1 mm between the pin hole and pin core diameter will be an ideal percutaneous implant. A radial preloading and tapered pin design is based on the observation that bending moment at the pin–bone interface in the distal cortex is smaller than that at the proximal interface. This is why a pin of smaller diameter can withstand bending forces at the distal cortex better than at the proximal cortex. For manufacturing reasons and in-use versatility, the tapered self-tapping pin commonly has a 9 mm diameter on the smooth cylindrical non-threaded part and tapers from 6 mm to 5 mm on the threaded section. This pin provides a better grip: tightening adjustment is easy in the event of loosening. The taper also makes for painless removal, which is always performed without an anaesthetic. The thread pitch and the shape have been obtained, through experimentation, after considering features such as the density, structural homogeneity and strength of both cortical and cancellous bone. These pins are available in two thread types: self-tapping and cutting thread at a pitch of 1.75 mm for cortical bone, and self-tapping and compressive thread at a pitch of 3 mm for cancellous bone.

RING FIXATORS[14]

The components of a ring fixator system are divided into two categories: a main and secondary one. The main parts are the standard elements used to correct skeletal deformities: rings, wires, wire fixation bolts and buckles, pins, and pin clamps.

The secondary parts of the system consist of the elements necessary for the assembly of the fixator: rods, plates, supports, posts, hinges, washers, sockets, bushings, bolts and nuts. To assemble the numerous pieces of equipment various types of wrenches and wire tensioner are needed. There are no screws in this system and screw drivers are not needed.

Rings

A ring with a flat surface and multiple holes is the principal component of a circular external fixator (Ilizarov).

The ring encircles a limb segment: two or more rings are connected to make a frame. The flat surface of the rings supports the heads of the bolts and nuts. The surface–bolt or surface–nut interface guarantees firm fixation of the wires, threaded rods and bolts during the treatment. The flat surface of the rings is important for achieving a secure wire inclination and plane orientation. All rings in a frame are aligned perpendicular to long axis of the bone. A ring is made of stainless steel or carbon fibres, provides strong support for the frame and is designed to bear high stresses of the tensioned wire, up to 150 kg. The internal diameter of a ring measures from 80 to 240 mm. A complete set has rings of 12 different diameters to suit various limbs thicknesses.

A ring fixator set has a number of half and full rings. A full ring is lighter, has more holes than two connected half-rings and does not require connecting bolts and nuts. The holes in the ring are used for introduction of a threaded rod, a hinge or a connecter plate. On the negative side a full ring must be positioned before introduction of wires. If clinical situation demands removal of a full ring during the treatment tenure, then it must be cut with specialized instruments.

Each half-ring, depending on its size, has 18–28 holes in the mid-segment of the flat surface. The standard holes are equidistant (4 mm apart) and are of same size (8 mm in diameter). Bolts or threaded rods are affixed in the holes. Two half-rings are joined by bolts and nuts to form a full ring. The ends of the plate do not have standard sized hole, are offset and ledged to fit together on an even plane to make a full ring (Fig. 8.13).

The half-rings also can be connected to form an oval ring, three and four leaf clover rings and other specialized constructs with the help of additional devices to increase the space between the ring and the limb (Fig. 8.13D–H).

Function of rings
- Supports Kirschner wires and Schanz screws
- Builds a fixator frame connecting two or more rings
- Props up frame's supplementary parts

A five-eights ring facilitates joint motion and is commonly deployed near knee and elbow joints. Besides motion, these rings facilitate introduction of cross-wires, a distinct advantage near these joints. This ring may be used in the middle of regular frame to provide access for soft tissue management (Fig. 8.14); however, five-eights ring is weaker than a full ring: a three point connection to a full ring reinforces and strengthens it. Wires attached to a five-eights ring are tensioned only after such stable connection is established. These rings are available in several sizes from 130 mm onwards.

Half-Ring with Curved Ends

Half-ring with curved ends is a modified five-eights ring with ends curved outwards (Fig. 8.15). The configuration fits deltoid area of the shoulder. It needs a three-point connection to a full ring for stability.

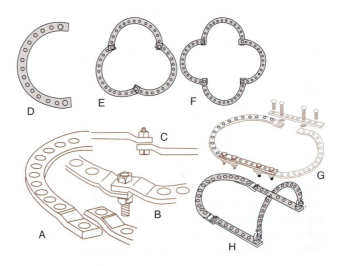

FIGURE 8.13

(A) Two half-rings being connected. (B) Ledged ends of the half-rings are offset but fit on an even plane. (C) Incorrect connection as the ring planes are uneven. (D) A half-ring is the basic unit. (E) Three-leaf clover (F) and four-leaf clover (G) rings enclose a larger space than a circular frame. An oval is fashioned by connecting two half-rings with long connection plates; washers are deployed to bring up the level in the ledged section. (H) Two half-rings are placed at right angle and joined by long connecting plate to make foot component of the leg frame.

RING FIXATORS

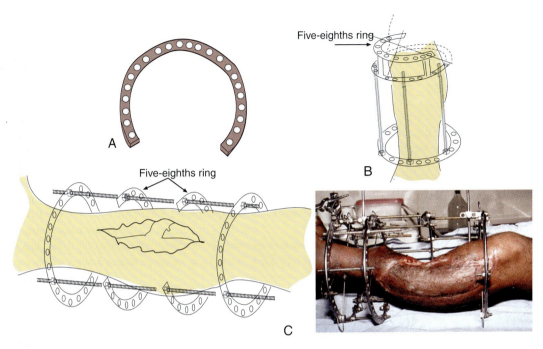

FIGURE 8.14
(**A**) Five-eights ring is used in around major joints like knee and elbow to facilitate range of motion. (**B**) It also provides more working space for introduction of K-wires in the region of tibial condyle. (**C**) At times this ring is used as a middle component of a stable full frame for access to open wounds.

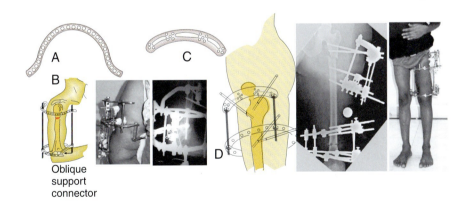

FIGURE 8.15
(**A**) Half-ring with curved ends. (**B**) This is a custom-made ring for deltoid area of the shoulder. Note a five-eights ring at the elbow to facilitate joint movement. (**C**) Clinical and radiograph showing similar frame. (**D**) 90° femoral arch. It is specifically used on the lateral side of the greater trochanter. Schanz screws are deployed to attach it to the bone. Radiograph and clinical pictures are of different subjects.

Arches

Arches are used in femoral trochanteric area as well as near the shoulder joint and are available as 90° and 120° units. Two or three Schanz screws are deployed with the arches (Fig. 8.15C and D).

Ring Connections

Bolts and Nuts

Various parts of the circular fixator are fastened together with bolts and nuts using wrenches; screws and screwdrivers are never used.

Bolts

A typical bolt has a hexagonal head of 10 mm and a threaded shaft that is 6 mm in diameter; the pitch of its thread is 1 mm. Bolts of lengths 10, 16 and 30 mm are often used. These are deployed to connect the threaded sockets and bushings to the rings, for connecting plates, for fastening the rods and half-pins through the socket's apertures. A 10-mm bolt is used for bushings and telescopic rods, but to connect all main parts a 16-mm piece is recommended. When three or more main parts are connected a 30-mm bolt is essential.

Nuts

Nuts have a diameter of 6 mm, but come in three heights: 6 mm (full), 5 mm (three-quarter) and 3 mm (half) (Fig. 8.16). The inside of the nut has thread of 1-mm pitch; i.e. the nut moves a distance of 1-mm when rotated through 360°. The turn of the nut is used as driving force in the Ilizarov system. One-fourth turn four times a day is the recommended distraction–compression rate. Often used 5-mm nut is weak for distraction–compression, and a 6-mm nut is recommended for this procedure. A 6-mm nut, that is a variation of the standard design and its four surfaces are differently marked, is on hand for distraction–compression action (Fig. 8.16E and F).

A 3-mm nut is used as a supplementary fastener. A nut with nylon insert, a 'stopper nut', is used in hinge assembly construction to maintain a desired gap.

All nuts and bolts are used on 'once only' basis. These work pieces are subjected to heavy loading during tightening and while supporting a treatment frame: a reused part may break and seriously weaken the frame.

Function of a nut
- Tighten the connecting bolt
- Stabilize the connecting rod
- Tighten the wire fixation bolt
- Driving vector for distraction-compression movement
- Lock socket and bushing onto a threaded rod
- Affix the pulling wire of a distraction device
- Achieve fixed positioning of male support
- Secure hinge clearance
- Secure a gap on the threaded rod

Rods and Plates

Seven types of connectors are used to link up the rings. Each connector is important and has a specific function.

Rods

A 6-mm thick stainless steel threaded rod is the main connector. Four rods placed at equal distance around a ring connect two neighbouring rings. A four-rod construct is stronger than a three-rod construct in negating bending forces. During construction of a frame, two neighbouring

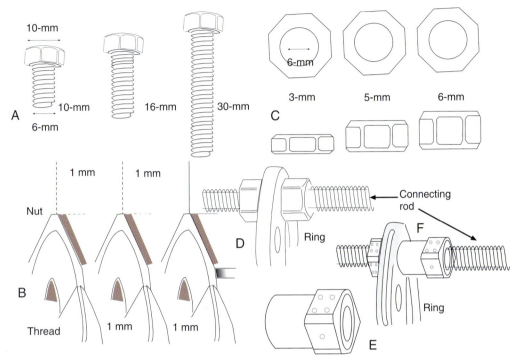

FIGURE 8.16

(**A**) Bolts have standard hexagonal head; shafts are of the same diameter, but their length differs. (**B**) With each full turn a nut advances by 1 mm over a bolt. (**C**) Internal diameter of the nuts is same; but their height differs. (**D**) Nuts are used to secure a long connecting rod to a ring. (**E**) A combined nut with quadragonal head for distraction–compression technique. (**F**) A section of a ring with two combined hexagonal nuts attached to the threaded rod.

rings must not be placed farther than their diameter. These rods also function as ring direction guides in the distraction and compression motion. Threaded rods can withstand high axial loading but are weak in buttressing bending forces. The rods are available in 10 lengths ranging from 60 to 400 mm. The pitch of thread is 1 mm.

A Slotted cannulated rod has a 2 × 2-mm slot extending the length of 20 threads. Its function is of a connecting rod and a pulling device. A cannulated threaded rod has an aperture of 2 mm at its end. K-wire can be attached to both the varieties by using a locking nut (Fig. 8.17).

Telescopic rod with partially threaded shaft is stiffer than a threaded rod and is employed to connect arches and rings. Partially threaded rods are used in combination with telescopic rods and provide a more stable assembly than one constructed using only fully threaded rods. Graduated telescopic rod is a further refinement that adds many safety features and prevents inadvertent over distraction (Fig. 8.18). This is a superior device for controlled distraction and compression.

Connection Plates are used to reinforce a ring fixator. More over these are also used to construct an oval ring for the foot and large frames for correction of angulation and pseudoarthorsis. Five types of connection plates are available (Fig. 8.19).

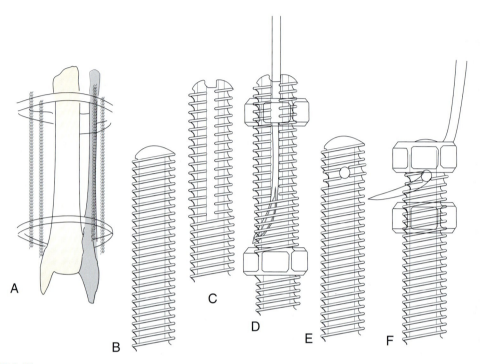

FIGURE 8.17

(A) Threaded rods have high axial load stiffness; however, shorter rods withstand bending forces better than longer rods. Four rods are used to connect two rings. **(B)** End of a standard rod: a close-up. **(C)** A slotted threaded rod: 2 × 2-mm slot extends the length of 20 threads. **(D)** A slotted threaded rod. With a K-wire. To tension and affix, the wire must be bent to 90° and locked in by two 5-mm nuts. **(E)** A cannulated threaded rod. **(F)** The same rod with a K-wire and locking nuts.

Threaded Sockets and Bushings

Threaded sockets and bushings are ancillary components that are used to reinforce a threaded rod (Fig. 8.19F). The cylindrical parts are hollow and threaded from inside. These also have a perpendicular, threaded hole running through the centre from side to side.

Supports, Posts and Half-Hinges

Supports, posts and half-hinges facilitate creation of different constructs (Fig. 8.19G–L). These versatile elements are placed virtually at any location and fixed at any angle. Supports and posts are thicker than other parts because they bear tremendous loads. Half-hinges have a supporting base with two flat surfaces matching the standard 10-mm wrench.

Wire fixation bolts are of two types: cannulated and slotted (Fig. 8.20). The slotted type has an oblique slit at the bottom of the head while a 2-mm hole in run-out area is the characteristic of the cannulated type. The hole has 0.5-mm groove to accommodate a wire. The bolt secures the wire on the ring. The bolt head is oval: 14 × 10 mm oval with two flat cuts on both sides to place a 10-mm wrench.

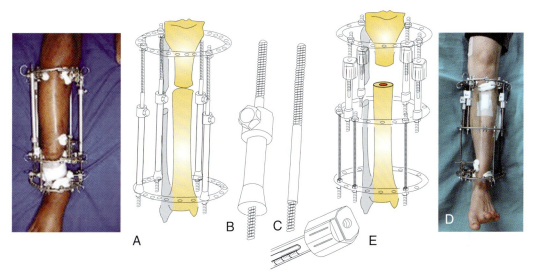

FIGURE 8.18
(**A**) Clinical photograph and sketch of an assembly with telescopic rod with partially threaded shaft. The rings are interconnected with four telescopic rods with threaded shafts. Turning the four pairs of nuts fixed to the upper ring produces compression. (**B**) Short telescopic rod assembled with a partially threaded rod. The bolt is fastened to the smooth portion of the rod. (**C**) Partially threaded rod with smooth middle portion, and one threaded area is shorter than the other so that rods of the same length could be used with telescopic cylinders of different lengths. (**D**) The proximal and middle rings are connected by four graduated telescopic rods that distract the bone. (**E**) Locking mechanism on the graduated telescopic rod.

The length of the head equals the width of the ring and provides maximum surface contact. The height of the wire-fixation bolt-head is twice that of a regular bolt head and is larger than a regular nut. This helps in tightening the wire fixation nut under all local circumstances. Cannulated wire-fixation bolt gives superior wire fixation.

Wire fixation buckle is used in location on a ring where there is no accessible hole. The buckle is attached to the flat surfaces of the ring with nuts and bolts. Dual-sided and detachable wire fixation buckle can hold wires at two different levels (Fig. 8.20B–D).

Washers

A washer fills space between a part and a ring and provides lock-tight fastening. All the washers have 7 mm holes in the centre but differ in thickness and diameter. The washer thickness ranges from 1.5 to 4 mm and a specialized conical washer-couple is also used to maintain an angulation of up to 15° (Fig. 8.21).

Wrenches

Many types of wrenches are used for constructing circular fixators. Wrenches are used in pairs, one for the nut, and one for the bolt: both are tightened simultaneously (Fig. 8.22).

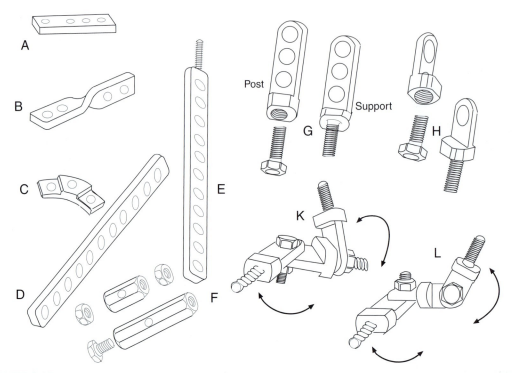

FIGURE 8.19

(**A**) Short connection plate comes in four sizes. (**B**) Twisted plate is used to connect two components positioned at right angles to one another. (**C**) A curved plate is used to increase the circumference of a half-ring and connect two half-rings. (**D**) Long plates are employed to reinforce large frames during bone fragment transport and as extension of the frame [illustration not to scale]. (**E**) Connection plate with threaded rod is deployed to support a hinge as well as a frame. (**F**) Small and large threaded sockets with nuts and bolt. All openings in the sockets have threading where rods could be connected to improve the stability. (**G**) Three-hole male support and three-hole female post. The base of the post is thicker than that of the support and it has an aperture for a bolt. (**H**) Regular size male and female half-hinges; small size half-hinges are available. (**I**) Two-axis hinge. (**J**) Combined-type hinge in diagonal and side views. It has a common base for two flanges at 90° to each other. Arrows indicate the direction in which the hinges turn.

Frame Assemblage

General

Two prevalent methods are complete frame construction before the surgery and application of a sterile frame at the operation. This requires experience but saves time at surgery. The other method requires assembly of the frame piece by piece at the surgery: easy for the less experienced but prolongs the surgical session.

Ring Position and Force Distribution

The rings form the main bulk of a circular frame and are described as of four types (Fig. 8.23).

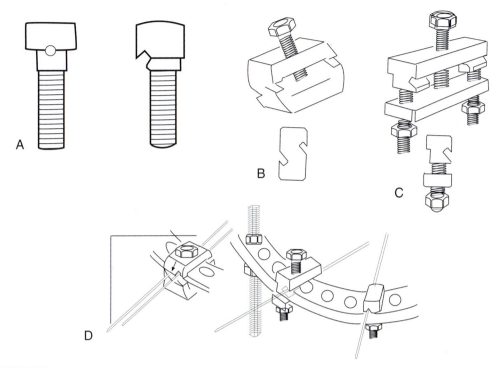

FIGURE 8.20

(**A**) Wire fixation bolts. Cannulated and slotted. (**B**) Dual sided buckle, assembled and in side view, which shows indentations for K-wires. The opposite facing indentations fasten the wires to the ring walls when the buckle is tightened. (**C**) The detachable wire-fixation buckle has indentation on one side. A rectangular base is attached by threaded leg and nut to the top piece. (**D**) A detachable wire-fixation buckle is attached between two holes; it is securing a wire on the upper side of the ring. Inset: Dual-sided fixation buckle is fastened between two holes fixing two wires on opposite walls of the ring. See arrow. A slotted wire fixation bolt is seen on the side where the wire is over the plate hole.

The main proximal frame-supporting ring is a stationary ring that is always at the base of the frame. It carries weight of the entire construction. Stationary, main supporting ring sustains the major load and must be located on the strongest and widest part of the bone that usually is the proximal end of a bone. When located 3–5 cm distal to the joint, it provides enough space for joint movements. The stabilizing frame-supporting ring located at the farthest point, may be stationary or moveable. The distal supporting is similarly located at distal epimetaphysis, 3–5 cm away from the joint space. The pusher–puller ring is movable and used for distraction–compression and is located 3–5 cm distal to fracture–osteotomy–nonunion (FON) site. Occasionally, two of these are used. The reference ring is used as a reference point for the supporting or distraction–compression rings. The reference or the free ring determines the distribution of the translational forces along the limb, and thus must be placed at the level of the intersection of these forces. In most cases this corresponds to the apex of the bone angulation.

The correcting ring determines the distribution of the forces in transverse or oblique directions (Fig. 8.23).

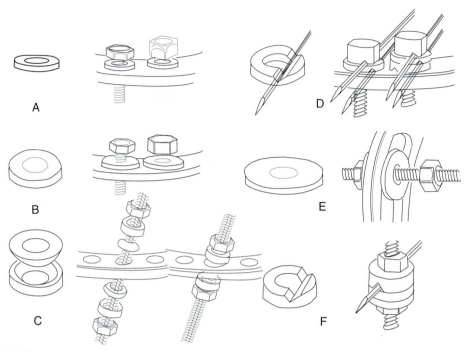

FIGURE 8.21

(**A**) Washers are vital in ring fixator because they provide lock-tight fastening and fill the spaces between the rings and the various parts. The 1.5-mm thick washer that has 12-mm diameter is used with nut and bolt head. It fits between two holes on a ring but is unsuitable for fastening a wire. (**B**) The 2.0-mm thick, 14-mm diameter is used with wire-fixation bolts and for support-post pairs adjustment. (**C**) The 3-mm thick, 12-mm diameter conical washer-couple consists of the two close fitting pieces and adjusts the parts positioned in an angulation of up to 15°. If it is locked in angulation by the nut, it remains stable. The conical washer can be used on both surfaces of the ring. (**D**) The 3-mm thick, 14-mm diameter washer with one flat and one slotted surface is used to adjust the wire-fixation bolt to the plane of an introduced K-wire. (**E**) The 2-mm thick, 20-mm diameter washer is used only for adjustment of a threaded rod to the femoral arch, always in pairs on either surface of the ring. (**F**) The 4-mm thick, 14-mm diameter with one flat surface and one slotted surface. It is used for same purpose as washer shown in D.

Ring Inclination

The ring inclination determines the direction of the forces applied to the ring. As a rule, the inclination of a ring is perpendicular to the bone segment fragment (Fig. 8.24). A minor inclination of 10° could produce large derangement at the farther end. To position the ring the surgeon must take into account the surrounding soft tissues, particularly muscle and subcutaneous fat. The ring is positioned around the anatomic bony centre of fixation.

Space between Skin and Ring

At the narrowest gap, a space of at least 3 cm should be maintained between the inner curve of the ring and skin: wider gaps at other levels are welcome. The gap protects the skin and soft tissue should

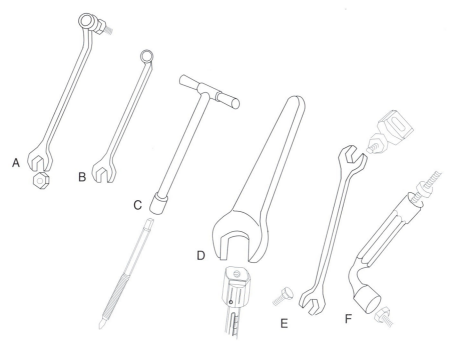

FIGURE 8.22

Wrenches. **(A)** A 10-mm wrench with open and angulated circular end – large size. **(B)** A 10-mm wrench with open and angulated circular end – small size. **(C)** T-wrench for Schanz screw. **(D)** A 19-mm wrench for telescopic rod. **(E)** The combined wrench, 13-mm and 10-mm open ends. **(F)** Angulated tubular wrench, 10-mm in size.

swelling occur, and permits wire tract care, manipulation of the bolts and nuts, introduction of threaded rods and attachment of all additional parts.

This is achieved in three ways (Fig. 8.24D–F). The limb is measured in two planes and largest diameter is considered. 6 cm are added to the figure to provide the necessary internal ring diameter, with a secure 3-cm space between ring and skin; Circumference ÷ 3 + 6 = Diameter of the ring. Second method is to attach the most anticipated size and seek a 3 cm space. From that point step-by-step addition of the rings ensures adequate spacing. Use of plastic template is the third method.

Ring Position at FON Sites

Closer the ring to the tip of a free bone fragment end, the more stable this fragment is during all necessary bone movements. Due consideration is given to the state of the bone that alludes to poor bone strength, like osteoporosis, avascularity, thinning of cortex and secondary damage from osteotomy, and ring distance from the FON site is increased.

Ring Orientation

Irrespective of the level, inclination or angulation of different rings of the same frame, the connecting parts of the half-rings must be aligned in a straight line (Fig. 8.25). This orientation puts the

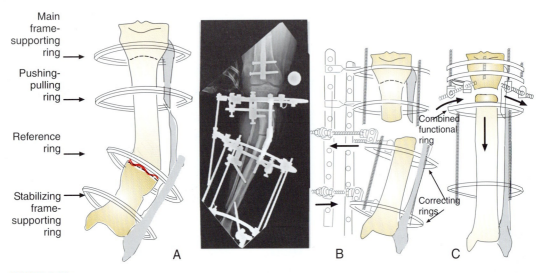

FIGURE 8.23

Four types of rings: main frame-stabilizing ring is the stationary ring. Stabilizing frame-supporting ring. Its position gradually changes as the correction progresses; this ring is considered 'moving ring'. The pushing–pulling ring is applied distal to the osteotomy site. It is parallel to proximal main ring. The reference ring is applied at the site of angulation of deformity at the site of osteotomy. (**A**) It is movable ring. (**B**) Correcting rings. (**C**) Combined functional ring.

corresponding holes of all rings along the same straight line thus making ring connection, especially with the threaded rods, relatively easy. After the correction is accomplished the rings arrive in a parallel position to each other and bone fragments in good alignment, however, the half-ring connections are in rotated location.

Kirschner wire is extensively used in circular fixators. It is elastic, but attains high degree of stiffness under tension. A tensioned wire withstands high magnitude of axial loading over long period. However, a small degree of elasticity persists and is of advantage because it boosts callus formation.

The surgeon predetermines a wire entry and exit points and the wire is inserted precisely at the desired site and in the preferred direction. As abundant caution, a wire is introduced at least 2 cm away from neurovascular bundle. A wire that is brought in gradually at low speed pushes aside a mobile neurovascular bundle: at times the wire may be hammered out.

The skin at the entrance and exit sites must be supported by finger pressure to secure the exact point of wire penetration. In a planned distraction manoeuvre the skin is pushed towards the corticotomy site while in compression it is pushed away from the site of the compressing ends. This manoeuvre prevents damage to skin by the wire and precludes pain and non-essential

Advantages of Tensioned Kirschner wires

- Inflicts minimal damage to bone and soft tissue during insertion
- Supports the bone, prevents damage to soft tissue and bone
- Least external contamination due to small diameter of the wire
- Nominal opening in bone on removal

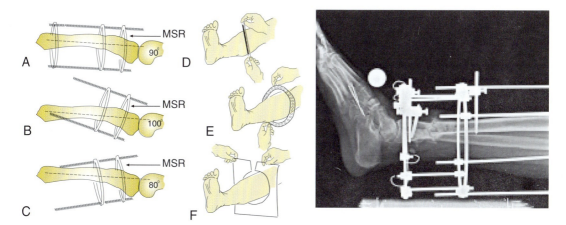

FIGURE 8.24

Ring inclination in three settings. **(A)** Line sketch and radiograph showing lateral view of tibia and a broken line along the long bone axis. Main supporting ring (MSR) is in a position of 90° inclination to the bone axis. The resultant angle is the same for all rings of the frame. **(B)** MSR is in a position of 100° inclination to the bone axis. The resultant angle puts the middle ring too close to the bone at the posterior side and totally deranges the attachment of the distal stabilizing frame supporting ring. **(C)** MSR is in a position of 80° inclination to the bone axis. The resultant angle puts the middle rig too close to the bone at the anterior side and again totally deranges the attachment of the distal stabilizing frame supporting ring. **(D)** Three methods to determine ring size for the leg. Measuring tape: add 6 cm to the widest part of the leg. Circumference ÷ 3 + 6 = Diameter of the ring. **(E)** Trial and error. **(F)** Proprietary template.

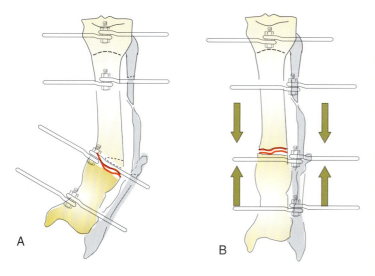

FIGURE 8.25

Ring orientation. **(A)** Rings at different levels and in different inclinations all are oriented so that the connections of the half-rings are aligned on the same straight line, say over the tibial anterior border. **(B)** After deformity correction, all rings are parallel to each other, and bone fragments are in good alignment. Note that the orientation of the proximal main stabilizing ring and the pulling ring next to it is now different and the other rings are in the same orientation as the pulling ring.

scar formation during the course of distraction–compression. At the time of wire insertion, the muscles in its vicinity must be kept at maximal functional length to prevent joint contractures. Multiple holes due several attempts at wire insertion damage cortical bone and 'one wire, one hole' is desirable.

Two wires sizes are used with circular frames: 1.8-mm for adults and 1.5-mm for children. A wire with a bayonet point is used in cortical bone while a trocar point tip is deployed in a 2 cancellous bone site (Fig. 8.26). Wires are inserted at least 3 cm apart.

Wire Positioning on the Same Ring

Wire is introduced on one side of the ring wall. Two wires criss-crossing at 90° to each other achieve the best stability. Lesser angles of insertion permit a degree of displacement; parallel wires permit free movement. Wires with olive-shaped stoppers are used to prevent side to side shift and to induce side ways re-location of a bone segment. Wires supported over the rings can exert distraction–compression forces and move bone fragments in the preferred direction. Stability of a ring can be enhanced by passing a wire at an offset level and connect it to the ring with two supports (Fig. 8.26F and G).

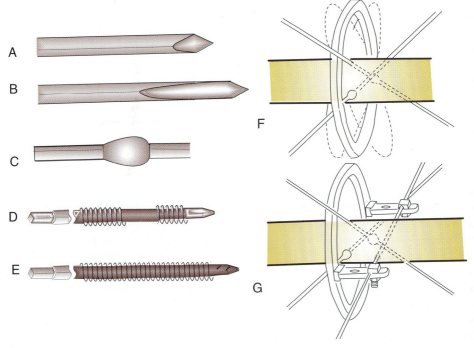

FIGURE 8.26

Wires and Schanz screws used in the ring fixator. (**A**) Trocar-pointed wire. (**B**) Bayonet-pointed wire. (**C**) Olive (stopper) wire. (**D**) Schanz screw with interrupted threaded section. (**E**) Schanz screw with continuous threading. (**F**) Two methods of ring stabilization through use of stopper and offset wires. Introduction of two olive-type stopper wires on opposite sides of the bone. Shearing of the ring (dotted lines) is still present. (**G**) An offset wire fastened to the ring by two supporters eliminates the problem.

Wire with Stopper

A wire with olive-shaped stopper is turned out of a single piece of stainless steel, and is used for bone fixation, for correction of bone fragment displacement, in technique of bone fragment pulling in an internal transport, in interfragmentary compression and in osteoporotic bone.

Wire Tensioning

Only a wire under tension can sustain the large loading forces and support a frame over long period. The degree of tension that can be put on a wire depends on local frame construction (e.g. half-ring or full ring), local bone condition (e.g. normal or osteoporotic bone), patient's weight and the functional wire loading (e.g. stabilization or distraction–compression). The tension on a wire could range from 50 to 130 kg and changes with movement of the frame. Decrease in tension causes pain and skin irritation at the wire site. Wire tensioning brings about a suitable balance in the stability and flexibility of the frame. The magnitude of wire tension dictates the quality of bone healing as well as of the bone regenerate.

A wire can be tensioned by several means. The nut and bolt are simultaneously twisted with wrenches to tighten a wire. Ilizarov used an efficient wire tensioner but that did not indicate the load on the wire. The scale of tension is only guessed in these two methods. As a practical guide, when stuck with a metal, a well-tensioned wire produces a high-pitched note; a loose wire emits a dull tone. Dynamometric wire tensioner is a sophisticated device that displays accurate wire tension (Fig. 8.27).

Good practices for wire tensioning
- Tension a wire on introduction and fixation
- Tension the wire from the end opposite the fastener
- Tension the wire from the end opposite an olive shaped stopper

Wire Fixation

A wire is never manipulated to facilitate its fixation to a ring. Rather a ring is brought up to a wire, using a washer, a post support or a half-ring (Fig. 8.28D–F), to fix it in the same position as it emerges from the skin wound. After successful insertion a wire end may be over the middle of a hole and is fixed with cannulated bolt, or near the edge of a hole is stabilized by a slotted bolt a wire between two holes is fixed using a buckle.

A wire may also be fixed away from the ring using other accessories described above (see Fig. 8.19). Wire is used to reduce displacement of the bone fragments. When employed for this purpose, it is called a reducing or correcting wire. Such a wire is curved or arched and is tightened to produce a shift of the bone towards the concavity of the arch to achieve correction on the table. If this is not possible, then a wire with olive-shaped stopper is deployed and attached to a pulling device to gradually shift the displaced fragments.

Recommended tension on wires
- Wire on a half ring 50–70 kg
- Offset wire depending on supporting post 50–80 kg
- Single wire on a ring up to 100 kg
- Two to three wires on a ring in young individual 110 kg on each wire
- Two to three wires on a ring in an adult 120 to 130 kg on each wire
- Wire with olive stopper 100 kg
- Wire with olive stopper for interfragmentary compression 50 kg

Wires that are fully tensioned at the conclusion of the operation tend to slacken over a period. Loose wires cause pain and inflammation of the surrounding tissue. Re-tensioning is performed by applying two wrenches simultaneously to the head of a fixation bolt and nut and slowly turning both of them a quarter or a half turn. Local anaesthesia or even short general anaesthesia should be administered at the wire tensioning session.

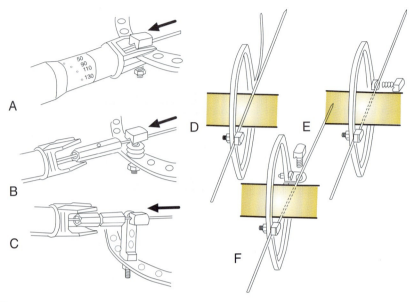

FIGURE 8.27
Wire tensioning. (**A**) Wire is on the same plane with the ring, and the jaw of the tensioner is attached to the ring edge. (**B**) Wire is raised above the ring with two washers; a hexagonal socket is introduced between the fixation bolt and tensioner. (**C**) The offset wire attached to the ring by a support; two hexagonal sockets are used as before. (**D**) Wire is never brought to the ring (interrupted line). (**E**) Ring is brought to the wire by using a washer. (**F**) Ring is brought to the wire by using a support.

Excess length of a wire is cut, bent and tucked under the ring. Failure to do so may harm the patient and physician.

Guide Wire
A guide wire is used to maintain desirable direction of the bone fragment that is being transported (Fig. 8.28). Such a wire offers axial stability to the moving fragment. The wire is drilled and buried in the proximal bone canal and the other end may be buried or attached to the opposite non-movable ring frame. It is never tensioned.

Pulling or Traction Wire
A K-wire can be used as a connecting device between the movable bone fragment and traction mechanism. Pulling or traction wires are of three types: olive stopper, Z-shaped wire twist and hooked end. Traction wires are introduced before the corticotomy. The distal end of the traction wire is connected to the traction device. Wire is removed in retrograde direction.

Schanz Screws or Half-Pins
This implant is used when a trans-osseous wire is likely to damage neurovascular structure, or an arch is used for support and as an additional hold in presence of wire fixation (see Fig. 8.26D and E).

RING FIXATORS

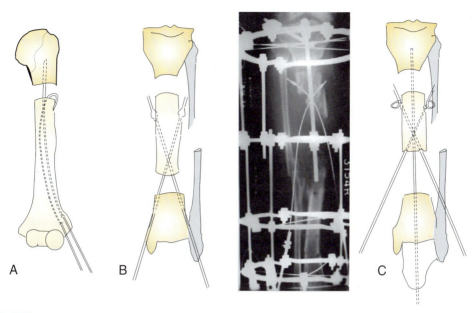

FIGURE 8.28

Traction wire techniques. **(A)** A smooth wire is introduced into the humerus and bent to hook the bone edge after being brought out at the FON site. A guide wire is introduced into the proximal fragment to prevent distal fragment deviation. **(B)** Line sketch and radiograph showing two olive wires, obliquely introduced below the FON site and exiting though the distal fragment, pull the bone in a balanced way and a guide wire is redundant. **(C)** Two smooth wires are introduced obliquely into the middle fragment with a Z-shaped bend to create stoppers. As they exit at the bone resection site, a guide wire introduced through the heel and drilled up to the proximal fragment prevents middle fragment deviation.

The Schanz screw is connected to the ring by threaded socket. When it is based on the same ring as a tensioned wire, it is essential that the wire be tensioned before the screw is attached: this prevents bending of the screw. The unwanted length of a Schanz screw must be cut off while the patient is under anaesthesia because it causes pain to a conscious patient. Use of a Schanz screw on a movable ring irritates skin and deep soft tissue, leaves a large scar, causes pain and predisposes to infection.

Hinges

Hinges give a ring fixator the capability to secure and establish angulation that is essential for correction of a deformity. The hinges are used as pivot (rotation) point necessary for straightening a deformity. Deployed in combination with distraction–compression devices, the hinges make it possible to gradually correct deformities, with simultaneous transformation of the bone and soft tissues. Hinges can promote straightening of an angulated non-union with concurrent compression, can achieve skin stretching, neovascularization and softening of a scarred area and thus influencing the local tissue orientation during deformity correction.

Advantage Hinge
- Hinge guides motion in a desired plane or planes
- Hinge makes available a fulcrum for calculation and control of angulation or displacement
- Hinge offers pivot for biologic adaptation of tissues to a new desired position

Edicts of hinge placement
- Place two hinges on opposite sides of the deformity site to ensure stability
- Align hinge axis in horizontal plane at the apex of the deformity
- Match the plane of hinges and deformity
- Set a hinge at concave side of a deformity to produces compression; one set at convex side generates distraction
- Execute corrections like opening wedge, distraction, compression, translation and derotation by hinge positioning
- The rings controlled by the hinges must be perpendicular to the bone axis: the rings must start at an angle and end parallel or vice versa

A hinge functions effectively when sufficient gap is created at the level of bone distraction and wires with stoppers are used to control and stabilize the bone fragments. Eight different hinge arrangements are shown in Fig. 8.29.

Hinge Function

Preoperative planning is mandatory for hinge application and working with X-ray paper tracings is an accepted modality. A hinge located on concave side of deformity produces open wedge correction. This is used frequently to straighten simple angular deformity. In principle, hinge position in relation to the shaft affects extent of opening of the wedge and compression of the cortex (Fig. 8.30).

A Distraction hinge is located on convex side of the deformity and opens gap on both sides of the bone as the deformity straightens. The magnitude of the gap is proportional to the distance of the hinge from the bone: within limits, the greater the distance the larger the gap. Use of distraction hinge is indicated in a deformity with bone shortening.

Fracture Healing with External Fixation

The mechanism of fracture healing is no different with an external fixator. As is well known, a fracture can heal by direct reconstruction of cortices (primary bone healing) or by external callus (secondary bone healing process). Primary or direct healing is a guided repair phenomenon, which does not guarantee quick healing of the fracture. Callus healing is physiological, and represents the natural reaction of the tissue to a fracture. In fractures treated by external skeletal fixation healing progresses by secondary (indirect) methods. Accurate reduction that will allow healing of the primary type is infrequent except under rigorously controlled experimental conditions.

Unilateral Uniplanar versus Bilateral Biplanar Frame

Comparison of the mechanical properties of unilateral uniplanar and bilateral biplanar fixation shows that the bilateral configuration significantly improves the rotational stiffness as well as the bending stiffness in the plane perpendicular to the plane of the half-pins of the unilateral fixation. The higher rigidity of the bilateral biplanar external fixation results in fracture healing with less callus formation. Bilateral fixation provides a healing pattern similar to primary bone healing.

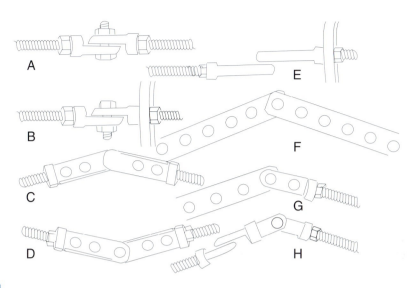

FIGURE 8.29

Assorted hinges. (**A**) Two female half-hinges. (**B**) One male half-hinge and one female half-hinge. (**C**) Two supports. (**D**) Two posts. (**E**) One support with one post. (**F**) Two plates. (**G**) One plate with one support of post. (**H**) Combined two-axis hinge with two half-hinges.

Unilateral Uniplanar Frame with Varying Rigidity

Very rigid external fixation inhibits periosteal callus formation whereas less rigid fixation results in enhanced periosteal callus formation, but at the same time, low initial stiffness of external fixation increases the potential for pin loosening and associated problems. An optimal degree of rigidity is essential for normal bone healing.

Effect of Fracture Type on Its Healing in External Fixation

Fracture healing can be achieved regardless of the pattern of fractured bone fragments as long as sufficient stability is guaranteed by the external fixator. Two-fragment fractures need a high stability in the external frame because all the displacement takes place at one fracture gap. Minor instability leads to a high tissue strain situation at this single-fracture plane, inhibiting fracture healing. Multifragmentary fractures are less susceptible to instability as the displacement is shared between several fracture gaps (Fig. 8.31).

Use of Minimal Internal Fixation

Additional internal fixation in combination with external fixation appears tempting but does not offer any important advantage. Use of a lag screw increases the stiffness of the external fixation and the fracture may mend by direct bone healing without much callus formation, as seen in compression plating. (The plate protects the callus until remodelling is complete while protection in external fixation is available only for a short duration.) A higher re-fracture rate is known after minimal internal fixation. A minor advantage of this method is the possibility of anatomical reduction; this is offset by increased frequency of skin complications.

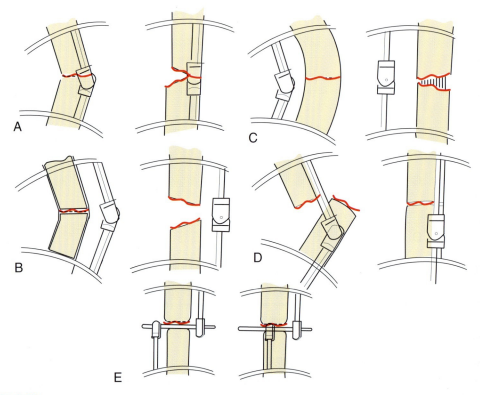

FIGURE 8.30

Hinge position. Interrupted line represents FON site. **(A)** Edge of the convex side of the deformity – for opening wedge. **(B)** Some distance out from the convex side of the deformity – for distraction. **(C)** Edge or outside the concave side – for compression. **(D)** Outside the level of the deformity apex – for translation. **(E)** No hinges; connected half-hinges – for derotation.

Compression versus No Compression under External Fixation

Although static compression can be applied through the external fixation frames, it is of little practical importance. Compression increases the rigidity of fixation to a small degree but does not promote bone healing.

Constant Rigid versus Dynamic Compression under External Fixation

Under external fixation, the fracture site is mechanically stimulated when the rigidity is altered to allow relative displacement of bone ends. The three possible Stimulation methods are as follows:

1. Static stimulation. The fracture site is compressed on weight bearing but the fracture gap returns to its previous state when the load is taken off: the bone contact is lost.
2. Dynamic stimulation of the fracture ends occurs when the clamp grip is adjusted to permit only axial displacement while bending and torsional stiffness is maintained. The fracture ends are under

uniform axial compression on weight bearing and remain in contact even when the weight bearing load is removed. Such stimulation is also called dynamization.
3. A computer-controlled actuator regulates the axial displacement. This is achieved either by load control or by displacement of the bone ends, and weight bearing is not required. Dynamic loading helps in formation of periosteal callus and hastens appreciable secondary bone healing.

Plate Fixation versus External Fixation

A plate-bone system is more rigid in all modes of testing than an unilateral uniplanar frame, except in lateral bending in the plane of the pins where the fixator is superior. The maximum torque and stiffness of the plate-bone construct is higher than the external fixator: A plate-bone system favours primary bone healing.

Dynamization

It is well known that some degree of micro-movement and loading of fracture callus is needed for progressive fracture healing. The term 'dynamization' embraces both the application of micro-movement and of loading to the fracture site without angulation, rotation or distraction of the fragments. Dynamization is effected by increasing the load placed upon the fracture, by encouraging patient activity and by one of the following methods:

1. The use of an elastic frame with overall low-axial stiffness
2. Progressive dismantling of the frame
3. Increased weight bearing in a low-axial-stiffness frame
4. Biocompression: the method uses a unilateral frame that allows free sliding. Weight bearing controls the axial strain on the fracture and it is believed that the patient's natural feedback mechanism ensures the most appropriate strain for healing.

In practice, one of the easiest ways to 'dynamize' the fixation as healing progresses is to loosen the pin clamps and slide them away from the skin, providing a longer pin span. In addition, or by itself, a reduction in the number of planes of fixation achieves greater flexibility in the fixation. Most alterations of pin span and bar configuration tend to increase the bending compliance to a greater degree than axial or torsional compliance.

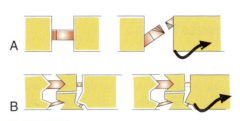

FIGURE 8.31

(**A**) In a transverse or short oblique fracture all displacement takes place at one fracture gap. Instability of the fixation leads to a high strain situation in the only fracture plane inhibiting fracture healing. Therefore, a high stability of fixation is required for fracture healing. (**B**) In a comminuted fracture the displacement is shared between several fractures gaps and low strain situation persists. Less rigid fixation is adequate.

External fixation — fracture healing

- External fixation favours periosteal healing.
- Unstable fixation and fracture gap advance pin loosening and failure of bone fixation, and delay healing.
- Rigidity of external fixation changes the speed of fracture healing. A less rigid frame promotes fracture healing by periosteal bone formation. When and how much to reduce the rigidity? Still unclear!

Reverse Dynamization

Changes in the mechanical environment of a fracture site alter the rate and quality of healing. At cellular level changes in tensile strain and hydrostatic pressure as well as in shear strain and fluid flow have been identified as the causative agents.[15] Timing of change of mechanical environment also speeds up bone formation and improves its quality. In animal studies it has been shown that low stiffness for first 14 days followed by high stiffness improved the quantity bone formation by intramembraneous ossification. The method is particularly effective in large bony defects. Conventional dynamization is initial high stiffness and lower stiffness towards the end of healing process. Reverse dynamization is initial low stiffness for first 14 days followed by high stiffness and again low stiffness towards the end of the healing process.[16] Changing the stiffness of an external fixator is simple, ambulatory intervention. It is anticipated that reverse dynamzation may eliminate the need for traditional bone-grafting techniques like micro-vascular surgery, harvesting cancellous bone grafts and vascularized bone grafts. It may also avoid the pain, discomfort and prolonged healing period associated with distraction osteogenesis.

Bone Grafting in External Fixation

Bone grafting in external fixation is used in two ways: to accelerate fracture healing in the early stages of consolidation and as an additional procedure in a delayed or arrested healing process.

Early bone grafting in external fixation, i.e. before any delay in fracture healing is noted, is a useful alternative to secondary internal fixation. Bone grafting is indicated in open comminuted fractures with or without bone loss and short oblique fractures with an intermediate fragment. Bone grafting results in early fracture healing.[17] Bone marrow injection has been used to prevent and treat delayed.[18] The method is less traumatic than standard bone grafting and holds promise.

Good pin insertion practice
- Make a liberal skin incision; spread deeper soft tissues with haemostat
- Lift periosteum with small elevator to prevent damage by drill bit
- Use trocar to mark pin insertion point
- Employ sleeve to drill a pilot hole and to insert a pin
- Use a power drill
- Sharp drill bit with simultaneous saline irrigation prevents thermal damage
- Clean drill bit flutes often
- Use depth gauge for accurate pin length
- Insert pin with hand instrument

FRAME CONSTRUCTION

External fixation pins are inserted without damaging neurovascular structures. Although the 'safe corridors' for all the limbs have been worked out, in reality there are no safe zones, only hazardous and dangerous zones; safe corridors should be followed with caution. As far as possible the pins are so inserted as to construct a stable frame with maximal access to the injured soft tissues.

The minimal distance between two single pins should be 3.5 cm. The pins should be prestressed (preloaded) in each fragment (Fig. 8.32A). When a clamp takes multiple pins, a pin-guide is used. The fracture is reduced and a frame is constructed. The first rod should be as near the body as possible allowing enough space for dressing the wound. The optimal skin–rod distance is 4 cm. The second rod significantly increases the rigidity of the frame. Rods longer than

FRAME CONSTRUCTION

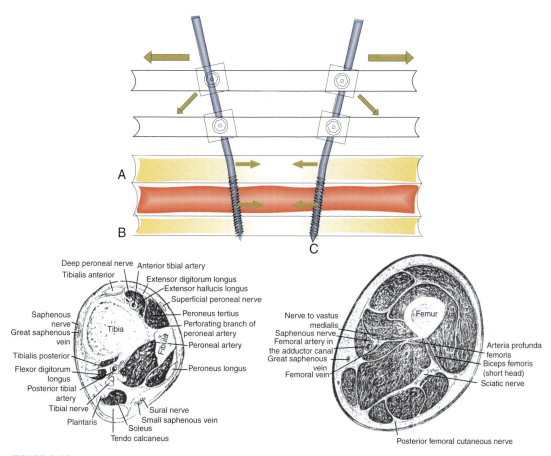

FIGURE 8.32

(**A**) of the pins within a fragment. The manoeuvre prevents pin loosening.[5] (**B**) Concentric limb segment. (**C**) Eccentric limb segment.

the limb tend to restrict the movements of the adjacent joints, e.g. dorsiflexion of ankle or extension of the knee. The stability of the reduction should be tested and radiographic films seen before the patient is out of anaesthesia. All connecting units, nuts and bolts are tightened.

Infection and Pin Loosening

Based on the distribution of the soft tissues, the limb segments are classified into two groups. In a concentric segment the bone is surrounded by muscle mass on all sides (Fig. 8.32B); the femur, the humerus, the radius and proximal phalanges are examples of this type. In concentric segments, the external fixation pin passes through a thick wad of muscles and other soft tissues. The movements between the pin shaft and the soft tissues predispose to a high incidence of pin tract infection, fibrosis of muscles and joint stiffness. Neurovascular complications are frequent. In these segments external fixation is used as a temporary stabilizer until the soft tissue healing is complete.

In an eccentric limb segment at least one border or surface of the bone is subcutaneous (Fig. 8.32C); the ulna, the tibia, metacarpals, metatarsals and the pelvis fall into this group. The pin travels through a minimum thickness of the soft tissues. Pin tract infection and other problems are minimal in eccentric segments and external fixation can be used as the definitive form of treatment.

Infection and pin loosening are two important issues in external fixation. Infection either presents as a soft tissue swelling, redness and tenderness around the pin or occurs as a moderate seropurulent discharge. Loosening is evident by tenderness on percussion of the pin or lucency around the pin on X-ray film. Infection and loosening occur in about 10% of pins. Pin problems are most common in the humerus and the pelvis and least common in hand and foot. The soft tissue thickness through which the pin passes affects the incidence of infection. Various known causes of infection and pin loosening are grouped below.

Pin-Related Causes

The pin thread should form quality bone threads that lay the basis of a firm pin hold. The thread profile influences the firmness of anchorage. Optimal pull-out strength is obtained when the threads are at right angles to the shaft of the screw. A smooth and polished surface finish of the pin facilitates its insertion and minimizes corrosion; poor surface finish causes thermal necrosis during insertion. Together with early corrosion, a poor finish also predisposes to loosening and infection.

Centrally threaded Steinmann pins are less prone to loosening because these have better grip on the bone than pins with a smooth shaft.

Soft Tissue-Related Causes

Pins in concentric limb segments are more predisposed to loosening and infection than pins in eccentric limb segments. Circumferential wrapping (bandaging) of the limb around the pin site reduces soft tissue movement and prevents its irritation and subsequent pin tract infection.

Surgeon-Related Causes

Good pin insertion practice should be followed. Adequate skin care is essential for long-term external fixation. The skin incisions around the pins are not sutured. A minor amount of discharge from the pin site is common. Petroleum-jelly-based ointments are best avoided as they block the discharges from flowing out. All dry discharge from the vicinity of the pin should be removed. It is best to educate the patient to keep the external fixator clean; this assures optimal upkeep.

Bone Regeneration with External Fixator[20]

Gradual mechanical distraction of a low-energy osteotomy spontaneously produces new bone from local host bone. This may be achieved by pin and ring fixators. Ring fixators are mainly used for regenerating bone in local deficiencies, alignment correction, intercalary gap closures, non-unions and osteomylitis. The regeneration is attainable in children as well as in adults. The bone can be regenerated over a distance of 18–20 cm from a single site; simultaneous lengthening at multiple sites is possible. The size and strength of bone regenerates equals the host bone. Although bone regeneration by distraction is highly successful, its clinical utility is limited by soft tissue growth and preservation of normal joint function. The distraction procedure may at times be used for stature lengthening in dwarfs and in stretching of joint contractures.

Histology of a low-energy osteotomy executed with care to preserve blood flow to each apposed surface, prior to distraction resembles patterns of fracture healing. When distracted at a regular, incremental rate of 1 mm/day by a stable external fixation system, new bone segment resembles growth plate and fills the osteotomy gap with normal bone. During distraction, the local histology transforms into five zones: a central radiolucent 'fibrous interzone' (FIZ), with immature collagen bundles and fibroblast-like cells arranged parallel to the distraction force spanning the entire cross-section of the bone gap and ranging from 4 to 8 mm in length. The next two adjacent zones are termed primary mineraliztion front (PMF) where collagen is rearranged in longitudinal columns by groups of osteoblast-like cells in vicinity of capillary buds. Close to this PMF on either side is zone of micro-column formation (MCF). In MCF zone primary bone units begin to mineralize, grow to maximal diameters of 150–200 microns, and cross-link to each other. These are surrounded by vascular sinusoids. MCF spans the cross-section of the gap. Host bone surface (HBS) is the fifth zone on either side of MCF. As the distraction progresses, the five zone bridge consolidates and remodels. The PMF traverses the FIZ followed by the MCF. Remodelling of a normal medullary canal by osteoclasts, condensation of the peripheral MCF into cortex and replacement of fibrovascular channels with bone marrow or fatty elements occurs late in the consolidation process. Distraction osteogenesis is intramembranous ossification in its purest form. The new bone grows at a rate of 300 microns per day during distraction osteogenesis. The bone growth in an adolescent distal femoral physis is 50 microns per day while the foetal femur grows at a linear rate of 400 microns per day; distraction osteogenesis approaches the growth rate of the foetal femur. Adequate regional and local blood supply is essential for regeneration of new bone. Metaphyseal zone has better blood supply, more cellularity and additional metabolic activity than diaphyseal sector. Osteotomies performed in metaphyseal segment produce better regenerate than diaphysis. Distraction should commence 7 days after the corticotomy for optimum results. The interval between corticotomy and commencement of distraction is called latent period, which may be between 5 and 10 days. Latent period varies and depends on age, quality of corticotomy, blood supply and any pathology such as chronic osteomyelitis. Rate and rhythm of distraction are important. Distraction rate of 1 mm/day at regular rhythm of 2,3,4 or more increments per day produces satisfactory regenerates. Rhythm can be increased to more than 4 (even up to 6 or 8) in children. Distraction rate slower than 1 mm/day leads to early consolidation while a rate of more than 2 mm/day produces non-union as the vascular elements fail to keep pace. Common causes of inferior regenerate are traumatic corticotomy, excessive distraction rate, irregular rhythm, initial diastasis, unstable frame or bone–fixator interface, distraction rate of greater than 2 mm/day, inadequate consolidation period and poor regional or local blood supply.

EXTERNAL FIXATOR, WHAT NEXT?

Once the soft tissues have healed there are two options (Table 8.2):

1. The external fixator is used until bone union occurs, 'first and final external fixator'.
2. Alternatively it is later replaced by an internal fixation, 'secondary internal fixation 'or 'sequential procedure'.

Table 8.2 Advantages and Disadvantages of 'First and Final External Fixator' and 'Sequential Procedure'

	Advantages	Disadvantages
'First and final external fixator'	No second operation Less risk of infection Implant removal without anaesthesia	Clumsy external device and long duration of external fixation Considerable rate of delayed union and pseudoarthrosis Pin loosening and pin tract infection
'Sequential procedure'	Short period of external fixation Earlier consolidation fixation Less risk of pseudoarthrosis	Risk of osteitis after internal fixation Further operation of internal and implant removal

Each procedure and concept has its advantages and disadvantage. If soft tissue healing is complete within 3 weeks, a change to internal fixation is more comfortable for the patient and is reasonably safe.

If soft tissue healing is not expected to be complete within 3 weeks, it seems safer to plan application of the fixator as the first and final device and to adapt its configuration accordingly.

Pin loosening does not mean that a change to internal fixation is mandatory. Often the pin is placed at a fresh site and the treatment continued. If the change to internal fixation is considered at a later stage or becomes unavoidable, the pins are removed a few weeks earlier to allow the pin tracks to heal under appropriate antibiotic coverage. This step lowers the risk of infection. Definitive data are not available; the literature on the details of these intervals and duration of antibiotic coverage is elusive.

Removal of an External Fixator

The decision to remove the fixator is often governed by screw loosening or screw tract infection, rather than by fracture healing. The external fixator should be removed after the fracture has solidly healed, unless the decision is taken to perform secondary internal stabilization or treatment in a functional brace, once the soft tissues allow such a step. Assessment of fracture healing is usually done by radiographs. Reading of radiographs may become somewhat subjective: an external fixator may thus be left in situ longer than is necessitated by the fracture healing.

REGIONAL CONSIDERATIONS

The Tibia

External fixation is a boon for tibial fractures; the tibia is the bone most frequently treated by external fixation. The percutaneous border of the tibia predisposes it to compound injuries. Plate fixation in this region is fraught with complications. A compound injury may be definitively treated by external fixation with minimal risk of joint stiffness and pin tract infection. A unilateral uniplanar frame is useful in management of fractures of the tibia (Fig. 8.33A). The modular version is simple to construct and

REGIONAL CONSIDERATIONS 353

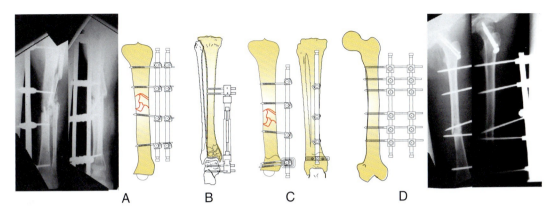

FIGURE 8.33

(**A**) Radiograph and schematics of unilateral uniplanar external fixation for tibia.[5] (**B**) Stabilization of periarticular fracture of lower tibia by ligamentotaxis.[1] (**C**) Pins in horizontal alignment held with a clamp to stabilize a small distal fragment. (**D**) Montage when it is necessary to treat a femoral fracture in External Fixation and radiograph of a clinical application.[5]

is versatile in stabilizing a variety of tibial fractures (see Fig. 8.9E). The two pins are placed according to local soft tissue conditions in each fragment and are connected to a short tube. Reduction is achieved by adjusting the fragments, and a third tube is attached using tube-to-tube clamps to maintain the reduction. The frame is easy to dynamize when indicated.

Periarticular Fractures of the Lower Leg

In extra-articular, metaphyseal fractures of the tibia the joint surface is still intact and the main problem is of implant anchorage in an often short, metaphyseal fragment. The distal fragment is too short to place two pins in the long axis. One solution is to bridge the ankle joint with a trans-articular external fixator, which is later replaced by an internal fixation (Fig. 8.33B). A better solution is to place two pins in transverse axis and hold them in a special clamp, ensuring a mobile ankle joint (Fig. 8.33C). Wide access is available for bone grafting.

The Femur

The femur has an anterior curve that tends to get straightened in external fixation: this makes it difficult to get a good alignment. Temporary external fixation is an option for early treatment of open or closed femoral fractures in polytraumatized patients (Fig. 8.33D). Long-term treatment in external fixation is uncomfortable and loss of knee flexion is frequent. The femur is enveloped by strong

External fixation – indications
- Compound fractures
- Closed fractures with severe associated soft tissue injuries; compartment syndromes
- Limb injuries requiring plastic and vascular procedures
- Ligamentotaxis
- Stress shielding device to protect internal fixation
- Infected non-unions
- Polytraumatized patients
- Selected fractures of pelvis

muscles on all sides and soft tissue complications of external fixation are frequent in this region. Delayed union is a frequent complication. However, femoral fractures may be healed by external fixation alone when conditions such as warfare make it impossible to use any other method.

The Radius and Ulna

External fixation is rarely used in the definitive management of open forearm fractures (Fig. 8.34A) because of a high risk of pseudoarthrosis and malrotation. When a primary external fixation is used, sequential procedures with early secondary internal fixation are the usual course of treatment.

The Wrist and Hand

External fixation with distraction between the radius and second metacarpal exerts steady traction on a comminuted fracture of the lower end of the radius by ligamentotaxis (Fig. 8.34B). This helps in maintaining the fracture reduction. The secondary loss of reduction with external fixation is minimal. Kirschner wire fixation of the fracture is an excellent adjunctive measure.

The Humerus

The humerus is wrapped in thick muscles. Three important nerves wind around the bone and are at risk during pin insertion. Operative stabilization of humeral shaft fractures in general is controversial but open fracture is often treated with operative fixation as it is unstable and difficult to manage with

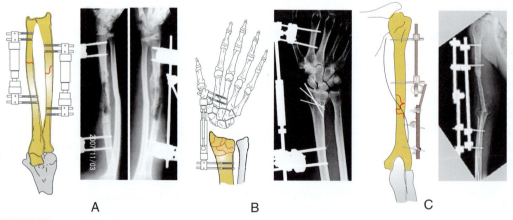

FIGURE 8.34

(**A**) External Fixation of forearm bones; accompanying radiograph of an infected non-union of radius after removal of a bone plate. (**B**) External Fixation of lower end of radius is a very useful treatment method; clinical example of fixator application for additional support. (**C**) Modular frame is the preferred configuration for External Fixation of humeral fractures.[1]

non-operative treatment. Similarly, humeral fracture in a polytraumatized patient should be treated by the operative method. Application of a modular frame on the humerus (Fig. 8.34C) is safe because tube-to-tube clamps allow placement of pins in two different planes, preventing the feared damage to the radial nerve.

The Pelvis

Pelvic injuries often tear the pelvic veins, causing massive haemorrhage. Reduction of the intrapelvic volume with external fixation can save lives. Early external fixation and reduction of the pelvic volume to the normal size before a large haematoma collects may produce tamponade in the restricted soft tissue spaces and reduce further bleeding. The fixator stabilizes the mobile hemipelvis and cuts down fresh bleeding from the cancellous bone surfaces. It helps to protect the newly formed clot against further dislodgement.

Screw Placement in the Pelvis

Pins placed in the strongest part of the bone have a good purchase on the pelvic bones. Common sites are the iliac crest, the ilium in the region of the anterior inferior iliac spine and transiliac placement.

The bone pins can be applied trans-cutaneously but it is safer to expose the bone and insert the pins in the correct direction under direct vision. Pin pressure on the skin is to be avoided as it leads to skin necrosis and early pin loosening.

The pins are driven in up to 5–6 cm in the thicker parts of the ilium for good grip. Various pin insertion sites in the ilium are shown in Fig. 8.35. The approach to the ilium around the anterior inferior iliac spine needs a wider incision. The anterior edge of the ilium here is rather sharp and the pin slips; a pin sleeve is used to stabilize the point during insertion. An image intensifier should be used to avoid accidental penetration into the hip joint. When the iliac crest is underdeveloped (in children) or fractured, this approach may be the only alternative. Trans-iliac pin fixation is a demanding and specialized technique; a jig is required for accuracy.

The connection between the two sides of the pelvis is achieved in different ways (Fig. 8.36). A detailed discussion of these frames is beyond the scope of this book; the general rule is the greater the number of bars and frames, the greater the stability.

Polytraumatized Patient

Early bone fixation is very important in improving the vital prognosis of the polytraumatized patient. When internal fixation is not practical because of the long operating time and inadequacy of post-operative intensive care, external fixation may be carried out swiftly and effectively. Major fractures of

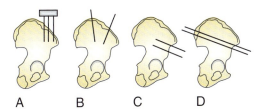

FIGURE 8.35

(**A**) Pins are placed in a cluster (**B**) or singly at an angle (**C**) in the iliac crest. Ilium near the anterior inferior iliac spine (**D**) and transiliac location are other two sites of pin placement in the pelvis.[21]

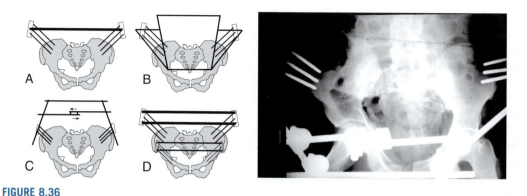

FIGURE 8.36

Various frames are in use. **(A)** Single bar frame **(B)** and double frame. **(C)** Double cluster connection can compress the bones together. **(D)** Transiliac pins provide full circumference fixation. **(E)** Radiograph showing application of external fixator to unstable pelvis.[21]

the long bones and joints may be fixed using modular external fixation frames without much loss of blood. This is a satisfactory solution for the early management of highly complex injuries in both children and adults.

Use in Children

External fixation is useful in the management of open and closed fractures, fractures associated with burns and multiple trauma, as well as in those children with increased motor tone and spasticity (Table 8.3).

Special attention must be paid to avoid injury to the growth plate; it is important to remember that its width is 4–6 mm. Moderate temperature changes due to drilling occur at 2.5–5.0 mm from the drill point and the area beyond 5 mm is a 'safe drilling' zone. However, because of its undulating shape it is necessary to allow a gap of at least 1 cm to avoid thermal damage. It is recommended that the most distal as well as the most proximal external fixator pin be placed 2 cm away from the growth plate (Fig. 8.37). The pins are inserted under fluoroscopic control.

Table 8.3 External Fixation in Children – Indications

Compound fractures	Grades II and III
Closed fractures	Polytraumatized patients
	Head injury, burns, unstable pelvic fractures
	Failure to maintain the reduction by closed methods
	Spasticity
Osteotomies	In obese children in whom internal fixation is tenuous and in whom the abnormal shape of the extremity precludes castings
Lengthening and deformity correction procedures	Congenital and acquired conditions

The external fixation of fractures in children is simple and elegant, but it is not without considerable complications, and the presumed advantages are not always obtained. Callus formation can be substantially slower in external fixation, with greater occurrence of delayed and non-union than in plaster immobilization.

There is a sizable incidence of continuing morbidity, such as pain at the healed fracture site, restriction of sporting activity, joint stiffness, cosmetic defects and minor leg length discrepancies. Open tibial fractures in general, and grade III injuries in particular, are associated with early and late complications. Hospital stay is sometimes longer than expected.[23, 24]

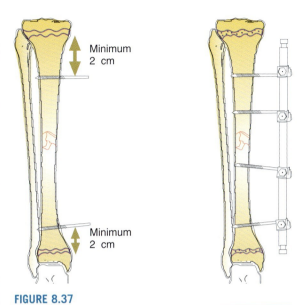

FIGURE 8.37

Pins are placed at least 2 cm away from epiphyseal plates to avoid thermal damage.[22]

THE DEVELOPING COUNTRIES AND EXTERNAL FIXATION

External fixation is an important tool in developing countries where the operating room environment is often far from ideal. The risk of infection for open reduction and internal fixation is usually high. Often a full set of the necessary instruments and implants is not available. This makes external fixation a relevant therapeutic option. The procedure is less demanding and the infection risk is low. The loss of fixator equipment is infrequent and a high retrieval rate has been reported by many centres in the developing countries.

Experience has taught us that using cheap and imperfectly made external fixators is more expensive in the long term than using good quality items. The developing countries need economical and properly constructed external fixators.

Such a new fixator is now available, which is low cost, has scientific base, executes reverse dynamization efficiently in technically simple steps[25] (Fig. 8.38). It can change construct stiffness as desired. Recent research has shown that the state of mechanical stability of fixation affects bone healing[16] Some degree of movement in early phase of bone healing (up to first 10 to 15 days) helps the differentiating factors spread out from the surrounding bone to provide signals to the proliferating cells in the fracture zone to turn themselves into bone forming cells. Thus, initial movement promotes convective mass transport of biological factors out of the bone driving the differentiation process of bone formation. After this early period, however, once the initial organic matrix for bone has been produced and the mineralization starts to set in, excessive movement prevents bridging of the gaps between the nuclei of mineralization and disrupts the healing process. High stiffness of the construct is now important to facilitate a safe and thorough process of mineralization. However, in the final stages of fracture union reduction of construct stiffness permits full physiological loading that promotes callus maturation.

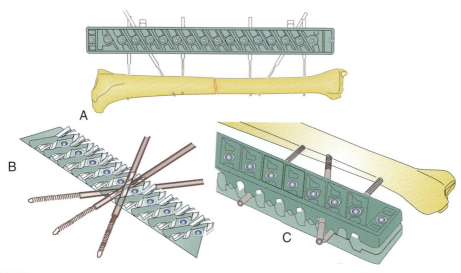

FIGURE 8.38

This external fixator facilitates 'reverse dynamization', which is stepping from low to high stiffness of the construct.[25] Modulation of a construct's stiffness involves loosening the adjacent bolts, followed by insertion or removal of shims, a washer like packing material. The two bars of this external fixator frame are identical parts made of autoclavable fibre-reinforced polymer that may be reused. When opposed to each other like two halves of a seashell (clamshell) and held tightly by nuts and bolts, they form a strong and stiff frame for holding the bone pins. The bone pins are placed either perpendicular or oblique to the frame. Clamping the two halves of the frame locks the perpendicular pins. The oblique bone pins can be locked only upon insertion of shims between the bone pins and bars of the frame. This mechanism allows for modulation of the construct stiffness at a chosen time. **(A)** Two parallel and one oblique pin is inserted in each main bone fragment. In the initial phase the oblique pin is left unlocked. After 10–15 days the oblique pin is locked and locking doubles the construct stiffness. When bone healing nears maturity, the oblique pin is loosened to reduce the stiffness. **(B)** Close-up of inner face of the fixator bar showing possible pin positions **(C)** side view of the fixator.

WAR, NATURAL CATASTROPHE AND EXTERNAL FIXATION

The medical situation in a natural catastrophe or during war is much similar. There is a sudden rush of severely injured patients, overloading the available facilities. These patients have to be treated on arrival in casualty by young and less experienced surgeons in far from ideal conditions. What should be the choice – internal or external fixation? In such situations, it is rarely possible to keep track of all the instruments and implants required for open reduction and internal fixation. A simple, user-friendly external fixator frame consisting of only a few elements that are quick and easy to insert is certainly preferable to conventional internal techniques. The external fixator enables a surgeon to fix multiple fractures quickly and atraumatically. A modular frame is an excellent choice in these situations.

REFERENCES

1. De Bastiani G, Aldegheri R, Renzo Brivio L, Trivella GP. Dynamic axial external fixation. Automedica 1989;10:235–72.
2. Catagni M. Fractures of the leg: the tibia. In: Bianchi Maiocchi A, Aronson J, editors. Operative principles of Ilizrov. Baltimore: Williams & Wilkins; 1991. p. 200.
3. Wikenheiser MA, Lewallen DG, Markel MD. In vitro mechanical, thermal, and microstructural performance of five external fixation pins. Transactions of the 38th Orthopaedic Research Society Meeting 1992;17:409.
4. Burgess AR, Poka A, Browner BD, First KR. Principles of external fixation. In: Browner B, editor. Biomechanics of fractures in skeletal trauma-fracture, dislocation and ligamentous injury. Philadelphia: WB Saunders; 1992. p. 231–42.
5. Hierholzer G, Riiedi Th, Allgower M, Schatzker J. Manual on the AO/ASII tubular external fixator. Berlin: Springer-Verlag; 1985.
6. Lazo-Zbikowski J, Aguilar F, Mozo F, Gonzalez-Buendia R, Lazo JM. Biocompression in external fixation: sliding external osteosynthesis. Clin Orthop 1986;206:169–84.
7. Dell'Occa AA, Castagnetto JJL. Actual state of military external fixation. Med Corps Int 1990;4/5:30–40.
8. Heim D, Regazzoni P, Perren SM. Current use of external fixation in open fractures. External fixators: what next? Injury 1992;23(Suppl. 2):1–35.
9. Fernandez Dell'Occa AA. External fixation using simple pin fixators. Injury 1992;23(Suppl. 4):1–54.
10. Tencer AF, Johnson KD. Biomechanics in orthopaedic trauma: bone fracture and fixation. London: Martin Dunitz; 1994.
11. Latta LL, Zych GA. Biomechanics: lower limb Part II. The mechanics of fracture fixation. Curr Orthop 1991;5:92–98.
12. Behrens F, Johnson WD. Unilateral external fixation methods to increase and reduce frame stiffness. Clin Orthop 1989;241:48–56.
13. Perren SM. Biomechanical aspects of the prevention of pin loosening in external fixators. AO/ASIF Dialogue 1988;1:11–13.
14. Golyakhovsky V, Frankel VH. Operative manual of Ilizarov techniques. St. Louis: Mosby; 1993.
15. Morgan EF, Gleason RE, Hayward LN, Leong PL, Palomares KT. Mechanotransduction and fracture repair. J Bone Joint Surg Am 2008;90(Suppl. 1):25–30.
16. Glatt V, Miller M, Ivkovic A, Liu F, Parry N, Griffin D, Vrahas M, Evans C. Improved healing of large segmental defects in the rat femur by reverse dynamization in the presence of bone morphogenetic protein-2. J Bone Joint Surg Am 2012;94:2063–73.
17. Thakur AJ, Patankar J. Open tibial fractures. Treatment by uniplanar external fixation and early bone grafting. J Bone Joint Surg 1991;73-B:448–51.
18. Connolly JF, Guse R, Tiedeman J, Dehne R. Autologous marrow injection as a substitute for operative grafting of tibial nonunions. Clin Orthop 1991;266:259–70.
19. Williams PL, editor. Gray's anatomy. 38th ed. New York: Churchill Livingstone; 1995. p. 872–83.
20. Aronson J. Basic science and biological principles of distraction ostogenesis. In: Rozbruch SR, Ilizarov S, editors. Limb lengthening and reconstruction surgery. Boca Raton, FL: CTC Press; 2007. p. 19–42.
21. Olerud S. External fixation of pelvic fractures. Curr Orthop 1990;4:33–9.
22. Alonso JE, Horowitz M. Use of the AO/ASIF external fixator in children. J Pediatr Orthop 1987;7:594–600.
23. Hope PG, Cole WG. Open fractures of the tibia in children. J Bone Joint Surg 1992;74-B:546–53.
24. van Tets WF, van der Werken C. External fixation for diaphyseal femoral fractures: a benefit to the young child? Injury 1992;23(3):162–4.
25. Tepic S. AKESO External fixator (Akeso AG, Zurich.) - a low cost frame for reverse dynamization. Personal communication 2014.

CHAPTER 9

SPINAL INSTRUMENTATION

Goals of Instrumentation
  Stabilization
  Deformity Correction
  Reconstruction and Replacement
Functional Modes
Implant Classification
  Rigid and Non-Rigid Implants
  Segmental and Non-Segmental Implants
  Constrained and Non-Constrained Implants
Spinal Implant Description
  Anchors
    Screws
      Pedicle Screws
  Gripping Implants
    Hooks
    Laminar Hooks
    Pedicle Hooks
    Transverse Process Hook
    Sublaminar Wires
  Longitudinal Members
    Three-Point Shear Clamps

    Lock Screw Connectors
    Circumferential Grip Connector
    Constrained Bolt–Plate Connectors
  Cross Fixators
    Semiconstrained Component–Rod Connectors
    Constrained Screw–Plate Connectors
    Cross-Connectors
    Accessories
  Struts or Abutting Implants
  Plates
  Rods
Mechanism of Load Bearing
  Simple Distraction Fixation
  Tension Band Fixation
  Three-Point Bending Fixation
  Cantilever Beam Fixation
    Fixed Moment Arm
    Non-Fixed Moment Arm
    Applied Moment Arm

In the early 1900s, Lange began to stabilize the spine internally. Early progress was slow, and it was not until the 1950s and 1960s that Harrington, Moe and others developed the first generation of modern spinal instrumentation. In the 1980s Cotrel and Dubousset first popularized rigid segmental hook-based fixation. Today rigid, segmental, posterior transpedicular constructs represent the most common forms of thoracolumbar instrumentation.

GOALS OF INSTRUMENTATION

Spinal instrumentations as a group are used to achieve one or more of the following goals[1]:

- Stabilization
- Deformity correction
- Reconstruction/replacement
- Facilitate fusion

Stabilization

Spinal instrumentation is used most often to provide stability. An illustrative example is the use of posterior segmental instrumentation for an unstable thoracolumbar fracture dislocation with ligamentous compromise. Instrumentation can help reduce the fracture and provides three-dimensional stability to the destabilized segments. Anterior or posterior implants are used to gain spinal stabilization.

Deformity Correction

Spinal deformity is produced by variety of reasons like trauma, infection, degeneration, tumour and idiopathy. Instrumentation is useful in achieving and maintaining spinal correction.

Reconstruction and Replacement

Anterior column reconstruction is indicated when vertebral body or intervertebral discs or both are compromised. Reconstruction of anterior column necessitates fusion across the reconstructedsegments. The device or implant must sustain the large compressive loads and provide a conduit for fusion.

FUNCTIONAL MODES

> **Functional modes of spinal implants[2]**
> - Tension banding
> - Buttressing
> - Neutralization
> - Lag screw
> - Deformity correction

Spinal implants work on one of the established principles (see text box), similar to other fixation implants. The buttress principle is used in anterior thoracic plating to prevent axial deformity. In this situation, the plate buttresses the spine, thereby reducing forces like compression, torque and shear. The Larger the contact area between the plate and bone, greater the support and more enhanced the buttressing effect. Removal of osteophytes from the vertebral body and contouring the plate increases the contact area and improves the buttress effect. Screw insertion in buttress mode implants begins in the area of greatest potential motion and moves away in both directions.

Tension band principle can be applied to the extension side of the spine; like in other fracture situations, an intact and load-bearing anterior column is mandatory for this to work. A translaminar facet screws in ALIF (Anterior Lumbar Inter-body Fusion) follows this principle; these screws resists tensile forces and bending moments only in presence of strong anterior column. An added advantage of dynamic compression effected by tension band effect is enhancing bone fusion, thus making posterior bone grafting redundant.

When the weight-bearing column is weak to resist compressive forces, a stiff, strong and rigid device works as a bridge across the weakened segment to maintain length, alignment and stability; an anterior cage is an example. Likewise, a long-segment posterior pedicle screw construct without formal anterior reconstruction is working in bridging mode. Short-segment anterior or posterior screw fixation placed after cage or strut graft reconstruction in treatment of a burst fracture, tumour resection, etc. works in neutralization mode.

IMPLANT CLASSIFICATION

The implants used in spine may be viewed as rigid and non-rigid, bridging and multisegmental, and constrained and non-constrained.

Rigid and Non-Rigid Implants

Sublaminar wires as anchors are non-rigid implants. The wires are wrapped around rods to get non-rigid segmental construct. Luque wires with pedicle screws and other bone anchors are used far more often. Another method is to wire the rod to the spinous processes; a button may be added to decrease wire cut through.

Screws, plates or rods, connectors and accessories create a rigid assembly or a construct. These resist forces in a superior way to non-rigid implants.

Segmental and Non-Segmental Implants

Implants used in spinal fixation work on non-segmental (bridging) and segmental (multisegmental) fixation principles; the term segmental fixation implies that bone anchors are placed at each site or many sites (multi) along the constructs. This contrasts with non-segmental fixation, which attaches to the spine at only two sites: one upper and one lower (Harrington instrumentation).

Constrained and Non-Constrained Implants

Constrained systems include a rigid locking mechanism between the individual components, e.g. the screw and rod. Maximum rigidity is achieved by segmental fixation of each vertebra to a constrained system. A non-constrained construct is fixed only at the ends of a multilevel construct or includes non-rigid connections between the screws and longitudinal member.

SPINAL IMPLANT DESCRIPTION

Anchors, longitudinal member and cross-connectors are elementary components of spinal fixation systems. An anchor describes the portion of the implant or construct that is fixed to the bone. Longitudinal member is that part of the implant that connects the anchors, a plate or rod. A cross-connector fixes longitudinal members to enhance their stability.

Anchors

Anchors affix to a single spinal level and are of two types: penetrating and gripping. Penetrating implants are of two types: those with pull-out resistance, e.g. screws, and those without pull-out resistance such as nails, spikes and staples. Examples of gripping implants are wires and hooks.

Screws

Screws are penetrating implants with pull-out resistance property. An extensive description on all aspects of bone screw is available in Chapter 3. A few pertinent points are recapitulated for convenience. A screw has four anatomical areas: head, core, thread and the tip. The head resists translational loads along the long axis of bone and is designed to abut the underlying surface of bone. The core of a screw affects its strength; the strength is proportional to the cube of its core diameter. The difference in strength between screws with a core diameter of 5–6 mm is nearly two-fold. The screw thread contributes to pull-out resistance; the thread depth is the screw's outer diameter minus the inner diameter (core) divided by 2. The pitch is the distance from a point on thread to the corresponding point on the next thread. A screw may be machine type (cortical) or wood type (cancellous); a self-tapping cortical screw is a combination of a machine screw and bone tap. Machine (cortical) screws are inserted in hard bone after tapping the threads with a bone tap; a self-tapping screw taps its own thread as it advances. Wood (cancellous) screws are used in soft bone. Cannulated screws are inserted over a guide wire for accuracy.

Screws are used in many locations: in combination with plates on vertebral bodies, compression osteosynthesis by screw fixation, transarticular screw fixation, translaminar fixation of spine, transpedicular screws, screws on their own, etc.

Pedicle Screws[1]

Pedicle screws offer superior biomechanical stability compared with other segmental constructs (Fig. 9.1). they offer excellent longitudinal compression-distraction, torsional and sagittal stability. Tapered screws fit the pedicle geometry better than cylindrical screws and allow improved bone compaction because they contact fresh bone with each turn thread. Variable pitch pedicle screws claim better purchase in the bone; their larger pitch in the distal shaft gains enhanced purchase in the cancellous bone of the vertebral body while the smaller pitch in the proximal shaft solidly engages cortical bone of the pedicle. The commonly used pedicle screws have a polyaxial head that allows angulation in multiple directions facilitate rod attachment. Conceptually, pedicle screws provide three-column stability, being anchored to the anterior and posterior vertebral bodies and the pedicle. Pedicle screw constructs are ideal for stabilizing spinal fractures and dislocation; they can be used to stabilize laminectomized vertebrae and have been shown to improve fusion rates.

Pedicle screws can be inserted into virtually any level of the thoracic and lumbar spine, and C7 vertebrae, provided that the screw can be accommodated by the pedicle. Pre-operative measurement of the transverse diameter determines the maximal diameter of the screw that may be inserted. The screw should be undersized in relation to the pedicle diameter. In general, lower lumbar spin has widest pedicles. The upper lumbar pedicles are usually smaller than the lower thoracic pedicles. The smallest transverse pedicle diameters are found in the mid-thoracic region (T4-7, approximately). The upper thoracic pedicles, T1-3 usually are larger than their mid-thoracic counterparts.

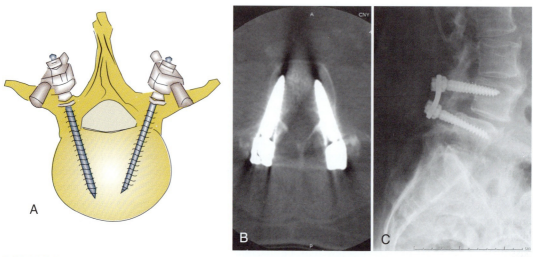

FIGURE 9.1

(A) Pedicle screw fixation. Triagulation of screws improves pull-out resistance (see Fig. 3.26). Longer the screw higher is the pull-out resistance. The triangulation effect requires cross-connectors (not shown). **(B)** CT-scan showing pedicle screw is safe position. **(C)** Radiographs showing application of pedicle screw.

Gripping Implants

Gripping implants provide a grip of the spine; they do not penetrate the bone surface. Hooks and wires provide greater functional surface area with cortical bone than the screws. They are an advantage to use in osteoporotic patients.

Hooks

Hooks are an effective and versatile method of stabilizing the spine. Hooks can be anchored onto the laminae, pedicles or transverse processes.

Hook placement is easier and quicker than pedicle screw insertion but their placement is critical. A pedicle hook inserted too deeply may cut into the pedicle and diminish the construct integrity (Fig. 9.2C); besides, hooks are intracanal space-occupying devices that have the potential for neural injury. A hook insertion to insufficient depth results in an improper engagement of the pedicle reducing its ability to augment torsional stability. Integrity of bone to which a hook is applied and magnitude and mode of force application for correction are important factors in successful use of a hook.

Laminar Hooks

Laminar hooks are used for segmental hook fixation. They can be inserted in as down-going or up-going hooks. For insertion, ligamentum flavum is removed and rectangular notch is cut in the inferior border of the lamina. Intrusion into the spinal canal is avoided. A trial hook is walked along the bone, keeping contact with undersurface of the lamina; this ensures snug seating of the final implant.

Pedicle Hooks

Pedicle hooks provide the strongest anchoring points but can be placed only in up-going fashion. The facet joint inferior to the pedicle is exposed. The articular capsule is removed with a curette. A hook trial is inserted into the facet joint walking it along the anterior surface of the inferior articular process of the upper vertebrae. The hook trial is advanced until the U-shaped end straddles the inferior surface of the pedicle, then the final implant is tamped into the place with a dedicated inserter. Lastly, a self-tapping screw is inserted to firmly fix the hook to the pedicle (Fig. 9.2C).

Transverse Process Hook

The transverse process is cleared off of soft tissue using specialized soft tissue elevator. A hook positioner is used to insert the implant around the transverse process.

Sublaminar Wires

Sublaminar wires are used in cervical, thoracic and lumbar spine (Fig. 9.3). Spinous process and interspinous ligaments are removed. A midline tract is created by releasing the ligamentum flavum to pass a wire loop in caudad to cranial direction in thoracic and lumber region. Braided cable is passed with the help of a malleable cable leader. Wires are tensioned to the rods in sequential fashion.

Wire constructs are economical and quick. They are superior to pedicle screws in porotic bone because the anterior aspect of the laminae are least affected by bone density losses. However, multiplanar stability obtained is limited.

Wires can be used individually or as multiple strands. The use of two wires doubles the contact surface with bone, thereby increasing the pull-through resistance. A twist in the wire weakens it.

Application of two full twists is the optimal method of wire-to-wire affixation; more that two twists do not bestow more security. Commercial wire tighteners provide consistent twists and inflict minimal

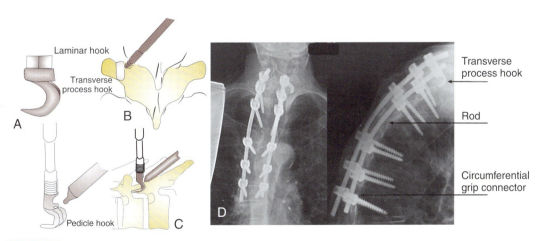

FIGURE 9.2

Hooks provide strong grip on the spine. (**A**) Laminar hook, (**B**) transverse process hook, (**C**) pedicle hook and applicator; its application to correct depth is critical for stability. (**D**) Radiographs showing transverse process hooks in position.

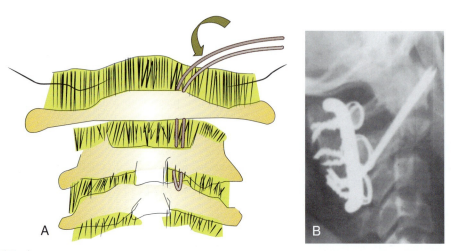

FIGURE 9.3
(**A**) Sublaminar wire in cervical region is passed from cephalad to caudal direction. (**B**) Radiographs showing sublaminar wires tensioned to a rod at three levels.

injury to soft tissue. Surface notch on a wire weakens it; titanium wires are more prone to damage than stainless steel wires. Cables are not affected by surface damage.

Longitudinal Members

Plates and rods are longitudinal members; they are connected by component to component connectors to anchors and cross-members. A brief description of these connectors is as follows:

Three-Point Shear Clamps
These clamps rely on friction between the component interfaces and provide resistance to axial, torsional and bending forces (Fig. 9.4).

Lock Screw Connectors
A set screw mechanism is deployed in a lock screw connector to provide half of the pincer mechanism to secure a rod; the other half of pincer is offered by a circumferential grip connector. The lock screw connector is positioned either end-on or in a tangential location (Fig. 9.5A).

Circumferential Grip Connector
Two types of circumferential grip connector are in use: one that provides two halves of the gripper mechanism and is in common use (Fig. 9.5B) and the other that allows truly circumferential force application.

Constrained Bolt–Plate Connectors
These are very rigid and are the strongest connectors; they yield only in failure. They are available as screw–plate or screw–rod systems (Fig. 9.5C).

SPINAL IMPLANT DESCRIPTION

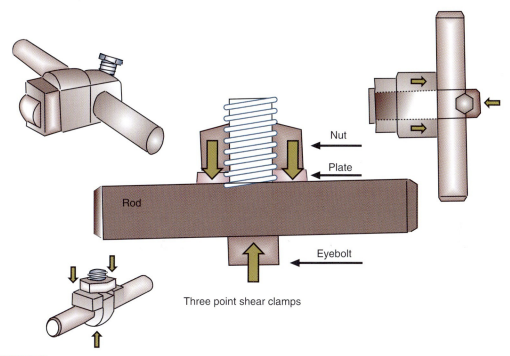

FIGURE 9.4

Clamps are simple mechanism based on three-point pressure system and are effective by creating friction at the interface.

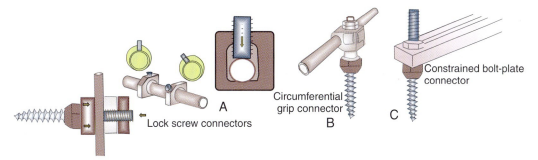

FIGURE 9.5

Connectors: (**A**) lock screw connectors; (**B**) circumferential grip connector; (**C**) constrained bolt–plate connector.

Cross Fixators

Semiconstrained Component–Rod Connectors

These connectors permit some degree of movement and are less stiff than the previous type; they allow some degree of toggle and are predisposed to fretting corrosion and loosening at the component–rod interface (Fig. 9.6A).

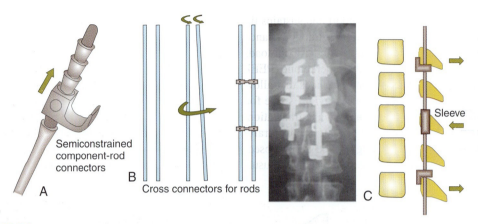

FIGURE 9.6
(**A**) Semiconstrained component–rod connector allows a degree of toggle. (**B**) Cross-connectors improve stability. Euler's calculations state that two cross-connectors increase the stability 16 times. Radiograph showing cross-connector in place. (**C**) Sleeve acts as spacer and helps application of force to extend the spine.

Constrained Screw–Plate Connectors

Constrained screw–plate connectors rigidly fix the screw to the plate or rod. Strategies to lock the screw to the plate include expansion head, cam lock, screw head securing mechanism, locking plates and modification of screw pitch near the head.

Cross-Connectors

Implants that provide rigid or semirigid fixation of parallel or bilaterally placed fixation devices like rods or plates are categorized as cross-connectors. Cross-connectors counter act the torsional stress that may cause twisting of the rods about each other (Fig. 9.6B) with subsequent implant failure.

Cross-connectors improve the stability of rod placed in parallel. The connectors should be placed at the junction of the terminal thirds of the rod with the middle third.

Cross-connectors improve stability in short and long constructs. The connectors reduce parallelogram deformation phenomenon, the incidence of sagittal plane translation and pull-out failure.

Hook–bone connectors, as and when they fail, do so one at a time; rigid cross-fixation prevents sequential failure of hook–bone assemblies and precludes a catastrophic debacle.

Accessories

Washers and rod sleeves are notable accessories; sleeves around the rod function as spacers for spinal extension enhancing force application and increasing extension (Fig. 9.6C).

Struts or Abutting Implants

Struts are structures placed between two vertebral bodies and function as spacer. A strut may be a bone graft, a cage filled with bone or rarely an inert material like metal, ceramic. Bone struts include tricortical bone grafts, rectangular and cylindrical bone grafts, bone dowels and threaded bone dowels.

A strut provides structural support and sustains the axial load until the bone graft remodels and fusion is achieved; bone graft mostly is autologous cancellous bone, rich in osteogenic substrates but poor in mechanical strength and buckles under axial load.

Cages are made of polyetheretherketone (PEEK), titanium and ceramic. A cage or spacer resembles an oval ring and has teeth on both sides that allows fixation into the end plate and prevent migration.[3] The large hollow, center space provides space for bone graft. The cages adequately resist axial loads and to a lesser extent the rotational and translational forces impacting on the spinal segment. Cages are also known by the face they present to bone graft bed; their labels, flat faced and round faced are self-explanatory (Fig. 9.7). The graft bed is composed of either an endplate or a vertebral body cancellous bone. A cage with a surface area of contact, usually oval in shape to approximate the vertebral body

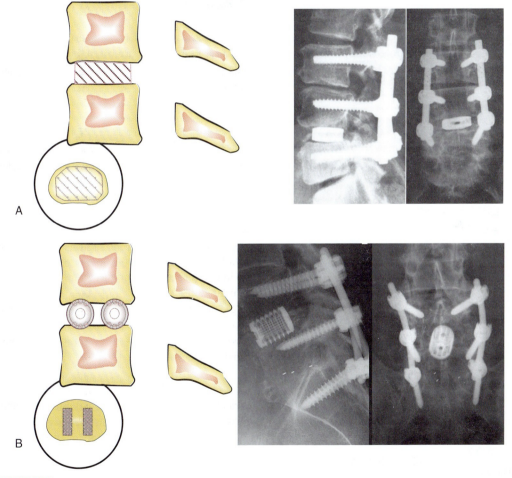

FIGURE 9.7

Illustration shows sketch and radiographs of (**A**) flat faced cage and (**B**) round-faced cage. The cage abuts the endplates, as shown in lateral projection.

wall circumferentially, is ideally suited to resist subsidence. A standalone PEEK cage with in situ screw insertion sites to engage in the caudal and cranial endplates in the cervical region to do away with anterior plate for support is also available.

Plates

Bone plates for application on anterior/anterolateral surface of the vertebral body are popular implants (Fig. 9.8). Plates buttress the spine in a corpectomy and prevent graft extrusion. Plates are fixed by screws in divergent pattern to improve pull-out resistance; a limited variation in insertion angle is possible. Conventional and locking screws are used for uni- or bicortical fixation. Conventional bone plates efficiently maintain axial and rotational alignment. A new version of cervical plate (dynamic plate) retains load-sharing characteristics; as the bone graft settles, the plate design enables sliding motion along the long axis of the plate in caudal direction; such movement maintains constant axial load on the graft. Use of locked screws precludes toggling at the screw holes and prevents hardware failure. Plates are more often used in cervical region than in the thoracic and lumbar region. Plates can be used on posterior surface of the spine for same purpose.

Rods

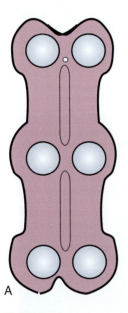
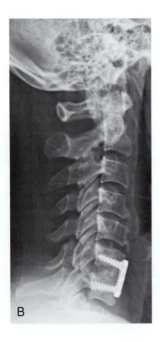

FIGURE 9.8

(A) Schematic presentation of a cervical spinal plate. (B) Radiograph showing its application.

Smooth rods used for spinal stabilization are made from titanium, cobalt–chromium alloy or stainless steel; titanium rods are preferred because their modulus of elasticity closely approaches that of the bone. Rods of varying thickness and stiffness are used in different regions of spine to support different levels of loads. The rods are available in many diameters (3.5–6 mm) and lengths (50–500 mm); special sleeves/connectors can interconnect rods of different thicknesses in transition zones. There are hard rods for fractures, tumours and deformity surgery and soft rods for low back surgery. Special instruments and templates are available to bend a rod as desired. Rods are used in both anterior and posterior locations on the spine. Special connectors that are used to create a construct have been described above (Fig. 9.9).

MECHANISM OF LOAD BEARING

A discussion of forces exerted by spinal implants helps in pre-operative planning of intended surgical steps. Six mechanism referred here are often involved in spinal surgery.

Simple Distraction Fixation[4]

A construct in distraction fixation applies a force in line with the instantaneous axis of rotation (see box); this is often located in the interbody region which is the neutral axis (Fig. 9.10).

Distraction effectively resists axial load; when distraction is applied in the line with IAR it does so without a bending moment (Fig. 9.11A). If distraction is performed ventral to IAR then spinal extension happens (Fig. 9.11B); conversely when distraction is applied on dorsal side the flexion and kyphosis results (Fig. 9.11C).

Tension Band Fixation

Tension band fixation applies compression at the application site (Fig. 9.12); this technique is often employed posteriorly but anterior application is possible. Dorsal application point results in extension of spine while ventral application effects in flexion of the spine (Fig. 9.12B and C). Increased bending load improves fixation; increase in the length of tension band construct does not make it any stronger.

Three-Point Bending Fixation

In three-point bending fixation similar force vectors exist at terminal ends and at the fulcrum (Fig. 9.13).

Three-point bending fixation is usually applied with an application of a distraction force. Three-point bending forces are affected by the length of the construct and not by the distance from the IAR; five or more spinal segments are essential to effectively apply this technique; the application of dorsal distraction forces to a lordotic spine may result in unexpected flexion (Fig. 9.14C).

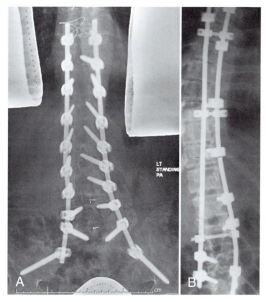

FIGURE 9.9

Radiographs showing application of rods for stability in thoracolumbar spine. (**A**) Pedicle screws and rods offer excellent stability. (**B**) Use of cross-connectors enhances stability many-folds.

Instantaneous axis of rotation (IAR)

(Also called 'instant centre of rotation)

When a rigid body moves in a plane, at every instant there is a point in the body or some hypothetical extension of it that does not move. An axis perpendicular to the plane of motion and passing through that point is the instantaneous axis (center) of rotation for that motion at that instant.

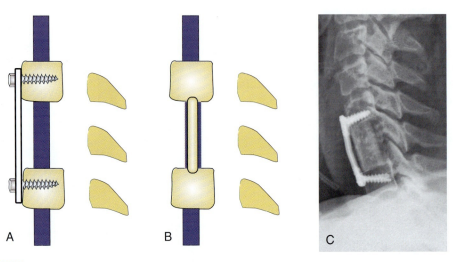

FIGURE 9.10

IAR is usually located in the interbody region which is the neutral axis. The neutral axis is depicted by blue area. **(A)** The interbody region may be buttressed by a rigid plate or **(B)** by an interbody strut. **(C)** Radiograph showing use of both, a plate and a bone strut for stabilization.

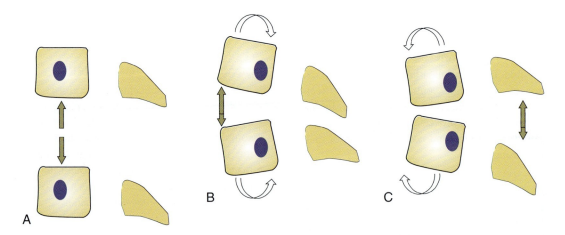

FIGURE 9.11

(A) Distraction of vertebrae in line with IAR does not cause a bending moment. **(B)** Extension of spine results when distraction is applied ventral to IAR. **(C)** Likewise, flexion of spine or kyphosis is observed when distraction is applied dorsal to IAR.

MECHANISM OF LOAD BEARING 373

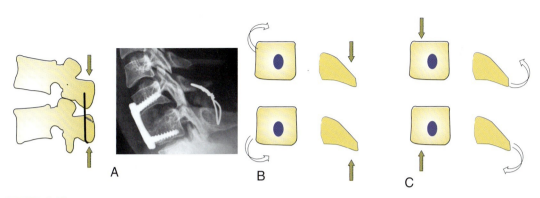

FIGURE 9.12
(A) Sketch and radiograph of tension band fixation showing compression at site of application. (B) Tension band fixation dorsal to the IAR causes spine extension. (C) Tension band fixation on ventral side of IAR produces spine flexion.

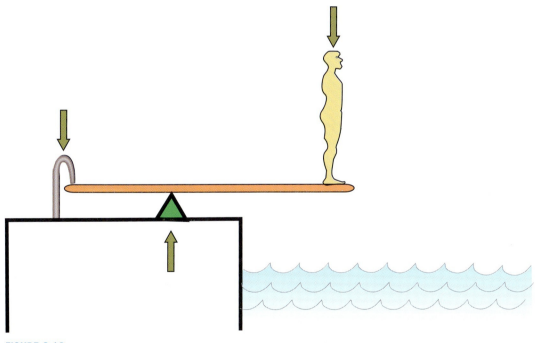

FIGURE 9.13
Three-point bending forces can be compared with the force vectors at work when a person is standing on the end of a springboard.

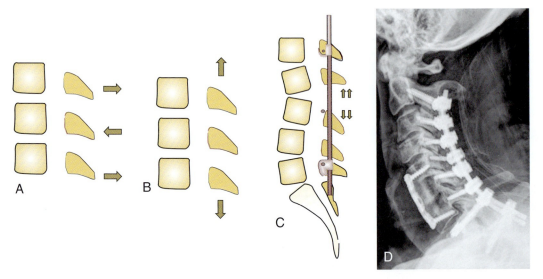

FIGURE 9.14

(**A and B**) Three-point bending is always applied with distraction. (**C**) It is applied over multiple spinal segments; unintended flexion may result. (**D**) Clinical application of the principle; note additional anterior fixation.

Cantilever Beam Fixation

Cantilever beam fixation bears a load over a space where support is not desirable or possible. Fixed moment arm, non-fixed moment arm and applied moment arm are three clinical types of application of cantilever beam principle.

Fixed Moment Arm

Fixed moment arm cantilever beam fixation rigidly supports the spine and bears an axial load without the assistance of other structures. This arrangement results in high stress at the point of maximum stress application (Fig. 9.15).

Non-Fixed Moment Arm

Non-fixed moment arm cantilever beam fixation assists an already present axial load-supporting structure with assistance of other structures like a vertebral body or interbody strut to bear an axial load. This technique is used only when spine is able to resist axial load. Screw toggling is permitted in the technique; the maximum stress is at the midportion of the screw where the maximum bending moment develops (Fig. 9.16); screw pull-out is a disadvantage. Lateral mass screw fixation is a clinical example of this technique.

Applied Moment Arm

Applied moment arm cantilever beam fixation can apply bending moment in flexion as well as in extension (Fig. 9.17).

MECHANISM OF LOAD BEARING 375

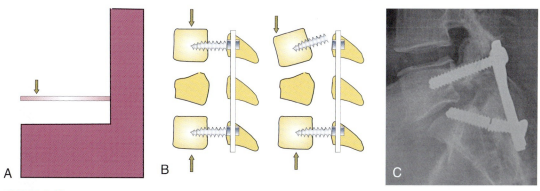

FIGURE 9.15

(**A**) Fixed moment arm cantilever beam fixation unbendingly supports axial load of the spine. (**B**) The construct is exposed to high stresses and may fail at the point of maximum stress application. (**C**) Radiograph showing a clinical example; compare the sites of breakage in Fig. 9.16.

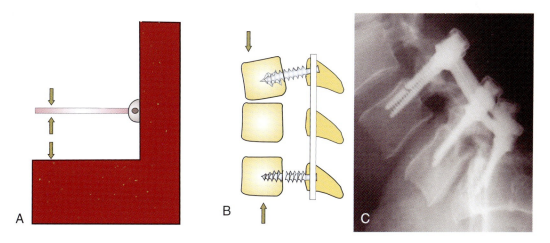

FIGURE 9.16

(**A**) Non-fixed moment arm cantilever beam fixation is similar to a cantilever beam fixed to a wall with a hinge. (**B**) The construct may fail with screw toggling and loosening. The screws are prone to failure at the point of maximum stress application. (**C**) Radiograph showing a clinical example; compare the sites of breakage in Fig. 9.15.

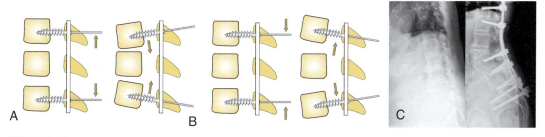

FIGURE 9.17

Applied moment arm cantilever beam fixation may be employed to manipulate the spine in desired direction. (**A**) Neutral spine and flexion obtained with dorsal distraction. (**B**) Neutral spine and extension obtained with dorsal compression. (**C**) Clinical application of the principle.

REFERENCES

1. Bono CM. Spinal instrumentation. In: Bono CM, Garfin SR, editors. Spine. Philadelphia: Lippincott Williams C& Wilkins; 2004.
2. Truumees E. Thoracolumbar instrumentation: anterior and posterior. In: Herkowitz HN, Garfin SR, Eismont FJ, Bell GR, Balderston RA, editors. Rothman-Simeone the spine. Philadelphia: Saunders; 2006.
3. Aebi M, Thalgott JS, Webb JK. AO ASIF principles in spinal surgery. Berlin: Springer; 1997. ISBN: 3-540-78109-9.
4. Lastra JJ, Benzel EC. Biomechanics of internal fixation. In: Vaccaro AR, Betz RR, Zeidman SM, editors. Principles and practice of spine surgery. St Louis: Mosby; 2003.

CHAPTER 10

MINIMAL INVASIVE OSTEOSYNTHESIS

Give us the tools, and we will finish the job.[1]

MIPO
  Advantages of MIPO
  Disadvantages and Shortcomings of MIPO
Fracture Reduction
  Direct Fracture Reduction
  Tools to Facilitate Direct Reduction
    Bump
    Mallet and F Tool
  Small Instruments and Implants
  Hohmann Retractor and Curved Impactor
    Bone Plate
    Reduction Screw
    Reduction Clamps
    Cerclage Wire

Indirect Fracture Reduction Methods
  Manual Traction
  Traction tables
  Push–Pull Method
  Handles for Minimally Invasive Reduction
  Plate Holder and Pusher
Useful Tactics for MIPO
  How to Locate a Plate Hole without Fluoroscopy?
  How to Insert Threaded Drill Guide with Ease without Exposing Hole of a Locking Plate?
  How to Measure Screw Length with Ease?
Fluoroscopy by C-Arm Image Intensifier

Minimal invasive surgery includes every operative procedure (damage to the integrity of the body surface), which can be performed without extensive incision (no large opening of body cavity), and with minor general body reaction of the patient, e.g. endoscopic, arthroscopic, laparoscopic or thoracoscopic interventions. What is minimally invasive osteosynthesis (MIO)? It is a philosophy of showing highest respect to bone and soft tissues. All forms of fracture fixation that use small soft-tissue window for insertion of implant or instruments. The procedures inflict minimal additional trauma to the soft-tissue and fracture fragments as they use indirect or gentle direct fracture reduction techniques. The procedures permit application of the biomechanical concept of relative stability or, exceptionally, absolute stability.

MIPO

Minimal invasive plate osteosynthesis (MIPO) means that a plate is placed through small incisions with as little dissection and stripping of the soft-tissue envelope as possible. It is also known as percutaneous (MIPPO), submuscular, minimal incisional and less invasive plating. Measures like smaller incisions, less soft-tissue dissection, less periosteal stripping, use of intra-operative imaging or intra-operative navigation preserve local blood supply, improve healing rates and reduce complications. Both conventional and locking plates can be applied through MIPO techniques. Locking plate technology and minimal invasive technique have evolved almost simultaneously but are different concepts.[2]

Advantages of MIPO

MIPO safeguards blood supply, as handling and direct reduction of intermediate fracture fragments is circumvented and direct friction over fracture zone is avoided. The method preserves periosteal blood supply and all other blood channels to the bone. The collateral advantages of maintaining blood supply are rapid bone healing and early recovery, reduced incidence of infection, less bleeding during surgery and reduced need for transfusion. Smaller incisions lead to improved cosmetics and less pain. MIPO should be performed at earliest opportunity, the earlier the better.

Disadvantages and Shortcomings of MIPO

The stability of the fracture fixation depends on the stiffness of the construct; this is tricky to judge and has a long learning curve; excessive flexibility or extreme stiffness delays bone healing. Similarly, closed reduction, minimally invasive plate application and intra-operative control of alignment are complicated techniques and take a while to master. Lack of useful but expensive reduction tools may compromise the quality of reduction. Bridge plating puts excessive demands on the implant as the bone does not carry any load.

> ### Critical steps in MIPO[3]
> - MIPO earlier the better; maintain length and good reduction if surgery is delayed
> - Precise surface anatomy landmarks is a requirement
> - Achieve indirect closed reduction; avoid exposure of the fracture; use special tools
> - Make small incisions for implant insertion
> - Deploy conventional plates/locked internal fixation plate (LIFP) as pure splints (always without the lag screw); prefer precontoured, low contact implants
> - Construct elastic bridging of the fracture zone (relative stability stimulates callus formation); often check alignment
> - Insert self-tapping locking screws for monocortical or bicortical placement

Achieving adequate reduction and plate fixation of fractures without inflicting additional trauma is the primary goal of MIPO and understanding the 'nature' of a particular fracture pattern is integral for successful plating procedure. A surgeon endeavours to avoid pitfalls of malreduction, which can potentially impact long-term prognosis. The choice of reduction technique should be made at the time of preoperative planning. Numerous closed or percutaneous reduction techniques can be employed to preserve fracture biology. However, in some fracture variants, meticulous open reduction strategies are acceptable to achieve a best possible reduction. Even with direct methods, there exist a variety of reduction aids and tools that minimize intra-operative trauma to the soft tissue surrounding the fracture. The key is to leave a small footprint or the least possible damage at the fracture zone.

FRACTURE REDUCTION

Fracture reduction may be achieved by indirect and direct methods.

Indirect reduction means that the forces and moments acting away from the fracture are used to manipulate and reduce a fracture, e. g. traction along the axis of the limb and the help of the soft tissues for the reduction manoeuvre (ligamentotaxis). The fracture line remains covered by surrounding tissue and is visualized with fluoroscopy or by only limited exposure. The necessary instruments and implants are introduced away from the injury zone.

Direct reduction is achieved by applying forces and moments directly in the vicinity of the fracture zone, i.e. the reduction is achieved by direct manipulation near the fracture. This may be done by surgical exposure of fracture lines, direct visualization of the fragments and manipulation by instruments close to the fracture line. Alternately, it may also be done percutaneously, fracture is not exposed and reduction instruments are applied through small incisions.

Direct Fracture Reduction

Direct reduction techniques are used when clinical situation demands that the fracture be reduced anatomically and absolute stability by rigid fixation is essential for sound healing. Indications are articular fracture, articular fracture with metaphyseal extension, irreducible fracture and non-union. Open reduction is indicated when closed and percutaneous strategies fail. Meticulous technique is employed to avoid disruption of fracture biology, and excessive stripping is often unnecessary to attain an adequate open reduction. Proximal femoral fractures that remain in varus after attempts at closed and percutaneous reduction should be reduced by open approach. Similarly, fractures extending in to the knee joint require precise articular reduction by open methods before plate fixation.

Tools to Facilitate Direct Reduction

Bump

Bumps fashioned from towels are primitive but effective aids in controlling the position of the fracture fragments. In fractures of the supracondylar region of the femur a recurvatum deformity is common; use of a bump at the level of the fracture counteracts the deformity and helps in maintaining the reduction (Fig. 10.1).

A bump is often used under the buttock to internally rotate proximal fragment of a hip fracture that has a tendency to rotate externally. In subtrochanteric fractures, the proximal segment is frequently flexed. A bump is often used under the distal main segment to draw it anteriorly; this move facilitates reduction and maintains the position of that fragment during plating. A bump also controls unwanted effect of traction applied by a distractor (see Fig. 10.13).

Mallet and F Tool

These instruments compress the surrounding soft tissues and help to pull off anatomical reduction by closed methods. Fluoroscopy during surgery directs application of the forces to achieve reduction. The same manoeuvres are necessary to gain successful guidewire passage and must be reproduced during the canal preparation/reaming process.

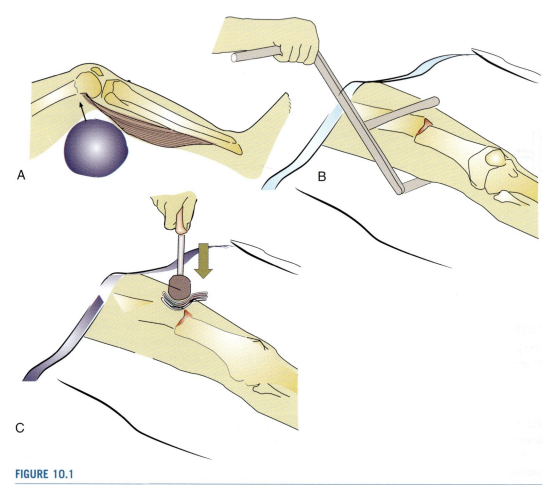

FIGURE 10.1

(**A**) Bumps are primitive but effective aids in fracture reduction. (**B**) An F tool is useful in closed fracture reduction in bulky limbs. (**C**) Mallet tool in use.

Small Instruments and Implants

A Schanz screw or a Steinmann pin mounted on a cannulated T-handled chuck is used as a joystick to control bone fragments in T-type supracondylar fracture of the distal femur (Fig. 10.2). To reduce and control the medial condyle through lateral approach, a Schanz screw is introduced through a stab incision on the medial side. The medially placed T-handle controls the rotation and varus-valgus position of the medial condoyle; the accuracy of the reduction is observed through the lateral operative incision. Similarly, a 3-mm Kirschner wire may be used to reposition a displaced head of the humerus.

A ball spike pusher and a bone hook are used with similar intent for femoral fractures (Fig. 10.3). A ball spike pusher is inserted through a stab incision. A unicortical hole in bone offers a firm footing

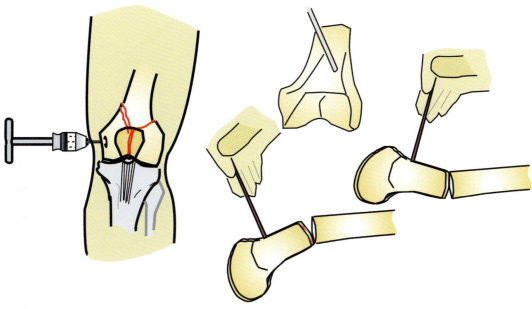

FIGURE 10.2

The joystick technique. A Steinmann pin or Schanz screw mounted on a T-handled chuck is placed in the medial condylar fragment, and used to derotate and control reduction of a supracondylar fracture with split, displaced condyles.

for the instrument and prevents any slippage off the bone cortex. A bone hook may be used to control bone fragments, especially to overcome sagging effect due to gravity.

Use of a curved Kochar's forces helps in achieving reduction of proximal fragment (PD Kothadia, personal written communication, 19 December 2014) (Fig. 10.4).

Hohmann Retractor and Curved Impactor

Hohmann retractor may be used as lever to achieve reduction. Its tip is inserted into the fracture, with the wider part of the blade abutting against one side of the fracture and the narrow pointed end levering out the other fragment (Fig. 10.5). The curve of the tip makes it a handy lever. Hohmann retractor may also be used percutaneously.

A Hohmann retractor is valuable in managing an irreducible variety of intertrochanteric fracture (Fig. 10.5). A curved impactor introduced percutaneously and through a small cortical window is useful to elevate a depressed fracture of tibial articular surface (Fig. 10.5D).

Bone Plate

A plate is useful in achieving reduction (Fig. 10.6). It can reduce a fracture as it is being applied. The plate is placed on the side of displaced fragment and screws are applied; as the screws are tightened, the plate comes in contact with displaced fragment and pushes it to a reduced position and maintains it.

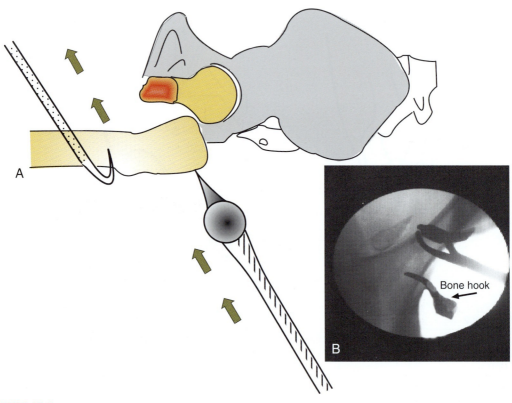

FIGURE 10.3

(A) A bone hook and a ball spike pusher to manipulate large bones. **(B)** A radiograph showing intra-operative use of bone hook.

Reduction Screw
A conventional cortex screw can be used as an aid to pull the bone towards the plate-reduction screw (Fig. 10.7).

Reduction Clamps
Collinear reduction clamp is a powerful reduction tool. It is useful in direct percutaneous reduction of difficult fractures (Fig. 10.8). It may be introduced through a small incision to grip bone and plate and its axial sliding mechanism achieves the desired reduction with minimum risk of soft tissue damage and bone stripping. Pelvic reduction clamp is useful in controlling reduction of fragments in knee and ankle (Fig. 10.8B). It may be used percutaneously or through small incisions.

Cerclage Wire
A cerclage wire is useful in reducing a severely displaced oblique or spiral fracture fragment or in maintaining a large wedge fragment in position (see Fig. 7.2). A wire passer is used carefully to place

INDIRECT FRACTURE REDUCTION METHODS 383

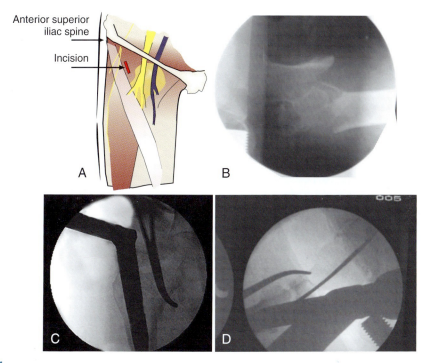

FIGURE 10.4

(**A**) A centimetre-long incision is placed 2.5 cm distal and 1.5 cm medial to the anterior superior iliac spine along the medial border of the Sartorius muscle. (**B**) Anteriorly displaced proximal fragment. (**C**) A long curved Kochar's forceps is passed obliquely and medially in the direction of proximal fragment towards the anteriorly displaced proximal fragment; radiograph of a different patient The fragment may be coaxed in the desired position under fluoroscopic control (PD Kothadia, personal written communication, 19 December 2014). (**D**) The curved forceps may also be passed through main lateral incision.

a wire around the fragment avoiding further damage to the soft tissue (Fig. 10.9). A wire tightener is helpful though not indispensable instrument in this method.

INDIRECT FRACTURE REDUCTION METHODS

Indirect reduction techniques are used in clinical situation when individual fracture fragments need not be anatomically reduced to regain normal function and just the restoration of length, axis and rotation to re-establish acceptable position of the adjacent joints is adequate. Indirect reduction technique is used in management of diaphyseal fractures. Aids available for the technique are manual traction, traction table, push–pull forceps, a distractor and external fixator.

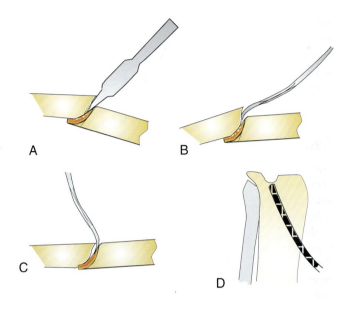

FIGURE 10.5

Reduction of a diaphyseal fracture with Hohmann retractor. (**A**) Select the retractor of a size that matches the bone. (**B**) Push the tip between the two cortices of a diaphyseal fracture. (**C**) The instrument is turned. The curved tip is a good lever to regain length. Another turn is often required to remove the Hohmann. (**D**) Percutaneous elevation of depressed bone fragment using a curved bone impactor.

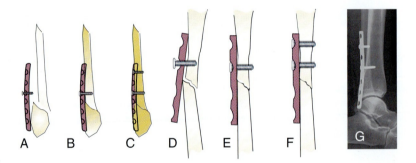

FIGURE 10.6

(**A–C**) A posteriorly positioned plate reduces the displaced fragment and prevents its redisplacement. In lateral malleolar fracture a screw in distal fragment may be unnecessary. (**D–F**) The reduction mechanism shown in detail. As the first screw is tightened, the plate pushes the displaced fragment in to position. (**G**) Radiographs showing application of the principle.

Manual Traction

The application of traction is an important natural step in achieving reduction by indirect means. Traction helps to gain length and restores rotational and axial malalignment. It is successful when two preconditions exist: the fracture fragments retain their soft tissue alignment for effective implementation of principle of ligamentotaxis and the fracture is relatively recent, as soft tissue contracture may prevent fracture reduction. For most diaphyseal fractures manual traction is effective; this is best carried out under fluoroscopic guidance on a radio-opaque operating table.

Traction Tables

Traction tables are widely used for convenience of applying longitudinal traction to gain a preliminary reduction through tension applied to the soft tissue envelope; it is a reliable assistant (Fig. 10.10). However, it has many disadvantages. The set-up is labour intensive. Length and rotation is typically prearranged before prepping and draping; the traction is applied across at least one joint; the surgical approach is frequently compromised and the surgeon is unable to

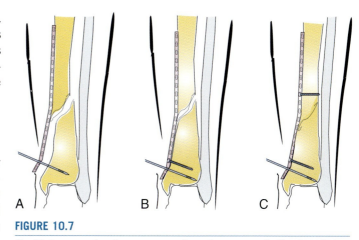

FIGURE 10.7

(A–C) A conventional cortex screw through an anatomically shaped plate pulls the bone to the plate and facilitates the reduction.

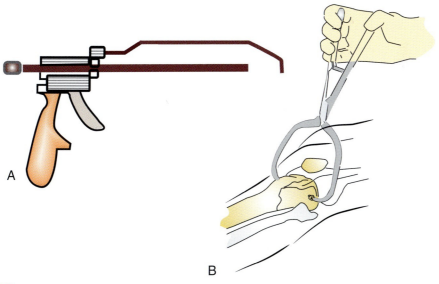

FIGURE 10.8

(A) Silhouette of a coaxial clamp[4] for femur fracture reduction. The clamp can be applied by mini-open procedure causing minimum disturbance of fracture biology. (B) A wedge fracture extending from the articular surface to the metaphysic must be reduced precisely; exacta reduction of metaphyseal spike leads to anatomical reduction of the articular surface without the need of arthrotomy. The pelvic reduction clamp maintains the reduction and may be used percutaneously or through mini-open protocol.

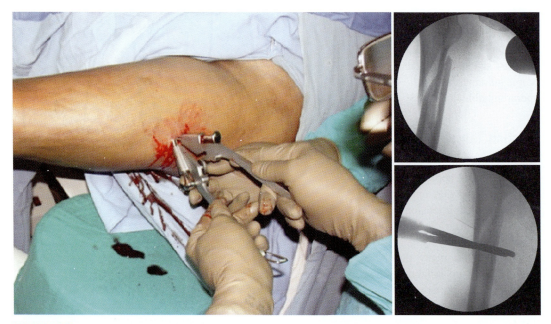

FIGURE 10.9

'Cerclage passer', designed for MIPO approach[4]; it has two limbs that are passed separately around the bone and locked to create a channel; a wire is passed without snaring the soft tissues.

easily move the limb. There is also difficulty in assessing the quality of reduction as comparison with intact side is not feasible. There are several risks in using this apparatus (see pages 220 and 264).

Posteriorly sagging distal fragment of an intertrochanteric fracture may be corrected by using a special device (Fig. 10.10). In managing a two-part intertrochanteric fracture the sliding hip screw may be introduced by MIPO technique. A guide wire is first introduced percutaneously (Fig. 10.11). After introducing the sliding screw, a short barrel plate is introduced with barrel face outwards; exercise caution in selecting barrel length.

Similarly, subtrochanteric comminuted fractures of the femur are amenable to biological fixation by MIPO. A 95° barrel plate is slid thorough small incisions with barrel facing outwards. After proper adjustment of length and reduction of the fracture, the barrel is turned over using a 4.5-mm screwdriver.[6] Introduction of a strong Kirschner wire as guiding device through the barrel and screw's cannulation helps in sliding the barrel over the sliding screw.

Push–Pull Method

A bone spreader, a Verbrugge clamp and an independent bone screw help indirect reduction of a fracture (Fig. 10.12). The technique is most useful to reduce a segmental fracture or where considerable comminution is present. A bone spreader is placed between a free screw head and the end of a plate. The fracture is distracted and reduced using pointed reduction forceps. Further compaction of

INDIRECT FRACTURE REDUCTION METHODS

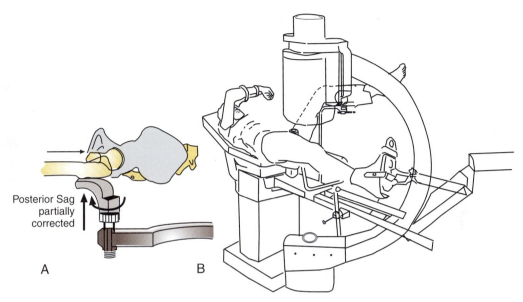

FIGURE 10.10

(**A**) An attachment for a conventional traction table can precisely correct a sagging trochanteric segment of intertrochanteric fracture.[5] It is a height-adjustable apparatus with radiolucent limb support at one end and a standard fixation connector to a traction table at the other end. (**B**) A traction table is used when closed reduction and maintenance of a fracture is possible; it is invaluable for a lone operating surgeon.

the reduction and compression of the fracture is achieved with a Verbrugge clamp. Its broad foot is centred on the far side of the screw; its small end fits into the end hole in the plate. It is then squeezed to apply tension to the plate, closing any remaining gaps in the fracture.

A distractor and external fixator are used to achieve reduction by ligamentotaxis. J Vidal (1979) coined the term 'ligamentotaxis'; he introduced the concept of reduction of comminuted metaphyseal and epiphyseal fragments by restoring tension in the capsuloligamentous structures that remain connected to the fracture fragments. Ligamentotaxis is useful in reduction of fractures of femur, tibial plateau, tibial pilon, os calcis and wrist. A distractor unit is used to create tension across the joint and fracture line to achieve reduction and maintain it till definitive plate fixation is completed. Distractors come in two common sizes: a hefty piece for femur and tibia; a mini fixator for foot and wrist. It is best to plan where and how to mount a distractor to avoid conflicts between the distractor and an implant as well as to anticipate and eliminate unforeseen problems of angulation. A distractor is applied directly to the main fragments to apply traction and achieve reduction. When a distractor is used it is possible to manoeuvre the limb during surgery. Angular or rotational corrections are difficult or even impossible with the distractor under axial load, and the construct at times may be cumbersome. A large distractor is a useful tool in indirect fracture reduction. However, with higher distraction forces the femur straightens out at the fracture site (Fig. 10.13). This leads to an undesirable posterior gap at the fracture site. A sheet is rolled to make a 'bump' and slid under the thigh at the fracture site during distraction. The gravity produces

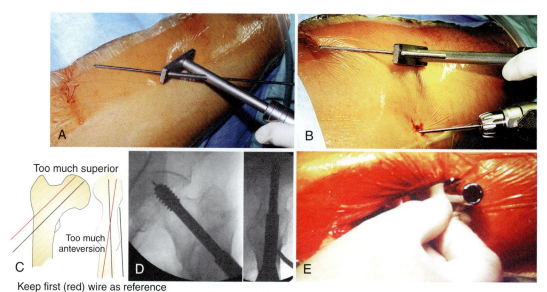

FIGURE 10.11

(**A**) Guide wire jig is placed in the fluoroscopy field to judge the direction (**B**) a guide wire is inserted free hand (**C**) first wire is retained even if it is not in correct position as a guide for subsequent attempts. (**D**) Sliding hip screw in correct position (**E**) the side plate for sliding hip screw is slid through a small incision with barrel facing outwards.

a slight anterior angulation while distraction is carried out. A plate is then fixed to stabilize the reduction.

In a simple transverse fracture that needs to be fixed with absolute stability, a compression clamp may be applied by mini-open approach (Fig. 10.13D).

External fixator is useful as a distractor but gentle lengthening is difficult to execute with the apparatus. When it is used to apply traction across a joint, ligaments and soft tissues around the fracture area help achieve reduction through ligamentotaxis or soft-tissue taxis. The external fixator is useful in management of multifragmentary metaphyseal or epiphyseal fracture, where the condition of the soft tissue or fracture fragmentation does not allow the use of open or direct reduction and stabilization techniques (Fig. 10.14).

Handles for Minimally Invasive Reduction

Schanz screws and conventional external fixation clamp and rod can be assembled to form a useful tool for minimally invasive reduction (Fig. 10.14A). However, specially designed reduction handles are more efficient tools for the procedure (Fig. 10.15). They are used with self-drilling threaded rods or guide wires. Their application is simple; they can be connected to support rods with clamps and serve as temporary external fixator and stabilize the fracture reduction. Planning is essential while inserting the rods in the bone to avoid interference with final plate application.

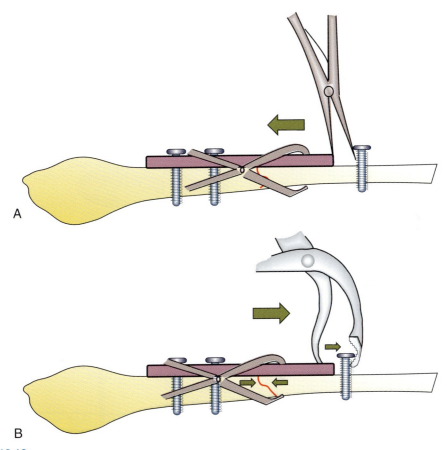

FIGURE 10.12

(**A**) A bone spreader is useful to distract the fracture to achieve reduction. (**B**) A plate holding clamp is used to compress a fracture.

Plate Holder and Pusher

A plate holder grips a plate at one end and has excellent control of the plate when it is under the soft tissue mantle (Fig. 10.16). A LIFP pusher temporarily moves the plate against bony cortex. It has a tip with threading that can be screwed in the threaded section of integrated hole. The heavy handles offer excellent points to apply a push to insert the plate under the soft tissue along the cortex.

USEFUL TACTICS FOR MIPO

How to Locate a Plate Hole without Fluoroscopy?

Fluoroscopy is not required to locate a plate hole. Place an identical plate over the subcutaneous plate and locate the holes; make stab incisions. Use small haemostats to locate the holes.

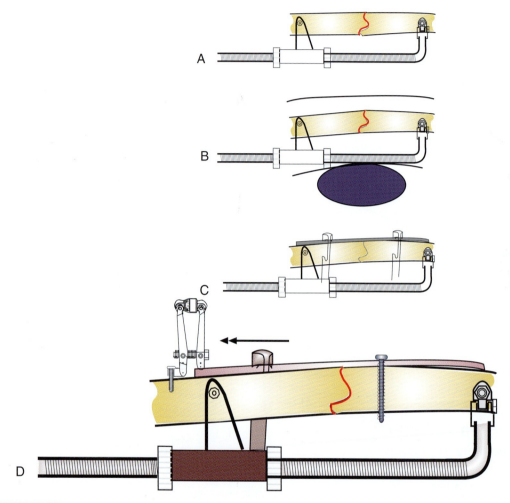

FIGURE 10.13

A large distractor and a 'bump' help in achieving reduction. **(A)** Posterior angulation of fragments **(B)** corrected by placing a 'bump' under the fracture site corrects the alignment **(C)** final stabilization achieved by plating. **(D)** When a simple fracture is to be plated compression from the femoral distractor is inadequate; though bone fragments are compressed, the plate is not preloaded. The plate should be fixed by a screw on one side of the fracture, and the articulating tensioner should be applied to the other end of the fracture; the plate is maximally tensioned. The femoral distractor should be maximally compressing the reduced fracture so that it is taking no load.

How to Insert Threaded Drill Guide with Ease without Exposing Hole of a Locking Plate?

Insert a 3-mm Kirschner wire as a stylet through the threaded drill guide. Locate the plate hole and then push the tip of the wire towards the threaded end of the hole. Once at the end, slide down the drill guide and turn to screw it into the threaded hole (Fig. 10.17).

USEFUL TACTICS FOR MIPO 391

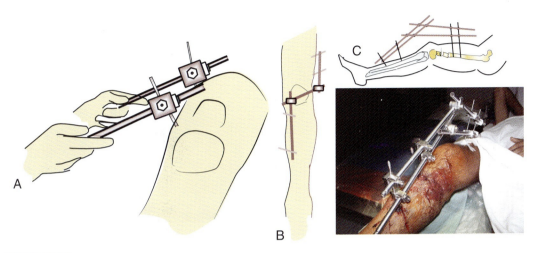

FIGURE 10.14

(**A**) Make-shift reduction tool from conventional external fixator elements. (**B and C**) Two schematics of temporary stabilization by external fixator. (**D**) External fixator in place to tide over soft tissue crisis.

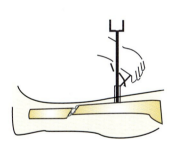

Self-tapping threaded rod inserted

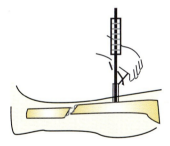

Reduction handle attached

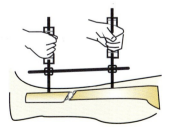

Reduction handles, connecting bar and clamps attached

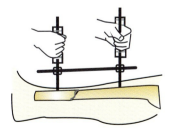

Fracture reduced and stabilized by securing the clamps to rods and connecting bar

FIGURE 10.15

Threaded rods get firm hold in the bone.[4] These are manipulated with handles to achieve reduction, which is then maintained by applying combination clamps and rods. Plates are applied for final fixation.

CHAPTER 3 MINIMAL INVASIVE OSTEOSYNTHESIS

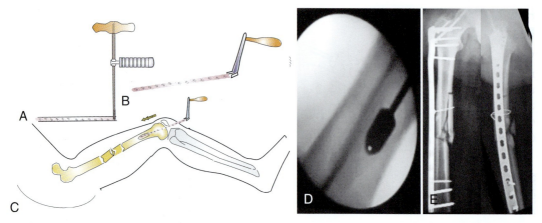

FIGURE 10.16

(**A**) A fixed screw driver, plate pusher and manipulator, a triple function tool for temporary stabilization of a plate; it taps and presses the plate against the bone. (**B**) A plate holder. (**C**) A schematic of use of a plate holder. (**D**) A tunneler in use; the hole near the tip is used to anchor strong thread to pull a plate though the tunnel just created. (**E**) A radiograph showing example of a bridge plating with use of cerclage by MIPO technique.

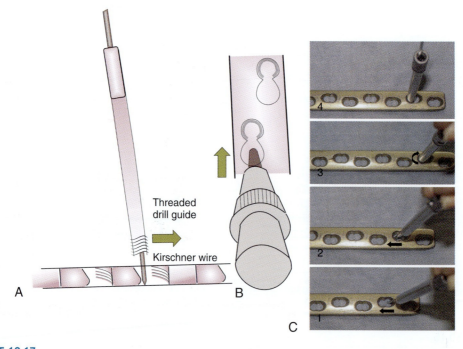

FIGURE 10.17

(**A and B**) Kirschner wire guides the threaded drill guide to the threaded end of the locking plate hole.[7] (**C**) Four-step photographic illustration to place a drill guide without exposing the plate hole.

How to Measure Screw Length with Ease?

When one reaches the far cortex, stop drilling and read out the marking on the drill bit. Alternately use a depth gauge/measuring device. Add to it approximate thickness of the cortex. This way one can quickly decide on the screw length (Fig. 10.18).

FLUOROSCOPY BY C-ARM IMAGE INTENSIFIER

In MIO fluoroscopy is the key tool in all stages of treatment to verify accuracy of reduction by multiple checks during surgery. There are many signs and procedures to carry out this task effectively. Three well-known fluoroscopic signs to verify precision of rotation in femoral diaphyseal fracture reduction are cortical step sign, bone diameter sign and lesser trochanter sign (Fig. 10.19).

All these signs, however, are arbitrary. Rotational malalignment of less than 10° is not detectable with any one of these methods. Use of electric cautery cable or alignment rod assists in intra-operative assessment of tibial or femoral axial alignment (Fig. 10.20).

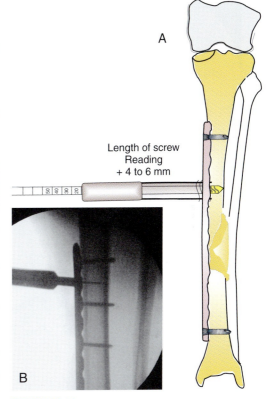

FIGURE 10.18

(A) Stop drilling at far cortex, note the depth and add 4–6 mm to the reading to arrive at required screw length.[7] (B) Screen shot showing use of screw length measuring device for the same purpose.

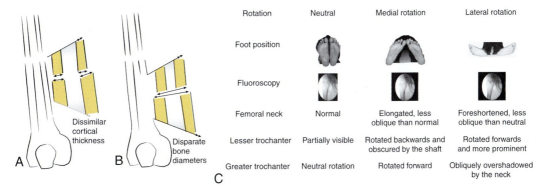

FIGURE 10.19

(A) Cortical step sign: the opposing bone ends have dissimilar cortical thickness. (B) Diameter difference sign: diameters of proximal and distal ends appear to be of different dimensions in presence of malrotation.[3] (C) Limb rotation alters the projection of the constituents of the upper end of the femur.

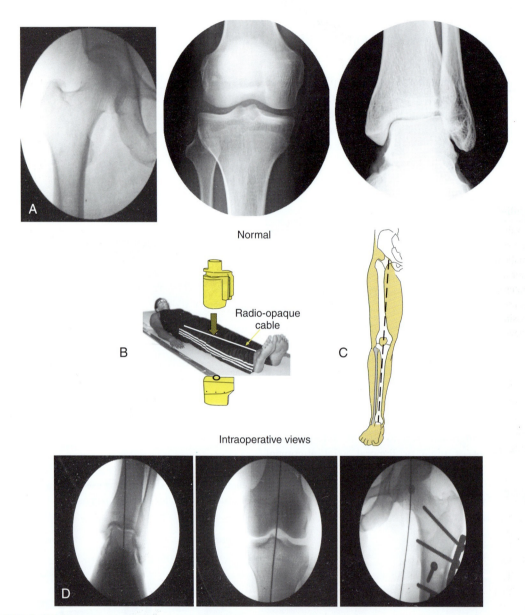

FIGURE 10.20

Cable technique is useful in intra-operative assessment of axial alignment in the frontal plane. **(A)** Before the surgery, with patella facing the ceiling, the centres of the femoral head and the ankle joint are marked under image intensification either on the skin or the surgical drapes. Another option is to place a disposable cardiac monitoring electrode over the hip spot. Its metal node is radiopaque and is palpable through the surgical drapes. An electrocautery cable is stretched between these two points with the image intensifier centred on the knee joint. Varus or valgus alignment could be determined by using the image of the cable as a reference line. The sagittal alignment is determined using a lateral view. **(B)** Arrangement of image intensifier. **(C)** Line sketch showing the alignment method. **(D)** Radiographs showing alignment assessment during MIPO.

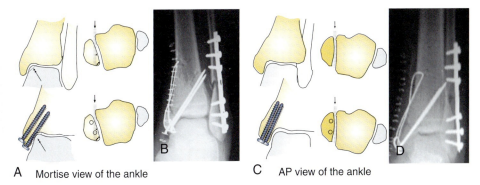

FIGURE 10.21

Evaluation of position of implants in medial malleolus. **(A)** The tracing of a mortise radiograph of the ankle shows the superior and lateral spaces well, but the medial space is oblique with overlap of the posterior margin of the malleolus on the talus (double headed arrow); the X-ray beam is at an angle to the medial joint space and the posterior implant incorrectly appears to be intra-articular. **(B)** Illustrative radiograph. **(C)** The tracing of a conventional anteroposterior radiograph of the ankle adequately shows the medial and superior joint spaces, but the lateral space is not visualized. The X-ray beam (arrow) is tangential to the medial joint space showing the actual intra-osseous position of the screws in the medial malleolus. **(D)** Illuminating radiograph of the ankle. Always use Anteroposterior view of ankle to evaluate position of implants in the medial malleolus.[8]

Characteristic positioning of the limb under fluoroscope facilitates in identifying transgression of joint space by screws in wrist (see page 185) and ankle. Conventional anteroposterior and mortise views are often used to assess the screw positions in ankle fracture fixation. Mortise view that shows the joint space so well, produces a faulty view of the implants; conventional ankle AP view is more reliable in this context[9] (Fig. 10.21).

REFERENCES

1. Sir Winston Churchill's message to President Roosevelt in a radio broadcast on 9 February 1941.
2. Anglen J, Kyle RF, Marsh JL, Virkus WW, Watters WC, III, Keith MW, Turkelson CM, Wies JL, Boyer KM. Locking plates for extremity fractures. J Am Acad Orthop Surg 2009;17:465–72.
3. Wagner M, Frenk A, Frigg R. Locked plating: biomechanics and biology and locked plating: clinical indications. Tech Orthop 2007;22(4):209–18.
4. Synthes®, West Chester, PA, USA.
5. The PORD™ Device Efratogo Ltd, Kiryat Bialik, Israel.
6. Rohilla R, Singh R, Magu NK, Sangwan SS, Devgun A, Siwach R. Technical aspects of the use of dynamic condylar screw in biological fixation of comminuted subtrochanteric fractures. Eur J Orthop Surg Traumatol 2009;19:33–7.
7. Bavonratanavech S. MIO – a new surgical culture for trauma. Guest lecture at Traumacon, August 16–19, 2012, Mumbai, India.
8. Thakur AJ. Strategic radiographic positioning for orthopaedicians and radiologist. New Delhi: Lippincott, Williams and Wilkins; 2010.
9. Gourineni, PVRKV, Knuth AE, Nuber GF. Radiographic evaluation of the position of implants in the medial malleolus in relation to the ankle joint space: anteroposterior compared with mortise radiographs. J Bone Joint Surg Am 1999;81:364–9.

Index

1-mm thick cable, 293f
8-plates, 191f

A

Abutting implants, 368–370
Adequate intracapsular fracture fixation, 271b
    implant removal, 271–274
Adequate trochanteric fracture fixation, 269b
Advantage hinge, 344b
Advantages of tensioned kirschner wires, 338b
Allogenic bone grafts, 40
Alloy F-90, 48b
American Wire Gauge (AWG), 277, 278t, 279t
Anatomy of a screw, 65–73
    head, 66–68
        function, 68
    shaft, 69
    tip, 71–73
Antibiotic impregnated intramedullary nail, 217–218
Anti-glide plate, 114f
Antirotation screw, 251
Application of wire, 280b
Applied moment arm, 374
Assorted hinges, 345f
ASTM F-136, 49
ASTM F-90, 49–48
Autogenous bone grafts, 40
Autologous platelet concentrate, 42

B

Ball spike pusher, 380–381
Beam, 3
    mechanical properties, 5
Bending and axial load, 127–129
Bending, 5
Biaxial compression plate, 254–255
Bilateral uniplanar frame, 320f
Bioactive glass ceramices, 45
Blocking K-wire technique, 174, 174f
Blocking screw, 214
BMD, 244
BMPs, 41
Bone graft substitute, 40–41
    bone-based, 40–41
    cell-based, 42–43
    ceramic-based, 43–45
    coral-based, 45
    growth factor-based, 41–42
    polymer-based, 45

Bone grafting in external fixation, 348
Bone healing after nailing, 202
Bone hook, 380–381
Bone marrow, 40
Bone plate, 108, 381
    biomechanics, 126–130
    classification, 109–115
        bridge plate, 113–114
        buttress plate, 112–113
        compression plate, 109–111
        condylar plate, 114–115
        protection (neutralization) plates, 109
        tension band plate, 112
    LIFP, 141
    paediatric applications, 188–191
    principles of plate fixation, 115–120
        bone-related factors, 117
        construct-related factors, 117–118
        double plating, 126
        effect of compression, 118–120
        plate bending, 126
        plate fixation of oblique long bone fractures, 125
        plate-related factors, 115–117
        prebending of plate, 123–125
        screw-related factors, 117
        tension band plate, 120–123
    regional considerations, 168–191
        clavicle, 187
        diaphysis of the radius and the ulna, 183
        distal femur, 171–172
        distal humerus, 179–181
        distal radius fracture, 186–187
        distal radius, 183–185
        femoral shaft, 169–171
        fractures of radial head, 181
        hand, 187
        preshaped plates, 168–169
        proximal humerus, 179
        proximal tibia, 175–176
        proximal ulna, 182
        rib, 187–188
        shaft of humerus, 179
        subtrochanteric fracture, 169
        the calcaneus, 177
        the condylar plate, 172–173
        the humerus, 177–181
        the radius and ulna, 181–187
        tibia, 174–177
        tibial locked internal fixator plate, 176–177

Bone plate *(Continued)*
  relative stability and bone plate, 139–141
  removal, 162–167
Bone regeneration with external fixator, 350–351
Bone response to nailing, 198–202
  effect on circulation, 198
  side effects of reaming, 198–201
Bone spreader, 389f
Bone, 25
  as material, 25–26
  biomechanical properties, 25
  tensile strength and elasticity, 26
Blood supply, 279
  grafts, 348
Brittleness, 20
Bump, 379, 380f
Butterfly fractures, 9
Buttress plate, 113f

C

C type fracture, 187f
Cable and wire, 294t
Cages, 369–370
Calcaneus locking plate, 178f
Calcium hydroxyapatite, 44–45
Calcium sulphate, 45
Callus formation and internal fixation, 28
CalTAD, 267-269
Cancellous bone screw, 74
Cantilever beam fixation, 374
Cerclage passer, 282f, 386f
Cerclage wire, 382–383
Cerclage wiring, 289–292
  regional application, 291–292
    patello-tibial cerclage, 291–292
    tibia and femur, 291
Cervical spinal plate, 370f
Clamps, 367f
Clavicle plate, 187
Clinical conditions delaying bone healing, 35–38
  ageing, 37–38
  chronic inflammation, 36
  diabetes, 37
  hypovitaminosis, 37
  NSAIDs, 38
  polytrauma, 38
Closed and open nailing, 218–219
Closed reduction of radial head fracture, 303f
Coaxial clamp, 385f
Collagen, 42–43
Collinear reduction clamp, 382
Column loading and tension band principle, 15–16
Combinations of different screws, 157
Components of external fixator, 316f
Compression versus no compression under external fixation, 346

Compression, 17
Connectors, 367f
Constant rigid versus dynamic compression under external fixation, 346–347
Conventional plate and bone vascularity, 136–138
Conversion table, AWG to metric, 278t
Coralline hydroxyapatite, 45
Core diameter, 69–70
Corkscrew phenomenon, 232
Corkscrew tip, 72
Corrosion, 60–62
  crevice, 61
  fretting, 61
  galvanic, 60–61
  intergranular, 61–62
  ion release, 62
  pitting, 61
  stress, 61
Cortical bone screw, 74
Countersink, 67–68, 90
Critical steps in MIPO, 378b
Cruciate head, 66
Curved impactor, 381
Cutting and helix angles, 82t

D

Definitive fixation, 299
Demineralized bone matrix, 41
Depth gauge, 89f
DEXA, 244
Diamond concept, 29–30
Diamond point, 296
Distance between bone and support column, 324
Distraction plating, 186–187
Divergent or convergent locked screws, 151–152
Drill bit failure, 86
Drill bits for orthopaedic use, 85t
Drilling, 80
  bit, 80–81
  common drilling terms, 82t
  depth, 87
  drill bit failure, 86–87
  drill guide, 87
  drill size nomenclature, 82
  drill sizes, 84t
  drill sleeve, 87
  effects of heat on the bone, 84
  factors affecting heat production, 84
  heat generation, 82–84
  mechanics, 85
  power drill, 87
  principles, 81
  techniques to minimize heat production, 85
Ductility, 20
Dynamic locking screw, 164f

Dynamic locking, 212–214
Dynamic plate, 370

E

Eccentric screw placement, 113f
Edicts of hinge placement, 344b
Effect of forces on a conventional plate screw construct, 127–129
Effect of fracture type on its healing in external fixation, 345
Effects of bending and axial loads on a locked plate, 151f
Efficiency of screw insertion, 91
Elastic stable intramedullary nailing, 229–236
    biomechanics, 229–232
        ball-tiped guide rod, 220
    regional considerations, 232
        femur, 232–234
        humerus, 235
        radius and the ulna, 234–235
        tibia, 235–236
Elasticity, 20
Electromagnetic stimulation, 46
End cap, 233f
Endochondral bone formation, 26
Enhancement of bone healing, 38–39
Epiphysiodesis, 191
Eschew unicortical screw, 155t
ESIN, 229
External fixation – indications, 353b
External fixation – fracture healing, 347b
External fixation frames – classification, 319t
External fixation in children – indications, 356t
External fixation pin, 316
    core, 317
    shaft, 317
    thread, 316–317
    tip, 316
External fixator frame designs, 319f
External fixator vs locked internal fixator plate, 147–148, 150t
External fixators, 313–359
    classification, 314–316
    mechanical properties, 322–327
    polytraumatized patient, 355–356
    regional considerations, 352–357
    removal, 352
    the developing countries and, 357
    use in children, 356–357
    war, natural catastrophe, 358

F

F tool, 379, 380f
Fabrication of implants, 59–60
Facia iliaca compartment block, 266f
Factors affecting hip fixation, 244b
Factors affecting sliding of a screw in a plate–barrel, 248f
Fan blade effect, 167

Far cortical locking (FCL) screw, 162f
Fixation of a spiral fracture, 102
Fixed moment arm, 374
Fluoroscopic evaluation of locked screw placement, 185–186
Fluoroscopy by C-ARM image intensifier, 393–395
Force components acting on a body, 4f
Force, 1–3
Forces acting on the plate-screw interface, 130–131
Forces on a locked screw-plate construct, 149–151
Forces on the hip, 240b
Fracture compression, 267
Fracture fixation construct, 16
Fracture healing with external fixation, 344–346
Fracture impaction, 267
Fracture patterns, 11f
Fracture reduction, 379–383
    direct, 379
    indirect, 383–389
    tools to facilitate direct reduction, 379
Fragment-specific implants, 185
Frame construction, 348–351
Frames, 318–321, 356f
    bilateral biplanar, 321
    bilateral uniplanar, 319–321
    modular, 321
    unilateral biplanar, 319
    unilateral, 318–319
Function of a nut, 330b
Function of rings, 328b
Functional gradient, 55
Functional modes of spinal implants, 361b
Functional segments of a fixation device, 246–247
Functionally graded material, 55–57

G

Gartland type 2 or 3 supracondylar fracture, 300
Gene therapy, 43
Goetze-Rhinelander-Böhler method, 291f
Good drilling practice, 87b
Good pin insertion practice, 348b
Good practices for locking screw, 102
Good practices for traction table, 222b
Good practices for wire tensioning, 341b
Good practices in ESIN, 235b
Gotfried's percutaneous compression-plating device, 254f
Guide wire, 262–263

H

Half-ring with curved ends, 329f
Handles for minimally invasive reduction, 388
Hazards in unicortical insertion, 153–154
Healing of a treated fracture, 26–30
Healing process, 28–29
Heat production in drilling, 84b

Helical nail, 204–205
Helix, 20
Hex head, 66–67
Hinge function, 344
Hinge position, 346f
Hip fixation devices – expectations, 244b
Hip fixation, 239–275
Hip, 239
    anatomy and forces acting on the hip joint, 239
    causes of hip fracture and associated forces, 240–242
    classification of hip fractures, 242–243
    comparative features of fixation devices, 261–262
    factors affecting fracture fixation, 244
    fixation devices, 244–260
    hip fracture and osteoporosis, 264–265, 265b
    need for fracture fixation, 243
    protector, 240–242
    regional considerations, 265–274
    traction table for fixation of proximal femur fractures, 263
        acute pain control in hip fracture, 265–266
        extracapsular fracture, 267–269
        intracapsular fractures, 269–271
Hohmann retractor, 381
Holding power of screw, 95–99
Hooks, 365f
How to insert threaded drill guide without exposing hole of locking plate, 390
How to locate a plate hole without fluoroscopy, 389
How to measure screw length, 393

I

Image intensifier adjustments, 226f
IMFN good practices, 258–259b
Implants for proximal femur fracture fixation, 253f
Inadequacies of compression plate, 140t
Indications for compression plating, 126b
Indicative zones of tibia, 236f
Infection and pin loosening, 349–350
    pin-related causes, 350
    soft tissue-related causes, 350
    surgeon-related causes, 350
Insertion of lag screw with a short intramedullary nail, 266–267
Insertion, 90–91
Instant centre of rotation, 371
Instantaneous axis of rotation, 371b
Insufficiencies of compression plate, 138–139
Insufficient lag screw–plate barrel engagement, 251f
Interfragmentary strain, 27f
Interlocking nail, 211–212
Intrafocal pinning, 304
Intramedullary nail, 197
Intramedullary pressure changes during nailing, 201t
Intramedullary sliding hip screw, 255–259

Intramembranous bone formation, 26
Irreducible intertrochanteric fracture, 265f
ISHS, 255–256

J

Joining ends of wire, 281f
Jones view, 301
Joystick technique, 381f

K

Kapandji technique, 305f
Kirschner wire pattern, 300f
Kirschner wire, 298–299

L

Lag screw practice, 99b
Lag screw, 99–102
Lead, 70–71
LIFP for clavicle fracture fixation, 189f
Limb lengthening and bone transport, 188–191
Load bearing structures, 6f
Load transfer mechanisms across a femoral neck fracture, 261f
Loading modes and fracture patterns, 6–9
Loading modes, 6–9
    bending and axial compression, 9
    bending, 7–9
    compression, 7
    tension, 7
    torsion, 9
    torsion, bending and axial compression, 9
Load-sharing and load bearing constructs, 130
Locations of callus, 31t
Locked K-wires, 306
Locked internal fixator plate, 141–162
    advantages, 158
    biomechanics, 147–152
    contraindications, 158
    disadvantages, 158–160
    far cortex locking, 160–162
        flexible fixation, 160–161
        load distribution, 161
        parallel interfragmentary motion, 162
        progressive stiffness, 161–162
    in combination of two methods, 157
    in compression mode, 156
    in splinting mode, 157
    indications, 154–157
    lag screw and protection plate, 156–157
    limitations, 158
    paediatric applications, 188–191
    pros and cons of fixed and variable angle locking systems, 145–147
    types, 141–142

Locked internal fixator plate *(Continued)*
    fixed angle plates, 142
    variable angle, 143–147
  undersurface of a locked hole, 147
Locking plate for proximal femur fractures, 252–253
Long connection plate, 328f

M

Mallet tool, 380f
Mallet, 379
Manual traction, 384–385
Mass moment of inertia, 12
Materials in fracture fixation, 46–51
Measurement of screw length, 91–92
Mechanics of transmedullary support screw, 214–217
Mechanism of load bearing, 371–374
  cantilever beam fixation, 374
  simple distraction fixation, 371
  tension band fixation, 371
  three-point bending fixation, 371
Medullary reaming – safe practices, 219b
Medullary reaming, factors affecting heat and pressure generation, 200f
Metal failure, 56
Metal removal, 56
Metal working methods, 57–60
  annealing, 58
  broaching, 58–59
  case hardening, 58
  casting, 57
  cold working, 58
  forging, 57
  machining, 58
  milling, 58
  rolling and drawing, 58
Metals in orthopaedic use, 47–50
  cobalt–chromium alloys, 48–49
  nickel–titanium alloy, 50–51
    nitinol, 50
  stainless steel, 47–48
  titanium alloys, 49
Methods of achieving compression, 110–111
Minimal invasive osteosynthesis, 377–396
Minimal invasive plate osteosynthesis, 141, 377–378
MIPO, 141, 377–378
  useful tactics, 389–393
    advantages, 378
    disadvantages, 378
Mixing of implants, 56-57
Modular frame – advantages, 321b
Modular sliding hip screw, 252
Moment of inertia, 12
Moment, 2f, 12
Multiple lag screw fixation, 260b
Multiple lag screws, 259–260

N

Nail design, 202–208
  cross-section, 202
  curves, 203–204
  ends of the nail, 207
  helical nail, 204–205
  length, 205–207
  material, 208
  nail diameter, 203
  working length, 205–207
Nail removal, 222–223
  bent nails, 223
  intact nail with failed extraction device, 223
  removal of broken solid nail, 223
Nailing, regional considerations, 225–229
  femur, 225–227
  humerus, 228
  radius and ulna, 228–229
  retrograde supracondylar intramedullary nail, 226–227
  tibia, 227–228
Near and far cortex, 18
Nerve palsy, 222
Nishiura technique, 266
Nitriding, 59
Non-fixed moment arm, 374
Non-self-tapping tip, 72
Number of pins, 322–323

O

Optimized plate anchorage, 151–152
Orthobiologics and tissue engineering, 39–45
Orthobiologics, 39
Orthogonal plating, 179–181
Orthopaedic alloys, 48f
Osteonal and non osteonal healing, 29

P

Parabolic flute, 85t
Parallel plating, 181
Parathyroid hormone therapy, 39
Parts of a bone drill bit, 81f
Patankar method, 307f
Patient positioning on a traction table, 221f
Patterns of load, 3f
PcCP device, 253
Pedicle screw fixation, 364f
Pedicle screws, 363
PEEK, 55
Pelvic reduction clamp, 382
Percutaneous compression plate, 253
Perfect anatomic reduction, 270f
Perineal post and soft tissue pressure, 264f
Perren hypothesis, 27–28
Phillips head, 66

Pilot hole, 88
Pin diameter, 323–324
Pin fixation techniques for metacarpal fractures, 306f
Pin fixator, 316–318
    components, 316–317
        central body, 317
        clamp, 317
        compression–distraction system, 318
        pin, 316
Pin–bone interface – stress-reducing factors, 324b
Pin–bone interface, 324–325, 326f
Pin–clamp interface, 324
Pins, 296–310
    regional considerations, 299–308
        femur, 353–354
        humerus, 354–355
        pelvis, 355
        periarticular fractures of the lower leg, 353
        radius and ulna, 354
        screw placement in the pelvis, 355
        the tibia, 352–353
        wrist and hand, 354
    Steinmann pin, 309–310
    technique of medial pinning, 302
    technique of pinning, 301
    use, 298–299
Pitch, 70
Plasticity, 20
Plate and bone vascularity, 30–35
Plate application to well apposed transverse fracture, 118f
Plate fixation of subtrochanteric fracture, 170f
Plate fixation versus external fixation, 347
Plate holder and pusher, 389
Plate length and number of screws, 138f
Plate length and plate working length, 131–133
Plate length and screw density, 130–136
Platelet-rich plasma, 42
Plating of humeral shaft, 181f
Polar and area moment of inertia, 13–14
Polishing and passivation, 59
Poller screw, 214–217
Polymers, 51–55
    bioabsorbable, 51
    biodegradable, 51
    bioerodible, 51
    bioresorbable, 51–55
    fracture fixation, 54–55
    mechanical properties, 54
    PEEK, 55
Polymethylmethacrylate (PMMA) beads, 217–218
Poor bone healing, 37t
Position for Kirschner (K) wire, 297f
Prebending plates, 123b
Precise insertion technique, 266–267
Predictors of instability, 183t
Preloading, 326–327
Prerequisites of tension band fixation, 123b
Pressure distribution in the fracture gap, 124f
Principle of bilateral cable tension banding operation, 295–296
Principle of eccentricity, 294–295
Principle of splintage, 197–198
Provisional fixation, 299
Proximal humerus locking plate, 180f
Push–pull method, 386–388

R

Radial column plate, 185f
Rake angle, 81, 82t, 83f
Reamed and non-reamed nails, 210
Reamed nailing, 210
Reamer–irrigator–aspirator, 40, 201–202
Reaming, 219–220
Recess, 66–67
Recommended tension on wires, 341b
Reduction of a diaphyseal fracture with hohmann retractor, 384f
Reduction screw, 382
Relative stability with conventional self-compression plate, 139–141
Reverse dynamization, 358f
Rib fracture fixation, 190f
Rib plate, 190f
Rigidity, 19
Ring fixators, 327–348
    arches, 330
    dynamization, 347
    frame assemblage, 334
    guide wire, 342
    half-ring with curved ends, 328
    hinges, 343–344
    pulling or traction wire, 342
    reverse dynamization, 348
    ring connections, 330–333
        bolts, 330
        nuts, 330
        rods, 330–331
        supports, posts and half-hinges, 332–333
        threaded sockets and bushings, 332
        washers, 333
        wrenches, 333
    ring inclination, 336
    ring orientation, 337–340
    ring position and force distribution, 334
    ring position at FON sites, 337
    rings, 327–330
    Schanz screws or half-pins, 342–343
    space between skin and ring, 336–337
    wire fixation, 341–342
    wire positioning on the same ring, 340
    wire tensioning, 341
    wire with stopper, 341

T

Tapping, 88–89
β-TCP, 44–45
Tension band fixation, 371
Tension band principle, 122f
Tension band wiring of the greater trochanter, 288f
Tension band wiring of the medial and lateral malleoli, 288f
Tension band wiring, 282b, 283–289
    general principles, 283–284
    regional considerations, 285–289
        arthrodesis of the thumb, 289
        arthrodesis of the wrist, 289
        arthrodesis, 308
        diaphysis of metacarpal and metatarsal, 289
        distal radius, 304–306
        forearm bones, 303
        greater trochanter of femur, 286
        greater tuberosity of humerus, 286–287
        intra-articular fracture, 308
        lateral end of the clavicle, 287
        medial malleolus, 286
        metacarpal and metatarsal, 306–307
        patella, 286
        radial head, 303–304
        supracondylar fracture of the humerus, 300
        tibial plateau, 299–300
        traction, 308
        ulna, 285–286
Thread design, 71
Thread diameter, 71
Thread, 69–71
Three-point bending fixation, 371
Timing of plate removal, 166t
    removal of LIFP, 167
Tip-apex distance for SHS, 268f
Tissue engineering, 39
Torsion, 5
Torsional load, 129
Toughness, 20
Traction table in fractures of upper end of femur, 263–264
Traction table, 220–222
    complications, 220–221
        nerve palsy, 222
        soft-tissue injury, 222
Traction table: good surgical practices, 263b
Traction tables, 385–386
Traction wire techniques, 343f
Tricalcium phosphate, 44–45
Trocar point, 296
Trocar tip, 72–73
Trochanter supporting plate, 251
Types and effects of loading, 3–5
Types of clamps, 318f
Types of rings, 338f
Types of screw tips, 72f

U

Ultrasound, 46
Uniaxial dynamization, 255f
Unicortical screw, 152–154
Unilateral uniplanar frame with varying rigidity, 345
Unilateral uniplanar frame, 320f
Unilateral uniplanar versus bilateral biplanar frame, 344
Unstable intertrochanteric fracture patterns, 259f
Use of minimal internal fixation, 345

V

Verbruge clamp, 113f
von Mises Stress, 22

W

Washers, 90, 336f
Wire cables, 292–296
Wire fixation bolts, 335f
Wire tensioning, 342f
WIRE, 277–282
    cerclage wiring, 289b
    classification of sutures, 278
    effect on blood supply of the bone, 279
    factors affecting the strength, 278–279
        effect of time, 279
        twisted wire, 279
        kinks and knots, 279
    instruments to handle wire, 280–281
    methods of fastening, 280
    size nomenclature, 277
    tension band wiring, 283–289
    uses, 281–282
Wire, cable and pins, 276–312
Wires and Schanz screws used in the ring fixator, 340f
Wires passers, 282f
Wolff's law, 21–22
Working length and strain, 137f
Working length of a nail, 207f
Working length of fixation constructs, 161f
Working length, 20–21
Wrenches, 337f

Y

Young's modulus, 13f

Z

Z-effect, 257f

Ring inclination, 339f
Ring orientation, 339f
Role of compression, 110
Run out, 69

S

Schanz screw, half-pin, 316
Sciatic and Common Peroneal Nerve palsy, 222
Screw drives, 67f
Screw failure, 96–99
Screw insertion, 80–91
Screw position, 137f
Screw removal, 92–93
   broken distal screw tip, 93
   screw with stripped head, 93
Screw type and placement, 133–136
Screw types, 73–80
   cannulated screw, 76–77
   cortical and cancellous screws, 74
   fully and partially threaded screws, 76
   Herbert screw, 79–80
   locking buttons, 79
   locking screw, 77–79
   machine screws, 73
   non-self-tapping screw, 75–76
   self-tapping screw, 74–75
   wood screws, 73
Screw vs bolt, 103
Self-drilling self-tapping tip, 73
Self-tapping tip, 71–72
Shape memory alloy, 50–51
Shock wave therapy, 46
Short connection plate, 334f
   combined-type hinge, 334f
   with threaded rod, 334f
SHS dimension, 249
SHS, 247
Side effects of reaming, 198–201
Single and multiple nails, 208–209
Single slot head, 66
Sliding hip screw – optimum, 249b
Sliding hip screw and intramedullary sliding hip screw, 261–262
Sliding hip screw and multiple lag screw, 261
Sliding hip screw, 247–251
Sliding hip screw: common causes of complications, 251b
Slotted and non-slotted nails, 210–211, 211t
Small instruments and implants, 380–383
Soft-tissue injury, 222
Spinal instrumentation, 360–376
   functional modes, 361–362
     goals, 361
       deformity correction, 361

Spinal instrumentation *(Continued)*
       reconstruction and replacement, 361
       stabilization, 361
   implant classification, 362
       constrained and non-constrained implants, 362
       rigid and non-rigid implants, 362
       segmental and non-segmental implants, 362
   spinal implant description, 362–370
       accessories, 368
       anchors, 363
       circumferential grip connector, 366
       constrained bolt–plate connectors, 366
       constrained screw–plate connectors, 368
       cross-connectors, 368
       gripping implants, 364–366
       hooks, 364
       laminar hooks, 364
       lock screw connectors, 366
       longitudinal members, 366
       pedicle hooks, 365
       plates, 370
       rods, 370
       screws, 363
       semiconstrained component–rod connectors, 367
       sublaminar wires, 365–366
       three-point shear clamps, 366
       transverse process hook, 365
Spiral, 20
Splintage, 197
Stable fixation, 18–19
Stable wiring configurations for the distal radial fracture, 305f
Standard locked construct, 163f
Standards organizations, 57
Static and dynamic compression, 110
Static compression using a plate, 124f
Static locking and bridging fixation, 212–218
Steinmann pin insertion, 310b
Steinmann pin with cove (niche) point, 309f
Steinmann pins, 309
Stem cells, 42
Steps of fracture healing, 26
Stiffness, 17
Strain, 12
Strength, 19
Stress risers, 15
Stress shielding, 15
Stress, 12
Struts, 368–369
Submuscular plating, 188–191, 191f
Supplementary fixation devices, 207–208
Supplementary fixations for SHS, 251
Suture sizes, 278